How To Survive Middle Age

Best wishes to you my friend!
Franklin Ross Jones

How To Survive Middle Age

Franklin Ross Jones

iUniverse, Inc.
New York Lincoln Shanghai

How To Survive Middle Age

iUniverse books may be ordered through booksellers or by contacting:

iUniverse
2021 Pine Lake Road, Suite 100
Lincoln, NE 68512
www.iuniverse.com
1-800-Authors (1-800-288-4677)

ISBN-13: 978-0-595-36864-8 (pbk)
ISBN-13: 978-0-595-81275-2 (ebk)
ISBN-10: 0-595-36864-6 (pbk)
ISBN-10: 0-595-81275-9 (ebk)

Printed in the United States of America

CONTENTS

Preface

This work is the culmination of several aspects related to my career. These included teaching and research on the psychology of human development, which resulted in numerous articles and studies, and the publication of three editions of a textbook. In addition there were several years of radio programs dealing with the problems of the middle years. Many listeners of that program encouraged me to combine the talks into a volume and make it available. The idea for this book came from my radio audience.

All of the areas or issues covered in the chapters have touched my life, which is not unusual as they are basic elements of existence in the lives of many persons. The ideas, a compendium of them, along with data and suggestions as well as the resources given, are designed to enable people to survive middle age successfully i.e., to age seventy. The increasing length of life has made it necessary to redefine what is middle age. Female babies born today in America will likely live 80 years—with men around seventy-six years. So when I speak of middle age or middlescence (my word) the term has three divisions for me—younger middle age 40-49, middle middlescence 50-59 and older middle age 60-69. Increasing numbers of people in America are living to be 80 and 90 even 100. This work is not principally concerning nomenclature but the substance of living—its fabric and structure as it interacts with the total environment in the broad middle years.

The information enclosed focuses on a volume comprising a number of salient features of survival in middle age. It contains a plethora of critical concepts and suggestions and resources enabling one to survive middle age (or middlescence). It is designed to help people who do not have the wherewithal, time or who do not know where to go for help in resolving problems and framing issues of important life affairs and make them understandable. It touches base with all the major areas in middle life that have to be dealt with by the genre. I believe the material in this book will provide answers to some troubling questions or provide the location of needed help in solving or understanding some problems in living.

This work begins with a chapter, which presents the current status of middle age people—cultural circumstance, longevity prospect, societal expectations and developmental tasks. Continuing in this book sections discussing stress, physical health, career responsibilities toward parent, money and future retirement, recreation and leisure, love, sex and marriage; more somber topics as divorce and afterward and death are included. Finally a chapter on the author's idea of the good life! The writing is straightforward and understandable by readers at the senior high school college freshman level. An exception perhaps exists in the chapter on health where terminology may interfere; however, means are taken to make it comprehensible. It should be remembered that the verities of today become tomorrow's suspect data due to the fluctuation of events that brings change frequently seen in taxation, economy, medical discoveries, the social climate, etc.

The opinions and ideas found in this volume are those of the author. It is intended to provide helpful information and material dealing with those topics presented here. It is provided with the understanding that the author and publisher is not engaged with rendering aid in specific ways, i.e., financial, psychological, health, counseling in marital affairs or any other adult problems. Before any serious decision is made by the reader, advice from one's own broker, physician, psychologist or psychiatrists or relevant consultant should be sought. The responsibility, loss, risks, liability, personal or otherwise is disclaimed by the writer and publisher. This volume is presented as a guide but definitive decisions by an individual should be made with an appropriate specialist.

ACKNOWLEDGEMENTS

The list of all those involved with the creation of this manuscript and those who contributed to its fruition would be difficult. Why, because information and experiences spoken of here have been generated from the multitude of circumstances, over time, schooling, family and friends, media, research over the years and environmental influences. The fear in recognition giving is that some persons who made a contribution will be overlooked nevertheless protocol impels me to make such enumeration.

Not given in order of importance but essential in bringing this work to publication was my assistant, researcher and aide Betty Levin. Specialists of numerous fields have received the outline and read the chapters found in this volume. They are Attorney, Al Teich, J.D.; Brokers Jim O'Brien and Christopher Doyle; Linda McDonald, H & R Block Tax Specialist; Dr. Lanny Hampel, Ph.D., Gerontologist Specialist; Elisabeth Mason, M.D., Researcher, Endocrinologist and Associate Professor at the Eastern Virginia Medical School; A. J. Ciccone, M.D., Family Practitioner; Dr. Peter Stewart, Ph.D., Historian and Researcher; Susan Richardson, Hospital Administrator; Steve Buchberg and Dave Hala, Pharmacists, the latter also a college instructor; Julia Whaley, Chemistry Professor; Dr. Chris Lovell, Ph.D., Counseling Consultant; Dr. Ray Morgan, D.Ed., Reading in the Content Area Specialist, Morton Jones, Scientist and Reader; Zebulon Hites, Writer; Paul Griffey, M.D., Ophthalmologist; Peggy Knight, Graphic Specialist; Dr. Venkat Reddy, M.D., Retinologist; and Robert Lanoue, M.D., Neurologist.

Many agencies and institutions also assisted through providing data, ideas and information such as the National Institutes of Health, U.S. Department of Labor, U.S. Department of Statistics, Virginia Social Welfare Commission, Duke University, U.S. Bureau of Census, County and Urban Nursing Homes Information, Harvard Medical School publications, Old Dominion University Library, U.S. Department of Health and Human Services, Medicare and Medicaid Services, U.S. Chamber of Commerce, National Parks Services and Cone Hospitals, Greensboro, NC.

CHAPTER I

THE MIDDLESCENT YEARS

"The Way We Are!"

"Middle aged!" hell (excuse me) I answered, responding to the nurse who asked my age as she took a blood sample. Forty-five, really forty-eight, but I do not feel really old! After all, most of the time I feel young—play tennis, stay up late at night, dance and do other youthful things. At times, we are forced to ponder the question—is age basically a matter of chronology or role? As is said in the preface the middle years I call middlescent are those somewhere between 40 and 69. Forty is about half of the life expectancy currently for female babies born today. For men only a few years behind. This suggests a beginning level to middle age. Sixty-five has marked the usual time of retirement for many, for others 50 or as late as 75. I think that middle age is some where between 40 and the late 60's. We can further break down the years into divisions for convenience: younger middle age 40-49, middle middle age 50-59, and older middle age 60-69. Certainly some are old psychologically, socially and physically at 50 or 60.

There is some evidence suggesting various classes view age differently. A study some years ago asking social classes at what point are women most beautiful found that lower-class persons as a group said women are most beautiful at twenty-five. On the other hand, middle class persons thought those around thirty should get the honor; the upper-middle class persons thought the age should be at thirty-five. This may be understandable, for those of less means typically have more stress than those of upper class people. The critical life-cycle events as a rule are experienced earlier—birth of the first and last child. There is general agreement that the upper class has been better cared for and have had considerable help to relieve worry and assist with various obligations.

However, today some would say outstanding beauty is found among those even 50 or beyond.

Classifying people into stages and divisions may be basically a matter of role and personality. Certainly if I were 35 or even 40 I'd object to being classified as middle-aged. Some play the role of the forty to fifty year old at sixty-five or even seventy—they're active—play golf or tennis, manage business, dress in the fashion of those twenty years their junior, are participants in community and social affairs. Others thirty years old or so dress, act, and are as inflexible as some sixty-year-olds. One thing we note is that the roles of men and women are no longer static. Walter Pitkin, a number of years ago, in his *Life Begins at Forty* advanced the years 40-60 as the in-between years. The in-between years of middlescence should be characterized by change and development—new roles, new perspectives and new lives; integration and restructuring. One thing is sure! Middlescence is younger than it used to be. Even with the increase in the life span there is some evidence that years between youth and aging are expanding. Civil servants are retiring as early as 55, (the average retirement age is 62) the average couple completes childbearing by 28-29 so that the last child is in his adolescence wile the parents are in their forties. Rose Franzblau in her book, *The Middle Generation*, says middle age is between 25-55. This is obviously too low. Demographers like 45-64 as the middle years. There are many individuals in their mid-sixties and older who refuse to accept the traditional stereotype role of "old folks" and for good reasons—they are in much better physical condition than their counterparts in the World War II era. They take more trips, play more games, participate in more sports, are still vitally engaged in occupations and/or avocations and there is evidence that this will increasingly be the case. Indeed, and importantly they should not play dead or be retiring, for women today at age sixty-five can look forward on the average to more than eighteen years of life. And men some twelve or thirteen years. Eighty-three and Seventy-eight—no wonder the middle years are extended! Adult aging starts early for some and physical changes, as presbyopia (old-sightedness) overtake those in their twenties and thirties, weight problems begin early, the cessation of the menses in some as early as 30-35, and other disabilities occur. Developmental changes occur in the thirties, but these incidences are ameliorated by the general conditions and health of thousands of people.

The Middle years are those times characterized by the establishment of a life style, a work pattern, definite views about the world at large, a sense of inner philosophical solidarity, the worth of things and ideas especially new meaning and vistas in life. For many, crises will mark the passage of early middlescence. The most general one will involve the psychological aspect of reassessing identity. The settling on one's identity in the mid-stream of life may for some precipitate the rites de passages to a different kind of life involving changes, marriage, work, life style. For many others, comes the acceptance and recognition of change with some discomfiture—for women a more adventuresome role and less of the nurturant quality that characterized their earlier lives looms; and for men less aggressive behavior and, increasingly, roles involving more understanding and sympathy for others and consolidating their economic status.

Clearly the benchmark for those in the middle years is general activity. Those who are too busy to notice the years piling up undoubtedly think of themselves as being younger. The idea of the middlescence relates to characteristics that make up a whole cluster of factors—physical, social, psychological, spiritual and philosophical. These factors compose the "in-between" age syndrome. An examination of the lives of men and women should help to introduce a positive element in their assessment of ourselves and our adjustment. Now let's turn our attention to who we are; eventually we will look at a variety of suggestions which could assist you in living.

Who Are We?

There are those who feel that "middle age" may be the dirtiest word in the English language. Despite being overlooked by the government, placed in limbo by America's youth cult and being ambivalent about their own identity, the middlescent goes forward without missing a step. Although, as a group, the middle aged are not as strong physically as the young, nevertheless a few years ago the healthiest man in the nation, judged by a health organization, was a forty-four year old farmer.

Testimony everywhere confirms the importance of the middlescent person. Some have called this group the command generation or the "take charge" generation. In fact, without exaggeration the world would bankrupt itself is such persons were eliminated. Their voting records are better than the young. Their attendance on the job is better. Though they represent only a third of the population, the age group 40-69 earns more than half of the money. Dr. Bernice Neugarten, professor of Human Development at Northwestern University in her book *Personality in Middle and Later Life*, says "Middle aged men and women are the norm-bearers and the decision-makers of our society." And while they live in a society which may be oriented toward youth, it is controlled by the middle-aged. With the increase in longevity they are likely to maintain control for even longer periods.

A new phenomena exists today as 78 million "baby boomers" born between 1946 and 1964 begin to turn 55. They are turning fifty at the rate of 10,000 a day. As Tim Smart of *U.S. News and World Report* states they've changed life as we know it in recent decades—from music to marriage to mutual funds—this healthy, wealthy and wise bands of "zoomers" he calls the boomers is charging toward retirement at its own breakneck speed. He reports they have transformed the suburbs, bringing about the "soccer moms" phenomena. The "boomers" will be a force to reckon with as they make up close to a third of the U.S. population. Already 14 million are 50 and up. Many are retiring before 55. Ninety percent have graduated from high school and more than 25% have a college degree. More than three-quarters own homes and 73% have some form of investment. The AARP on the 50 plus generation shows those in the top one fourth had a median income of $100,000. The median income is not distributed evenly as those in the bottom fourth had a median income of only $10,000. These were disproportionately women.

The most common trait of the boomer generation is that they have been a very distinct group throughout their lives, says William Frey of The Milken Institute. This demographer says "they had broken the mold in every conceivable way." I can't image them really changing as they age. A discussion of their financial prowess and outlook will be discussed in the chapter on money and future retirement.

Retirement experts say the "zoomers" as they are called are: independent, youthful, with prospects of a long life ahead and well off. Their bank accounts fattened by two wage earners in many families, their bodies strengthened by years of exercise, their minds stimulated by college and some times postgraduate educations, are generally far better equipped for retirement than their parents were.

Still there are millions of middleagers born in the war years and before and those after the 1964 boomer period, in fact, nearly 25 million between the ages of 55-64 plus other millions from 65-69-our upper older middlescent group.

Many consider the middle years to be the vintage years. Barry Goldwater, at eighty said that "too many people over 40 feel that the best years of their lives are behind. They don't realize that an individual's growth does not or should not stop at 40 or 50 but should continue to reinforce itself throughout his entire life. Not only do the middle-aged do themselves an injustice when they picture themselves on the verge of decline but they fail in one of their most important and challenging contributions, the transmission to the young of what is best in our society."

Identity Crisis

In the book *Faces People Wear*, the authors name the crisis of identity as one of the principal difficulties besetting our troubled society. To put it simply, many of us are not sure who we are and are struggling with the task of finding ourselves.

In the situation is analogous to being an adolescent again. Dr. Erik H. Erikson, a former Harvard professor of psychiatry, states that identity confusion is the principal developmental problem of the teenager. The confusion of adolescent identity relates to physical changes and the attending psychological shifts. In youth, this quandary is seen in such questions as what role should I play—that of leader, follower or experimenter. Whose basic identity do I take—mom, dad, teacher, TV star, rap singer, athlete or friend? Am I free as a bird to go and do what I want? To get a job or not, to be titillated by sex and drink or whatever!

The middle years suggests Dr. Erik Erikson, is a period characterized by either activity (production) or stagnation. Activity refers to the productivity of work, ideas, planning and creativity—raising a garden, painting a picture, sewing, being nurturant to others, and being a positive role model. Stagnation is the opposite situation where the person does nothing more than routines of work and necessary activities. Such persons pursue no projects or seek new vistas, but by and large are preoccupied with self.

Edmund Bergler, a psychologist, wrote some years ago in his *Revolt of the Middle Age Man* that with the second emotional adolescence comes a confusion of identity. For the first 40 years a man has been unrolling fresh scroll that bears the story of what he is and his aspirations as a worker, father, husband, lover, doer-everything. All he has achieved or failed to achieve is there, even his most fantastic dreams like imagining being the president of his company, winning the Nobel Prize or being Julia Robert's lover. The woman, too, considers being sought after by Tom Cruise, dreams of professional or occupational success, and fantasizes of being fabulously rich and the owner of a palatial mansion. However, there usually comes an event which forces him or her to see what and is really happening. At the same time, they see the scroll beginning to yellow and fade. For women, dramatic physical changes and though less dramatic men lose potentia and develop wide girths together with the "blahs" of life force an evaluation.

In the middle years, one frequently poses the question to himself of "What's the use?" With all the years behind, it would seem that the person in midstream would know who he is, but the subtle shifts of ground belie this. The individual is under the heaviest burden of responsibility, with increased physical and psychological distraction and with a decrease in strength and drive. Because of self-doubt, the question arises: Will past values sustain me for the remaining years? What has my life been? Fish or foul? Just who am I? How shall I manage the rest of my life?

The crisis of identity is compounded by the necessity of serving a middleman function of relating to other generations—one's parents and children—and at the same time forwarding one's own personal fulfillment. This is sometimes called the general squeeze. Sinclair Lewis wrote in *Babbitt*, "I'm sick of it!" He rages…

> Having to carry these generations. Whole damn bunch lean on me. Pay half of mother's income, listen to Henry T., listen to Myre's worrying, be polite to Mart, and get called an old grouch for trying to help the children. All of them depend on me and picking on me and not a damn one of 'em grateful! No relief, and no credit, and no help from anybody. And to keep it up for—good Lord, how long?

The claims of time and energy are unrelenting, and although men and women reach the peak of their influence upon society at this time, it is also true that society makes its maximum demands upon them. These pressures, along with those of biological change, environmental impact, and individual self-realization, make the task of easy transition through this stage one of considerable magnitude. By 40 most adults have parents 60 to 80 years of age probably most 65-70. For these younger middleagers many becoming care takers or giving assistance to parents although only 10% of elderly couples live with children while 17% widows and widowers will live with children (Rice, 2000). Besides the care of aging parents the demand to help children become emancipated becomes a paramount concern.

Societal Expectations: A Perspective

In the western world, certain expectancies for the various periods of life exist. They have arisen partly out of the historical adherence to the Protestant and Hebrew ethic and the pragmatic philosophy of America. These expectancies are called "Developmental Tasks" by Robert Havinghurst, a former social scientist of the University of Chicago. These tasks that follow serve as a guide for the middlescent in comparing his life to others; these are significant priorities.

- Establishing a standard of living.
- Assisting teen-age children to become responsible and adjusted persons,
- Developing adult leisure time pursuits,
- Relating oneself to one's spouse as a person,
- Accepting and adjusting to the physical changes of middle age,
- Adjusting to the emancipation of children, and
- Adjusting to the aging of parents and kinspeople

The emphasis is on the word "adjustment," unlike the task of the child and adolescent, where the key words are "formal learning," "developing," and "achieving." In the young adult, the task is mainly preparing and beginning—and education, a marriage or love relation, a family, a home or occupation and civic responsibility.

The overlay of roles both from the past and those anticipated in the future combine to add muddy waters to life just when one shakingly ponders, "What's in it for me?" Tasks tend to accumulate, jeopardizing those remaining to be learned (like the development of an ethical system values and sense of the right behavior). All of this delays adult maturity and creates problems when the middlescent is focusing on essential issues. For Erikson, personality develops across a series of stages that occur from childhood to old age. Each stage incorporates a central crisis or conflict, which is psychosocial in nature. There are eight stages beginning with the first year of life—involving trust versus mistrust as the social crisis. For the middle age person the central problem is generativity (<u>production</u>) as opposed to stagnation (vegetation). Generativity means the commitment to care for others, a willingness to guide and counsel and a positive outlook on life in general. <u>Stagnation</u> represents over-concern with self, rejection of a positive outlook, and perhaps the manifestation of destruction impulses toward ones family, social heirs and the community.

Carl Jung divides development into two phases, the first from birth to about 40, involving preoccupation with meeting obligations revolving around family and society. The second phase, 40 years and beyond, relates to the recognition of the inner world and bringing parts of this world to consciousness. It means giving up the image of youth and recognition of the finiteness of life. A person must find the meaning of one's inner self. Jung has said "what youth found and must find outside, the man of life's afternoon must find within himself." This balance of opposites is often rejected by people who would elude it, preferring to retain inappropriate life-styles. You need an example here? I know a forty-year-old man who is still living in his teens and early twenties through athletics. He is consumed by playing flag football and sports events. In Raleigh, North Carolina, there are a number of persons now in their forties who graduate from the local State University who are still pursuing the social life of the undergraduate. They are continuing to attend fraternity social activities with their round of cocktail parties.

Meeting the obligations of the first adult years imposes constraint on the developing personality in that men often focus on the instrumental (ways to get ahead) and achievement oriented aspects of personality, while women focus on the more expressive and nurturant areas of life. Completion of the transition to an inner orientation allows the person to continue to function with undiminished motivation and effectiveness. Jung believed one of the major causes of neuroses in the second part of life comes form the preservation of an inappropriate life-style, the playing out of model roles, "forever 25 years old, the continual partier, etc." A theme that is continually heralded by television and Hollywood.

There are a number of changes which take place during the early and middle period of middlescence which are significant. They do not necessarily precipitate crisis nor are they always traumatic, but they are of signal importance. People in this period of their life should not mistake changes that typically take place as a crisis of earth-shaking impact. Such changes as need to relocate, get another job, or having our son or daughter find suitable work, or get fat or lose our hair. Currents, ripples and eddies in the stream of life do not for the most indicate that the stream of life will burst its bounds and that it is time for us to bail out. Perhaps this is why physicians prescribe a deluge of drugs to their patients in hopes of calming knee-jerk reaction that could in time incur irrefutable damage. In most cases the storms of life do not shatter our foundations; they only help to purify and strength our lives. Perhaps due to longer life or greater self-honesty, it can be expected that erosions in many marriages will force their dissolvement. Altered patterns of ecology such as continued drought force people to move or alter their work and economic circumstances (job in the auto industry because of automation) and many small Great Plains towns due to curtailed railroads and loss of industry are vanishing, this will require new occupations and living locations.

Changes Take Place

Physical, environmental, and personal changes are common to nearly everyone. The physical changes—the decrease in physical strength, losses in vision and hearing, losses of hair in amount and color, loss of sexual potency, etc.—are paralleled by undesirable weight gains—increased sensitivity to noise (high decibels and cacophonous sounds), weight increases, higher blood pressure, and greater psychological distractions. The American people are mobile-nearly a third will move from their present place of living to a new home (if only a neighborhood away) every year. Distance separates families and often precludes available assistance in crises. During the middlescent period the need to take in an aging parent increases the complexity of the environment of people in the household. Also their children often need help in launching themselves into the world of college or work. Functioning as a buffer between the younger and older generations is difficult without the constant stimulus of one's psyche asking "what's in it for me?" and "how can I forward my own interests?"

Middlescence is a time when family and community responsibility is greatest; its only compensation is the cumulative wisdom of experience, and of course success of our children in their home and work places. Even that, at this period, becomes doubtful. For almost everyone comes at some point in the middle years to reevaluate his or her value system. Will the values I have thus far built my life upon sustain me the rest of my life? Do I need to reconsider my values?

Perhaps, you might say that you have found relating to the spouse an impossible task and opt for another alternative. Maybe you have no children or they are emancipated and living their own lives. Maybe other kin are not close by or you do not care to relate to them. What then? Try another life style or career? Why not? The problems people have are usually different and demand varied approaches. There are, however, some fundamental components that influence each of us.

People have viewed development in life as being complete when one reaches twenty-one. We now know that this is not true. Adult life does not plateau at an early age. Any individual's chronology concerns three dimensions of time: (a) "life time"—one's age; human development theorists think physical development in general is completed first (on average by 25) mental development (by thirty) and emotional maturation by 60; (2) "social time"—how age is graded, its status, etc., and the expectations society has for us (like the "developmental tasks" mentioned earlier); and (3) "historical time"—those political and economic circumstances into which one is born which dynamically affect the life that is lived. Many middle aged persons born in the 1920's and 1930's who were radically affected by the depression, lived lives handicapped by lack of economic resources for college educations, travel, special training, clothes, food and medical care.

David Gutmann suggests men change from active to passive mastery styles as they approach their fifties and are more interested in their feelings and ideas than the activity perhaps due to diminishing success in this mode. Women change in the opposite direction—from passive to more aggressive, active mastery styles as witness the dramatic entrance of women in the job market in this mode. My grandmother built a substantial dining room table when she was fifty after being promised one by my grandfather for a long time. Everywhere one sees evidence of women in middle age taking matters into their own hands where men formerly held sway—in such areas a politics, business, and law. Evidence for tentative acceptance of Gutmann's notion abounds.

Parenthood is the pivot around which adult life is organized—men traditionally the providers of physical security and women emotional security. This is not to say that "woman's destiny is her uterus." Child bearing, a basic function in evolutionary history, provides life for the race. Certainly the changing roles of women demand a broader rationale for theorizing a view which must, while not eliminating the importance of bearing children in our society, give increasing weight to the equal roles women play as leaders, heads of households, providers, protectors, and determiners of values in the world.

If sex role distinctions are evolutionary responses to the "parental imperative" and these account for making possible the survival of the young, does this radically change normal post-parental condition when the "look alike, do alike" syndrome erases traditional marriage roles? The answer is no. However we must make the roles of each partner more acceptable and understandable. What expectations do exist for the middlescent in our times if the major conception of adult life—marriage, children, emancipation of children, grandparentage, etc.—are replaced? Obviously, if the world is to continue some form of the birth cycle and parenthood must proceed. To help understand your time and place in life, what can be said as certain?

Certainty

The greatest certainty of growing older, of becoming middlescent, is that of change. The change is not the product of chance but a process imposed from without and from within. Somewhere toward the end the younger middlescent period 40-49 one reaches a plateau where it is possible to view life in backward perspective and forward in prospect. By this time one has lived for approximately half of his or her lifetime. For almost everyone this time is a period of evaluation and reflection. People feel the need to assess their lives. This often precipitates an identity crisis, often resulting in new starts—in marriage, in the work world, style of living, and a new view of ourselves. It does not in most cases destroy the foundations that one's life has been built upon.

In life, changes take place in three areas: the physical, the social, and the psychological. Much of life is physical—the forty-year-old is no longer like the twenty-year-old. As Dr. Campbell Moses of the American Heart Association, an authority on aging says subtle losses take place by the time man is forty—in the central nervous system, change in the alpha rhythms affect attention and the loss of nerve velocity along with cellular enzymes. At 20, the heart when needed pumps as much as 40 liters of blood in a minute. At forty, the heart under stress pumps only 23 liters. In addition, the kidneys have lost their reserve capacity to concentrate wastes. The thyroid has begun to shrink. The good news is that there is usually plenty left to carry one until he or she is seventy or eighty years old. Changes typically initiate greater body monitoring, particularly for men, than in the early adult period.

The social environment is a very important aspect of the life cycle. There are great demands placed upon us in our lives by society, especially in the western world. The middlescent person has to respond to society's ideal of and not unity and decide what direction he or she goes—retreat and consolidate, or advance and try new ventures.

The psychological aspect of maturing reflects one's ability to maintain a mental balance between goals, identity, the use of energy, and the reaction to crisis. At middlescence one's internal solidarity increases in importance—that the view of self and of life, both in its maturing aspects and the impetus given to important projects, is in synchronization, and one is largely at peace. A person does not easily reach this point in life.

Adult Stages

Development as adults is broadly related to different facets: (1) maturing physically and absolving the problems and illusions of childhood, and (2) adjustment to change as demanded by the life situation and one's self-consistency.

By the time a person is thirty or thirty-five, most adults have "settled down," have married, established a home or a love relationship, and have accepted community responsibility. Men during this period often have or have had mentors who serve alternatively as parents and/or peers who helped them to advance a career or clarify goals and prospects. As women's roles change and they become involved in a greater variety of occupations at all levels, they too will have more mentors. In the academic profession, especially at the doctoral level, this is commonplace today. The mentor is typically a man. Researcher, Victoria Djimidian has said that a major focus of professional women aged 33-40 is the relational time to a special other with whom an intimate bond has been established. Although Djimidian says that the work life is very important to women during this phase of life, she maintains that for many younger married women, family and children represent their major interest. These women find psychological value and pleasure in the growth of children. Somewhere between the ages of thirty-five and forty-five, women undergo a reappraisal of earlier notions of their lives. They reassess their lives and what re-orientation should be made. Often this ends up in a significant crisis, trauma or change. It requires a new integration, consolidation of values and r4estructuring of the new terms encountered in one's life.

Around the age of forty or later the identity crisis is one of a fractured ego or fractured identity. One questions whether he or she is effective, no longer viewing themselves as attractive, physically strong, or successful. In the middle age adult, the task of this period is to establish generativity. Generativity is achieved by investing in the product of one's creation, one's children or a humanitarian cause. In the latter part of middlescence (55 to 65 and beyond) often the emphasis is on integrity—the sense that one's life has been worthwhile. Failure of integrity leads to despair and fear of death.

The middlescent must adequately solve the problems of the developmental tasks found in each epoch or stage of life. At the same time the middlescent must overcome the problem of the illusion of childhood. People hold on to these illusions until the age of forty-five or fifty. Roger Gould suggests that some of these illusions are (a) if our parents live, we will be saved from unhappy lives, (b) that we will always be close to our parents and be their child, (c) that with our parents we are always safe from harm, and (d) that there is no death while our parents live. The first and perhaps the greatest source of the idea of happiness in life comes from childhood. The sense of well-being and safety is so great that it usually colors life until middle age and perhaps longer. When parents die, the last vestige of the illusion of safety may be destroyed. However, lesser events often break down the aura of invincibility of parents—parents could not make their children's business succeed, could not provide money to ease deprivations, or save them from failures in marriage or in other ways make their lives happy.

Many problems found in adult life (even in middle age) are rooted in childhood. Increasingly, human development specialists are treating many emotional difficulties as failure to resolve genuine adult problems rather than conflicts left over from infancy. Social and cultural factors are seen as the key to development; this should help to relieve parents of the burdens of ear and guilt impinging upon them. Parents no longer have to feel like villains if their children grow into troubled, disturbed adults. It should also be true that adults can no longer blame their troubles on their parents.

Even if the adult understands the developmental aspects of life, the transition from young adulthood to older adulthood can be difficult. What benchmark can be used to judge one's life or provide help in particular areas of life? This volume is designed to do simply that. What are the experiences others have had with love, marriage and divorce? How do you solve the problems that thousands have in the balancing act between the younger and older generations? Self-fulfillment and leisure time during the middlescent years are increasingly urgent issues. So you know about the prospects of a second career at forty-five? What should you do in preparation for retirement? What about physical and mental health? Finally, what are the necessary ingredients of the "good life?" The chapters in this book are designed to help you answer these questions and solve some of life's most stressing problems.

In this chapter, we have made the following points:

- The middle years, though they are often associated with the 35-65 are becoming older at both ends. Middle age starts later and ends later than it did fifty years ago.
- The middle years are those times characterized by the establishment of a life style, a work pattern, a worldview, inner solidarity and a sense of the worth of ideas and things.
- The middlescent in our time is the leader, the take charge generation and because of life's extension will be in command for longer than its predecessors.
- This period of life is a time for "assessing one's life," what has it been, what may it be? Is there a crisis to resolve we ponder? How best can we use the future!
- The middleager serves a "middle man functions" in that he or she relates to maturing children and the older generation of mom and dad, often placing a squeeze on one's own life's fulfillment.
- The key to successful life for those in the in-between years is adjustment, understanding the societal demands on us, the decision to be positive and to live productive lives.
- The individual chronology concerns three dimension of time—"Life Time"—one's age, "Social Time" how age is graded and "Historical Time" meaning the kind of economic and political environment of the present.
- Women in middlescence develop active mastery styles particularly in the larger world—work community—whereas men mainly develop passive mastery styles becoming more nurturance while women often become more aggressive.
- Adult life is unique; it is developmental. People who have emotional difficulties are not thought to have had them as a hold over from childhood but as a genuine adult problem. Cultured and social factors in development are the key.

CHAPTER II

STRESS AND TENSION AND MENTAL HEALTH

"Am I Crazy?"

Perhaps at no time is stress or tension more evident than during middle age. The young are protected by their ability to adjust more easily to stress due to their physical prowess, resiliency and increasingly effective organ and gland systems. In daily activity our body's cells are continually being worn out and replaced with new ones. In a medical sense, stress has been defined as all the wear and tear in the body caused by living. All emotions—from love to hate—involve stress. Even what we term play is stressful and so is physical exertion—swimming, golf, or just a brisk walk, even projects involving our jobs can be zestful and stimulating. These types of stress are good (called eustress) for us. The important thing is not the stress or tension created but its effect on us—in short, how we handle it.

Stress and Middle Age

The anxiety of middle age differs from that of a younger person who is striving to make a beginning in the work-a-day world and the establishment of a home. Major contributing factors to the middle years tension are: (1) physical strength erosion, (2) inability to control or favorably influence children, (3) children leaving home, (4) poor health, (5) job insecurity, (6) identity problems, (7) career limitations, (8) sexual ineffectiveness, (9) money problems, (10) death in the family, and (11) change. The person in the in-between years has less life energy and strength left to carry the thrusts of unrelenting competition, the baffled fury of change, and less time to reconstruct or rechannel old patterns than does the young adult. For these reasons it is much more important that the middlescent learn how to handle emotional tensions. In the first place, it is unhealthy to keep emotional tensions bottled up. Release can come through talking, playing, and working. It is important to learn how to handle our emotional tensions. To do this one must understand his or her physical emotional limitation. This is easier said than done. But understanding is the first step. By being knowledgeable of the common emotional stresses and recognizing them rather than ignoring them, we will see a reduction in those illnesses that strike us through our inner conflicts.

Childhood is not the happy, carefree time of life we may like to image. Most of us have forgotten or repressed many of our childhood tragedies because they were too painful for us to remember. But as a young child we can remember being left alone at camp for this first time or taken to a little known kinsman to stay while our parents took a trip. Or perhaps we remember our parents violently arguing in the next room night after night. Some have known the tension of having our parents separate and divorce. We can help our children by learning to become more sensitive to their needs and to see that they are free from excessive worry and tension. It is not emotions that are at fault when we refer to stressful problems. For an emotion, whether pleasant or unpleasant, is simply a person's response to a fact or a situation as he sees it.

Understanding Stress and Its Effects on Life

Most adults recognize that some stress is a part of daily life. Often pressure from the outside can make you feel tense inside. It is also true that pressure that comes from inside can make us feel tense. Wherever the source, these tensions can create anxiety. This anxiety is a vague fear that something unpleasant is going to happen often caused by holding back feelings we can't cope with or understand. It could be a conflict between what we would like to do and what we want to do. Depression is also fathered by tension, resulting in sadness or apathy. It may come from the inability to control our world, to cope with frustrations and the responsibilities of daily life. By examining some of the types of stress and their effect on the body we can have a basis for better understanding what can be done to relieve or adjust to stress. Let's examine external and internal sources of stress.

External Stress

This kind of stress comes from the environment. There are two kinds—physical and psychological. Certain actions are motivated by our demand to satisfy our hunger, to communicate, be involved in activities and to have sex.

The undue frustration of these needs creates stress. Psychological relates to adjustment.

In a rapidly changing society such as ours, there is an increasing number of choices to make. In primitive times choices were made for people—their occupation, their mate, religion, etc. The burden of adjustment now is often overwhelming. However, most people seem to be able to adjust to almost anything where the need of change comes slowly. When this is not the case, the demands for immediate adjustment often create a state of stress.

Financial problems, pressure to "keep up with the neighbors," worry over debt and inflation are major sources of stress. Many of these concerns are related to emotional and status needs—security, recognition, affection, power—all of which we associate with money. Lack of money creates real stress. The college student wants to go to medical school, a family is forced to live in sub-standard housing or a small apartment for lack of money. Teeth repair or other essential medical needs have to be foregone because of lack of ability to pay. A mother who is forced to work, leaving small children at home or sending the very young adolescent out to work, all create the conditions that are likely to tax our capacity to adjust.

Even physical objects become stressors. Their range runs from the baby whose pen limits the area of exploration and the mountain that stands between a city and a potential water supply. Acts of nature serve as stressors—floods, fires, winds and earthquakes. To a lesser degree, stress may result from ants getting into our food at a picnic. Rain canceling a ball game eagerly awaited. The stench of garbage and offensive odor where we work or play, unpleasing colors and discordant noise all combine to cause stress. The human organism is so constituted that it requires external stimulation to maintain equilibrium; otherwise, the efficiency of a person is disturbed.

Internal Stress

This kind of stress, often called psychological stress, is less visible and specific. We are often unaware or partly aware of what is bothering us when we feel anxious or insecure. When we have guilt feelings or feelings of being worthless, humiliated, and are insecure, it gives us a constant fear of failure in life. Unconscious conflicts often involve contradictions such as love and hate of the same individual or object (the school or a crooked curving road). Many conflicts are carried over from childhood but still persist. The child is constantly reminded of his physical and mental limitation. My sister had a smaller than usual head and was frequently hailed by other children as "little head" with little intelligence. This notion was never forgotten until she was required when she was 35 to take an IQ test for a job. After finding out her standing, she considered herself mentally normal. The fact that a child cannot pound a nail like his father, solve an algebra problem like his older sister, or throw a ball like big brother, may combine to harden within himself a view of constant shortcomings. Too great a feeling of limitation will affect his future efforts and inadequacy in achieving goals. Even adults have periods of limitations due to stress, an example some persons who watch violence on TV over and over, and are then afraid to venture outdoors.

Most of us find ourselves in some situations where we are bound to fail either because of lack of knowledge, strength, ability or talent. Some famous businessmen find trying one business after another business until they often are successful. One such person failed in six businesses and was 44 when he finally established a successful business. Ten years later he was a millionaire. These happen less in adulthood, not because we're grown or mature, but mainly because we have learned to avoid situations where we are likely to fail and to make the most of ourselves. As a youth I listened to a young lady singing a song with the notes in a key I thought she could not reach. Upon the approach to the final highest note she collapsed on the floor. I wondered then, but now know that she was escaping from censure by using avoidance as a defense adjustment; probably later she wouldn't have tried that high a note. Certainly any failure affects our self-esteem and status—hence its stress produces a reaction and often a defense mechanism.

The most stressful circumstance man faces, however, is frustration concerning personal needs. To be denied food, clothing, or housing is calamitous! If we are denied love, we are put under extreme stress, for this calls into question the fundamental worth of our existence. One should remember that needs are multiple and often in conflict with those of society. The rules and regulations of a complex society, though necessary for its survival, often become sources of stress for the people in society. There are more laws, restrictions, forms to fill out, growing taxes, increasing numbers of stoplights and red tape. Most people view these as sources of external pressure and stress.

Even other people become sources of stress. Sartre, the French philosopher-writer, has one of the characters in a play to reflect—"hell is other people." Stress coming from interpersonal relations may be imposed deliberately or accidentally; it may also be felt consciously or unconsciously. The boy who goads his little brother to tears because he is resentful and envious may know he is tormenting his brother but not aware of his reasons for doing so. The over-protective mother may hide from herself the reasons for babying her child, but may deny that she is a source of stress and frustration to him. Every child growing up is faced with frustration, criticism, demands, and aggression. This is part of testing the nature of the world or "reality testing." All parents put some demands on their children. The controls placed upon children by their parents serve to counter some of aggressive and sexual impulses. This aids in channeling behavior into acceptable outlets and to become responsible citizens. If the stress for the child is so that he can overcome it without too much difficulty, the child's ego will be strengthened, his self-concept enhanced and he will be able to meet future stress with greater confidence. If stress is more than a child can bear and adjustment cannot be made, the ego will be overwhelmed and less able to cope with later stress.

Stress in interpersonal relations is not always one-sided. In marriage conflicts, often each party puts the other partner under stress. A cycle is set up in which one of the parties fails to meet the needs of the other. Frustration and tension develop creating an additional barrier preventing the needs of either partner from being met. Though the presence of people causes stress, so does absence from them. Separation from supporting friends and loved-ones often upsets us. The sudden loss of love can be traumatic and where dependency is so great, even death can occur. This is seen in cases of elderly couples when, shortly after the death of a mate, the remaining partner dies.

Competing motives create conflict; this is seen when we involve ourselves in our demanding work requiring extra time but would like at the same time to be with friends pursuing leisure time activities—playing cards, fishing, camping, vacationing, partying and a variety of other things. Having talked about kinds of stress, the question arises of just how the body handles stress. It is pretty well agreed that the body takes care of stress under what is called the Adaptation Syndrome.

A Little Theory

Stress covers a wide range of characteristics—fear, exhilaration, frustration, injury, conflict, disease and even normal body operation. All of these in one way or the other are handled through the General Adaptation Syndrome theory developed by Hans Selye. Simply put, this involves three stages, which the body goes through to defend itself from danger, whether the dangers are real or imagined, external or internal. The stages through which this is handled are Stage 1—the alarm reaction, Stage 2—the resistance stage, and Stage 3 B the stage of exhaustion. This is diagramed as follows:

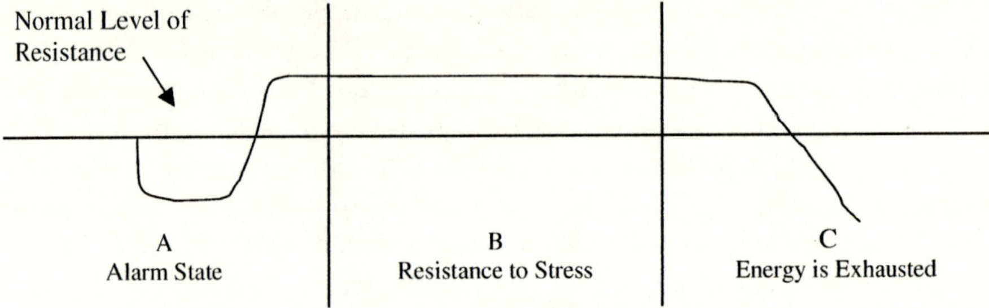

In response to stress the brain activates the hypothalamus glands in the base of the brain which stimulates the production of CRF (Corticotropin Release Factor) and other chemical messengers. These are sent along the parasympathetic nerve and the sympathetic nerves tracks. This is the alarm stage of Selye's theory. The first track leads to the pituitary where a chemical change into the hormone ACTH (Adrenocorticotrophin) is made. It enters the bloodstream and travels to the adrenal glands where ACTH initiates the production of cortisol, a chemical that increases the blood sugar and speeds up metabolism.

The second track begins with the hypothalamus, which triggers electrochemical impulses, and spinal cord until the signals reach the core of the adrenal. Epinephrine (formerly called adrenaline) is released supplying fuel to the muscles and brain with glucose. It also releases norephinephrine, which speeds up the heart and raises the blood pressure. In Selye's second stage both tracks feed back to the pituitary to regulate the stress response. Normalcy in time is resumed when ACTH is inhibited by the adrenal hormones.

If the stress continues until the energy of adaptation is used up then serious difficulty ensues which may mean loss of consciousness or coma even death. This is the third and final stage of Selye's theory.

In a study at Stanford University rats were forced to swim in 4 degrees Centigrade water for three minutes. Examination of their brain tissue afterward revealed that levels of norepinephrine had fallen 20% and epinephrine

30% to 40%. These triggers chemical changes in the brain. Sensitivity to emotional strain are potent chemicals called neurotransmitters (serotonin, epinephrine, norepinephrine, acetylcholine, dopamine) which act as messengers between the nerve cells. Depression has been associated with serotonin and norepinephrine. Schizophrenia seems to be related to excess dopamine. When the neurotransmitters become altered (usually under long-time duress) the following effects of stress on the body is likely.

If Stress Effects the

Depletion of Norepinephrine and serotonin then it causes endocrine disorders such as reduction of thyroid affecting metabolism and insulin production which controls sugar levels.	Autonomic Nervous System upsets the psychophysiologic pattern which leads to ulcers, high blood pressure, colitis (irritable colon) and asthma.	Hypothalamus then upper respiratory infections result.

(The area affected depends upon the individual.)

Withstanding Stress

How well an individual withstands stress depends upon a number of factors—their physical and mental health, their environment, their perception of a stressful situation and the number of acute stresses suffered over a given period of time. Drs. Holmes and Rahe (University of Washington Medical School), both psychiatrists found that though people (Sample: 5,000 persons from Japan, Canada, Europe and the United States) are different but there is agreement on the relative importance of stress events. On this chart below, those people who had scores of 300 or over in a year experienced significant health problems. Life events are ranked according to their stress value in the chart below. The top value of 100 is given the Life Change Units (LCU). Also small hassles which Holmes and Rahe believe can often mean as much as major events. Here's his list of hassles and uplifts which he sampled getting information from a number of men and women 48-52 for these lists. Holmes and Rahe found the daily uplifts do little to compensate for the hassles.

Rank	Life event	LCU value
1.	Death of spouse	100
2.	Divorce	73
3.	Marital separation	65
4.	Jail term	63
5.	Death of close family member	63
6.	Personal injury or illness	53
7.	Marriage	50
8.	Fired from job	47
9.	Marital reconciliation	45
10.	Retirement	45
11.	Change in health of family member	44
12.	Pregnancy	40
13.	Sex difficulties	39
14.	Gain of new family member	39
15.	Business readjustment	39
16.	Change in financial state	38
17.	Death of close friend	37
18.	Change to different line of work	36
19.	Change in number of arguments with spouse	35
20.	Mortgage over $100,000	31
21.	Foreclosure of mortgage or loan	30
22.	Change in responsibilities at work	29

Rank	Life Event	LCU value
23.	Son or daughter leaving home	29
24.	Trouble with in-laws	29
25.	Outstanding personal achievement	28
26.	Wife begins or stops work	26
27.	Begin or end school	26
28.	Change in living conditions	25
29.	Revision of personal habits	24
30.	Trouble with boss	23
31.	Change in work hours or conditions	20
32.	Change in residence	20
33.	Change in schools	20
34.	Change in recreation	19
35.	Change in church activities	19
36.	Change in social activities	18
37.	Loan less than $10,000	17
38.	Change in sleeping habits	16
39.	Change in number of family get-togethers	15
40.	Change in eating habits	15
41.	Vacation	13
42.	Christmas	12
43.	Minor violations of the law	11

<u>Hassles</u>

1. Concern about weight
2. Health of a family member
3. Rising price of common goods
4. Home maintenance
5. Too many things to do
6. Misplacing or losing things
7. Yard work
8. Property investment or taxes
9. Crime
10. Physical appearance

Additional hassles we add

1. Children's schooling—lessons, books, assignments and problems
2. A child that hangs up their clothes on the floor, helps little to keep his room in order.

<u>Uplifts</u>

1. Relating well with your spouse or lover
2. Relating well with friends
3. Completing a task
4. Feeling healthy
5. Getting enough sleep
6. Eating out
7. Meeting responsibilities
8. Visiting, phoning or writing someone
9. Spending time with family
10. Having a home pleasing to you

Additional uplifts added by the author

1. A good report card
2. A child or children who cooperate in keeping their room clean and in order.

Adapted from Holmes and Rahe

You can assess your stress. Recall what happened to you over the past year. Check the vents and add up the points. If your total was under 50, you will escape adverse reactions. A score of 150-199 indicates a mild problem. From 200-299, you have a moderate problem with a 51% chance of change in your health. Total points over 300 are a threat to your well being.

In all groups everywhere the scale has a grim usefulness as a tool for predicting stress-related illness—the higher the score the greater the likelihood of such illnesses. The difference in effect on people depends on those things previously mentioned (personality, health, etc.) but one important influence seems to be knowledge—an understanding of what is happening. Realistic and believable information—ideally in advance of a crisis can help soften the shock and reduce the after effects. A colleague had a score of 180 and six months later he contracted asthma. The score can be a fairly good predictor of future illness and problems.

There are no easy solutions to the problems of life which cause much tension and strife. Such problems are inherent in the system. In fact, life is impossible without some stress. By making an effort, however, we can find new and better ways of dealing with our tensions.

<u>Suggestions for Improving Every Day Stress of Living</u>

(1) <u>Balance work with play</u>. It is a must to schedule time for fun and recreation. Remember that a good hobby can be relaxing. Of course, work can be a cure for emotional situations that are hard to bear such as the death of a loved one, a divorce, or losing out in love.

(2) <u>Loaf a little</u>. Some people feel guilt when they're not constantly working, but the change of pace that comes from doing nothing but sitting and talking can bring renewed zest to life.

(3) <u>Get enough rest and sleep</u>. To be at our best we need generally to have between 7 to8 hours of sleep per night. Accumulative sleep losses contribute to nervousness and illness. If possible, take a nap or at least lie down sometime during the day. This slows down the pace.

(4) <u>Work off tensions</u>. When angry or upset we can blow off steam or work off our feelings with physical exercise. Jump into some activity like gardening, playing tennis, taking a long walk, swimming or playing some sport. This not only helps relieve anger but makes it easier to

face and handle irritating problems more calmly. Regular exercise is therapeutic in its own right.

(5) Talk out troubles. Those things that appear to be serious problems generating high degrees of strain can be discussed with clergymen or your physician. If warranted the physician will refer you to a guidance clinic or family service agency.

(6) Learn to accept what you cannot change. Many of us get upset over things we cannot control. We ask ourselves when people cannot be made to suit our ideals, "Isn't everybody that way—even me?" And in the long run, what difference does it really make if we cannot change a certain situation.

(7) Get away from it all. The diversion created by simply leaving a situation which has us in a quandary may be important. Go to a movie, visit a friend or take a few days off. These distractions help one to cope and allow us a chance to catch our breath and to regain the composure we need to face everyday problems. This may give us a new perspective. This

(8) Avoid self-medication. Do not use drugs or tranquilizers without consultation with your physician. Remember anything that reduces tension (drugs, alcohol, eating) becomes habit forming. Many physicians feel prescribing Valium or Meprobamate is of less evil than the potential tragedy of "nervous breakdown," heart attack, loss of loved one, divorce, loss of a job or catastrophic illness. Rarely do physicians have or take the time to develop a program for getting someone off a drug. CNS depressants such as Xanax, Valium and Ativan are the most commonly used for sleeping. Restaril and Ambien are most often prescribed. Newer drugs like EffexorXR and PaxilCR cover general anxiety. Drugs can reduce blood pressure and heart rate directly. They do not eliminate the actual stress, which caused the increase in heart rate or blood pressure, anxiety, or tension. Unless the stress is identified and corrected, however, the drugs that block the normal response to stress can cause more problems than they expect to relieve.

(9) Have regular visits to a physician. One's physical condition affects a person's outlook on life. The body that is fit can take stress, disappointments, and handle tensions more easily. A clean bill of health will also provide you extra peace of mind.

(10) Eat less. Americans are over-fed, over-weight, and under-exercised. All of this relates to stress. Emphasize foods that you like that are good for you!

Stress continued over a long period of time becomes intimately related to the sugar utilization in the body. The metabolism of sugar is an increasing problem for adults in the middle years. Sugar is associated with weight and unfortunately at every level of age from the middle 20's to the mid 60's, Americans on the average are overweight.

(11) Finally, take one thing at a time. It may seem impossible but make yourself, particularly when you feel the pressures of too much to do. Remember, of all the people in the world, you are the most important! So take charge of your life!! Everyone needs help, love, understanding and support in developing and maintaining a wellness life pattern. You should therefore have at least 2 persons you can count on for companionship and support when you need them. Beyond this one should set goals and priorities. Plan your work. Tension and anxiety really build up when work seems endless. Make a list of things to do and do them one at a time. Their completion will give you confidence. Finally, don't drift along with troublesome and stressful situations. If a marriage is bad, rehabilitate it or resolve it. Eliminate those friends who are really not your friends (where the exchange of attention and energy is unequal) and settle those matters that are bothersome to you, besides they give you needless worry. It's your life and you can manage it.

Burnout—A Special Problem With Stress

It happens to many people—executives, teachers, engineers, physicians, lawyers, nurses, people in business, high pressure types of work; it can also strike housewives or anyone who place stress on themselves. It also affects persons living or working in a stressful environment. Burnout often occurs in jobs where the work is extraordinarily repetitive. Burnout is frequently associated with high achievement and for people on the path to burn out or have or arrived as a defense against falling apart, or have developed ragged edges—they bristle at criticism, have little patience and are inveterate smokers, coffee drinkers, use uppers or downers, require constant excitement to charge them up to provide a euphoric moment.

Burnout describes a person who is fatigued and/or frustrated who are pursuing some goal or pattern of live or relationship that has failed to provide expected rewards. When one's expected level of success is miles away form its achievement resulting in frantic persistent and accelerated attempts to succeed, then trouble (burnout) is on its way. Friction is building with its inevitable drain of energy, vitality and ability to function. Said in another way, burnout means to deplete oneself, to exhaust one's physical and mental resources, to wear oneself out by excessively striving to reach some unrealistic goal imposed by one's self or by the values of society.

The following questions posed by Herbert Freudenberger can provide a clue to whether or not you're a candidate for burnout. Any long time problems at home, work, even with play where unresolved issues are chronic may herald negative affirmative to this quiz!

1. Are you working more now and enjoying it less whether it relates to marriage, your job, friendship or love?
2. Do you find it more difficult to confide in others?
3. Must you force yourself as a rule to do routine things?
4. Are you listless, bored, constantly seeking excitement?
5. Would you rather be somewhere else doing something else with somebody else?
6. Have you lost the joy of sex?
7. Do you think more than you used to within?
8. Do you need a tranquilizer to face the day? Need an upper?
9. Are you resigned about your future?
10. Is your need for a particular crutch increasing, like smoking, drugs, eating, nail biting?

The Two States of Burnout

There are two states to burnout. The first is the feeling state—the point in which tiredness, detachment, cynicism and hypersensitivity take over. At this stage the reserve energy, resources and functioning ability is going. The second state involves non-feeling—this is the stage in which the person denies anything is wrong in her life—friends may have given up on you and assume you'll muddle through.

The feeling state of burnout is characterized by chronic fatigue. One has been controlled by the way they interpret what they should do—at work, home in friendship or love—according to the environment. They have failed or have refused to stay in touch with their inner feelings. You need to think about your life, and get away from the crowd. In getting away, one needs to think about these areas: (1) what situations give you energy or drain you? (2) Are you involved in them or detached? and (3) Are you enthusiastic about them or cynical? (Jot down your answers to these questions for they will help you get in touch with yourself.) Your feelings about these questions can help you examine related emotions.

The non-feeling state of burnout involves a real danger—the denial that anything is wrong—for this follows the first stage exhaustion. If denial is seeping into your life—you can check this by remembering how many times you have said, "I don't care" or "that's not me." A review of these kind of denials may help at this point. These denials are: the denial of failure, the denial of fear, the denial of age and the denial of death.

The denial of failure is pervasive in our society. There is no room for failure, no provision for inadequacy when the taxes are due, inflation, to pay for the good life and good education for our children. Many set unrealistic standards for themselves—success however is a personal matter—some deem success to make a salary of $25,000 others feel themselves failures making $50,000. I can remember a millionaire businessman friend who had 6 businesses. Four of them failed in a two-year span. Even though two were flourishing, he was so despondent that he hung himself in his garage.

With others it is a status concern, of holding a certain position, it may be social—to be a member of a certain club or group—for those who have not made the dream some compensation is necessary. For some this means overcompensation—splurge by financial misspending or bolstering one's ego with extramarital affairs—for some reevaluation of the goals, abilities and basic interests.

The denial of fear—don't be afraid our parents tell us—the doggie won't bite, the water isn't deep, you will not fall! The normal fears we have are defense mechanisms designed by nature to make us cautious, conservative in order to protect our bodies and lives. Many of our parents have, at least among the boys, sent us back to fight the bully who just beat us up. Be brave, you can do it, otherwise you're a sissy. Many spend their lives trying to prove they're no sissy, they are good girls or that they're brave—no failure, no fear—damn the torpedoes full speed ahead!

The denial of age, oh, to be thirty again! But there are thirty-year-old people who deny they are that old. Everywhere you look the emphasis is on youth. Facelifts and tummy tucking is fashionable. Forty and fifty-year old men are turning back the calendar with affairs of the libido, some are making a last surge to compete with the younger, more ambitious persons moving up the ladder by working harder at their jobs. Unfortunately its true, that older men often take younger wives, older executives are often put out to pasture and it's certainly true that the fifty year old woman trying to get into the job market will experience difficulty. The overly made-up, youthfully dressed matron invites unflattering comparisons in a room with pretty young women. And in the denial of fear we often damage ourselves by point out our deficiencies and playing down our strengths. We exhaust our systems by placing the extra burden of fear upon them.

When fear predominates our lives unfortunately the very thing we try to forestall comes about. A physician, a senior member of a flourishing medical group, was looked upon by the group of doctors around him as the major source of diagnostic skill and judgment. At sixty he began acting like a novice, fighting for this job. He took every call he could, unfortunately making his services unavailable when his colleagues needed him. The end result was that the group finally asked him to leave as he was getting into everyone's territory, working unnecessarily long hours and generally disrupting the organization. He accused them of being goof-offs and forcing him to do all the work. But in reality this was not so, and in the end he lost out.

Denial of death is the most intense form of denial. From earlier times—childhood up we are subliminally aware of death. As we grow older we worry about death in another sense—will there be time to get all those things done I would like to do? But those who enter life vigorously are ruled by the life force, others by death wish. Most people are in the center of life's movements but some are haunted by the pervading aura of fatality. This coloration of life keeps them, at least to some degree or more, detached, ruthless and essentially disengaged. Some middle age persons when told to slow down, change their pace, take a vacation, react in denial, "there's nothing wrong with me." That's what the sixty-five year old woman with a broken collarbone said when her daughter asked her not to go canoeing. She went anyway disdaining (think I'm not up to it) the warning and ended up with a concussion and nearly drowning when the canoe turned over. A friend of mine, a man of forty, who was an executive in a paper company, had a fear of dying on his fortieth birthday—the time his father had died. For a year or two approaching his father's birthday he worried, so much so that his company passed him over for promotion. Of course he didn't die but his lack of concentration during this period on this job altered the course of his life. He went with another company but never had the success he had formerly achieved.

When people grow older they see some of their dreams fade and so become more susceptible to burnout. Many have been dominated by denials we just discussed above. They see their bodies aging, their loves growing colder, sex lives disappointing and their economic success less than they had hoped; still some remember wasted motion and time, no wonder they are susceptible to burnout. Assessment is painful, many just break loose—swinging in the wildest way—giving upon marriages of twenty and thirty years. Others begin health trips with a vengeance. These burnout's or partial burnout's typically are oriented by the work ethic therefore do "their thing" in the most compelling fashion.

What can help? Being knowledgeable of the things discussed here is a start. There are three things I believe that are essential to turn back burnout.

1. Understanding of the problems and your relations to it.
2. Getting sensitive to yourself—the inner self and your feelings and,
3. Developing a plan—assess your circumstance and recognize the false cures—and carry out the plan you make.

In developing a plan you can short-cut burnout by organizing your life somewhat better, and even if you are organized the following plan for allotting time and priorities will aid you in reviewing ways to change for the better your pattern. Some people cannot manage or translate suggestions for self help. These people need professional help either a psychotherapist or psychiatrist. Your physician can recommend one.

ORGANIZING YOUR TIME

1. <u>Assess how you spend your time</u>:	Represent Your <u>Present Time Allotments</u>
Sleeping	
At work, on the job	
On work you take home	
Shopping	
With friends	

Alone pursuing a hobby
Reading, watching TV
Chores at home
With the family
Miscellaneous activities

2. List the significant people in each slice. Your Ideal Time Allotments

Is time spent on your real interests?

List the most important people in your life. Rank according to time you invest. Do they invest the same amount in you?

3. Draw your ideal allotment of time.

4. What might you actually do to change the size of the various activity slices to make them more ideal for you?

____

____

____

____

____

____

____

Review your relationships and friendships as objectively as you can, considering what you are bringing to them. If things are not going too well, try to figure out in what ways you may be contributing. Don't place the blame on others. See first how much blame may be yours. Do you distance yourself from the other persons? Are you stingy about sharing yourself? Do you listen when others talk? Can you sympathize their problems? See if you can discover new ways of viewing other peoples' faults so that you minimize rather than magnify them.

Think about your work. Are you letting it devour you? Can you continue to do a good job without being so intense? Can you take a day off now and again? Can you delegate some of your responsibilities? Can you share your duties with someone else? Over commitment may be depriving a fellow worker of an opportunity. Be honest about your motivations for working so hard. Is there some other area of life you want to avoid? Marriage, home responsibilities, children or parents? Pursuits undertaken for the wrong reasons backfire, so be firm with yourself while you probe. If it's a subject that makes you uncomfortable, you'll try to wiggle out of answering. Don't let yourself. It will save you grief in the long run.

One of the best ways to desensitize your physical body and consequently the mind, is to involve yourself in an activity. The tendency and fact of burnout is to eventually make the person a paranoiac, neurasthenic, psychosomatic—colds that linger, backaches, headaches and finally an emotionally cripple. The best activity I believe is physical—swimming, jogging, tennis playing, dancing, riding a bicycle, walking, yard work and the like. Vigorous exercise will give you more energy, help metabolize your food, even help you reduce and/or firm up your body. This has to be done regularly and it won't be easy not just once in a while but at least three to four times a week. If you have not done anything new or different or met someone new, do it—new people are great for putting a new face on things. Set aside time to be alone and think about yourself. Some specific suggestions on reducing stress on the job is found in the appendix, also suggestions for various problems of ennui, feeling of being a failure, working with machines and repetitive jobs. Start your new life today! The old Ink Spots lyrics popularized by Perry Como.

> Alone night to night you'll find me too weak to break the bonds that bind me. I can't escape for its too late now. I'm just a prisoner of love.

You can break these bonds of stress and escape—with a program and will. Good luck!

<u>Mental Health and Personality Problems</u>

One's attempt to adjust to live situations sometimes results in abnormal behavior, which may become a serious matter. Although stress and tension do not cause abnormal behavior when they are excessive it can lead to it. The following list provides a number of important characteristics of normal behavior. Also, some information is given on the slightly and seriously disturbed person.

The normal adult is a person who has these characteristics:

1. Has realistic attitudes. The healthy adult faces facts both pleasant and unpleasant. He enjoys driving a car but recognizes the hazard involved so keeps his car in good condition and avoids driving in severe weather. Because he has taken precautions he doesn't constantly need to check his oil or brakes.
2. Is independent. The mentally well person forms and acts on reasoned opinions. He will seek advice, and once he has the facts, he is capable of making a decision and facing the consequence of his decision.
3. Has affection for others. This person takes pleasure in being loving and kind to others—spouses, children, relatives, friends—and is sympathetic to less fortunate people. He doesn't require great numbers of persons with whom to be intimate as the immature person does who has difficulty giving love and wants to be the center of attention.
4. Has reasonable dependence on others. The nature person can receive love as well as give it. Feels the need to receive love as well as give it. Feels the need to relate to and share with others.
5. Can make long-range choices. The normal person can usually forego short-range gratification for the sake of long-range goals, that is, turn aside more immediate pleasures for future consideration.
6. Reacts moderately. Most normal persons get angry and use hateful language and thoughts to express it. But normal persons do not do this for long. Although badly treated, a normal person doesn't develop a lasting vendetta with someone or an institution.
7. Is comfortable with himself. An adult so characterized has a relaxed conscience and is not constantly reminded of his failures. He or she recognizes that they sometimes fail at what they try to do or that they don't always do things as well as they like to, but they can still relax and enjoy leisure.
8. Adjusts well to work. Most normal persons are satisfied with their work and change their jobs only for good reasons. They recognize the

day to day grind and unpleasant tasks are part of the job but nonetheless take a positive view of it and persist.

9. Accepts adult roles of women and men. The healthy person treats the opposite sex with dignity and as an equal. They accept their sex roles, themselves, and those of a different race with equanimity. Good sexual adjustment is also a part of the normal person's life. The mature person is characterized by the ability to sustain a single relationship with a sexual partner, to enjoy sex and companionship.
10. Continues to be creative and allows for growth. The normal person has the ability to keep learning. A characteristic of our age is change. The tell-tale clue of the mature person is an acceptance of change—our environment, our friends, our jobs, our physical bodies—and all with a minimum of trauma.

No one person is expected to get a perfect grade on all ten characteristics cited above. To be normal is also to be human, which brings with it frailty of some type. Hence most normal adults are touched by fears and conflicts—so no one is 100% normal. And among the normal there are various types of people—some are introverts, some extroverts. Dr. Karen Horney suggests that there are three basic types: (1) those who move toward others, (2) those who move against others, and (3) those who move away from people. These might be successful teachers, professional football players, or writers. Unhappily they might be playboys, robbers, or a recluse.

The maladjusted person or individual who has a personality problem is termed a neurotic. This person typically lives with threats and anxiety, which may interfere with his normal functioning in day to day life. Usually, however, the neurotic's situation is rarely so bad that hospitalization is required. Their orientation to reality is usually good enough so that they can function fairly well particularly if they have a regular job. This structure provides a buffer and protection from the bizarre and volatile change. Some general characteristics of the slightly disturbed person are as follows:

1. They have fears, worries, tension, emotional discomfort usually exaggerated, continual, and they are not realistic. Anyone is afraid of catching a disease. The maladjusted person anticipates getting a disease, panics at the thought and frequently contrives a way to reduce this fear (phobia) as pairing it with a ritual. The normal person will worry about business but will rejoice when it's good; the neurotic under these

conditions emphasizes the negative and never the positive. Worries interfere with their work and with their relationships with people.

2. They exhibit exaggerated sensitivity, which is out of proportion to the situation. A well-adjusted mother knows her older children face certain risks (such as in driving an automobile for the first time) but she doesn't refuse to let them out of her sight on account of it. Criticism is never welcomed by most normal people but they can take it. However, the disturbed might quit their jobs over a mild reprimand or rebuke.

3. Frequently these persons have excessive worry, fear and depression but do not know why they experience these feelings. These feelings sometimes give a person the idea that they are crazy. The fact that they wonder may be evidence that they aren't crazy. Probably there is some truth in the statement that the best way to keep from going crazy is to be neurotic. It's not the best way, as that would be like saying the best way to keep your leg from being broken is to put it in a cast.

The problem of people with personality difficulties is rooted in the unconscious. The unconscious mind is like a storage room that houses all of our experiences and thoughts of the past. Part of this is released by the mind to the present gradually and tentatively because the human tendency is to forget what is unpleasant and hateful. Because of feelings of guilt or inferiority, the neurotic person behaves in peculiar and puzzling ways. He can no more look into his unconscious mind that you can gaze into a mirror to see how you look with your eyes closed. The unconscious of the healthy person is very seldom in serious conflict with his conscious desires; the conscious of the neurotic is constantly being forced to surrender to his unconscious. One might say the neurotic is under subjection to this closet of past thoughts.

Some common minor personality problems can be classified in the following categories:

1. Anxiety reaction—People with this problem are in a constant state of "anxious expectation" of some impending dreadful, often unnamed happening. They experience episodes of mild panic and show physical indications of this through sweating, dizziness, palpitations, diarrhea, difficulty in breathing, pain in the heart or chest. This is often associated with the fear of losing a loved one or a friend.

2. Phobias—These types of fears are usually divided into two groups called common and specific phobias. A common one would be claus-

trophobia, fear of closed places. Potamophobia is a fear of running water. Phobias represent exaggerated fears of things of which most people are afraid, like death. Often half forgotten experiences as being trapped in a cave-in, car wreck or in an over-turned boat.

3. Hypochondria—Mental difficulty is expressed through the preoccupation with body functions. The individual thinks he has a disease or is ill. He monitors his body very closely noting his feelings of fatigue or his heart beat B the sort of things normal people don't worry about. There is no physical basis for this but the typical physician, if consulted, will check this out for certain. This phobia is linked with fear, the feelings of tired-ness, etc. Many unmarried are afflicted with hypochondria. Marrying sometimes helps, for one is forced to think of other things beside himself.
4. Depression—This refers to depression that is normal as in the case of the person who has lost their job, a spouse or parent in death or has been divorced. These are normal reactions in experiencing grief and setbacks. Most people suffer the "blues" or lack of interest in their surroundings sometimes. They suffer from feeling of not being able to get ahead or think they're getting little out of life. They wake up and decide there are more bills than fun, more work than hours to find it.

Labeling behavior is a serious matter. Most psychiatrists prefer to talk about symptoms upon which a diagnosis is to be made in an individual case. Misapplied labels tend to stick, be harmful and sometimes become self-fulfilling prophecies. As emphasized earlier, the mildly maladjusted usually can function well enough to get by in their work and at home. They use a variety of defense mechanisms and tactics to survive. These may deter successful living in the highest sense, though they allow a meager existence. Most deviations in behavior are not considered diseases. There are two general types of these: the psychosomatic and the psychotic. In the former, an individual has a condition of mental life that affects the physical body of the person as in hypochondria. These usually affect those parts of the body under control of the involuntary nervous system such as the heart, digestive tract, the endocrine glands, lungs, urinary, bladder, and skin. The problem in psychosomatic illness is one of association of certain fear with abnormal ones, for example when emotional reactions stimulate the flow of digestive juices and there is no food. In the absence of food the acids irritate the stomach causing the possible development of an ulcer. Stress and emotional factors play an important part in the development of such physical difficulties as migraine headache, mucous colitis, ulcers, asthma, high blood pressure, abnormal thyroid activity, arthritis, rheumatism, skin allergies, and diabetes.

The well known Type A personalities (hard driving, aggressive, chronic hurriers who eat rich food, smoke and drink, get little exercise, and are combative) are subject to inordinate stresses. Research by Meyer Friedman and Ray Roseman indicates these types of men or women are three times as likely to get coronaries and Type B, the more easy going, relaxed temperate habituated type of woman or man. A serious problem is that long term stress effects the ability of the body's adaptive mechanisms, such as the endocrine glands, to function properly.

The Seriously Mentally Disturbed

The answer to the question am I crazy? This is a misnomer, for even a psychosis is a relative matter that may at least in part cause the problem. Remarkable cures for psychosis can be brought about by removing such a person from a restrictive environment, eliminating or reducing stressful situations, or by improving a person's physical health. We all may wonder as to the degree of sanity we possess at a given time. It is normal for people to feel that they are "as crazy as a loon"—the bird that is. The problem is that most people do not obtain help for milder forms of maladjustments even though they should. If individuals exhibit some of the following problems, then help should be sought. These problems are not matters for the do-it-yourself therapy. You should not muddle through with them; you should get expert help. In any event, check these suggested by Dr. Benjamin Miller:

1. Is the person's behavior suitable for the occasion? Does he pout or complain on every kind of occasion where frustration is faced in everyday situations? Inappropriate reaction to day to day happenings may be a signal that trouble is coming.
2. Major changes in traits or behavior? Does a person who has been an introvert suddenly begin to be very vocal, a careful housewife overnight becomes a poor one, the well-dressed person becomes careless and sloppy? Change from long-established patterns of behavior may provide a clue to abnormal behavior.
3. Is there a reason for the behavior? In response to why you do this or think that, the normal people usually have an acceptable reason. The

disturbed may not have a reason but may act things out imagined. If continued, this may be a sure hallmark of illness.

4. Does one have control of his actions? Sometimes we have urges that are crazy or are seized with an absurd idea to do something. Normal persons resist giving in to these but the mentally ill do not. They see no reason to control themselves and they may even think they can do the impossible.
5. Has one's emotional strength been lost? Many of us have at times been temporarily overwhelmed with shock or grief and periods of crisis which may be connected with our jobs or love affairs but we bounce back and regain our composure. The mentally ill go into depression for long periods of time and indeed may not come out of it without some help.
6. Is one's behavior destructive? Long term, chronic destructive behavior in an adult or child is an attribute of mental sickness. If a child continually damages property, mistreats animals (pets) or himself and others, the call for help is clear. Adults who do the same things are also suspect and if they beat up on their children, spouses and others, immediate assistance is needed!

Personality disorders like alcoholism, sex deviations and drug addiction may be the symptoms of problems that can be relieved by therapy. Therapy for any symptoms such as those mentioned above can usually be treated on an outpatient basis. Modern medicines and treatment can effect miracles in many cases mental as well as physical, so one should seek aid with mental problems. The seriously disturbed (those with psychoses) usually are classified as either functional or organic. The organic refers to those with brain damage, tumors, senility, poisons, etc. The functional psychoses are seen as (1) schizophrenia, (2) paranoia and (3) manic-depressive. Most physicians will recommend counseling centers for alcoholism, drugs, etc. or stress management programs where individual effort is not enough to bring wellness. New yellow pages provide action indexes for emergency help.

An interesting study was reported by P. Rosenhan in *Science* a few years ago. In the experiment eight normal well-established individuals with no previous history of personality problems got themselves admitted to different mental hospitals reporting that they had had auditory hallucinations. No other symptoms were reported and in all other respects they behaved normally. All except one were admitted to the hospitals and diagnosed as schizophrenic. The other "patient" received a diagnosis of manic-depressive psychosis. The original labeling colored all the subsequent review and nothing about their behavior was entered into the reports. We should not take this to mean mental illness is a joke. But it does suggest we should hesitate to label people as "sick," considering the difficulty of diagnosis through troubled behavior may be obvious and needs care.

In conclusion, you can evaluate for yourself and others by understanding the causes of stress and depression. The first step is recognizing the problem exists. You help yourself by talking it over with someone thereby keeping things in perspective—keep stress in bounds before it causes trouble and know where to go for help. Help from professionals keep minor problems from becoming serious ones.

Appendices

Appendix 1

LIFE STAGES AND STRESS EXERCISE*

Use the following descriptions of the issues commonly encountered in each life stage to see where you are in your own journey. Within the appropriate stages, cross out the issues you've already dealt with, and circle the issues that you're struggling with now.

Breaking loose (late teens): Leaving home, focus on peers, testing our wings, loneliness, attachment to causes, changing life style, throwing out family morals, conforming to friends.

Building the nest (twenties): Search for identity, intimate friendships, marriage, intoxication with own peer, great dreams, making commitments, taking on responsibilities, getting launched in a career, working toward goals, doing "shoulds," finding a mentor, having children.

Looking around (thirties): Raising question, recognizing painful limitations, gathering possessions, moving up the career ladder, declining satisfaction in marriage, settling down, desiring freedom, asking "What do I want to do with my life?"

Mid-life rebirth (around forty): Awareness of mortality, diminishing physical energy, emotional turmoil, parenting teenagers, finding new friends, deep questions, changing careers, second adolescence, sense of aloneness, divorce, remarriage, conflicting pressures, remodeling life structures, learning to play again.

Investing in life (fifties): Life reordered, settling down, acting on new values, focus on people instead of possessions and power, selecting a few good friends, last child leaving home, grandparenting, more financial freedom, enjoying life, empty nest, lost dream.

Deepening wisdom (later years): Softening feelings, mellowing wisdom, steady commitments to self and others, deepening richness, simplifying life, adjustment to limitations, loss of energy, financial pressures, retirement, quiet joys, self-knowledge, self-acceptance, facing death.

Twilight years: Loneliness, freedom from "should," dependence on those who once depended on you, mind sharp/body failing, body fine/mind failing, loss of mate and friends, preparing for death, sense of peace and perspective.

- In what stage of adult development are you in right now?
- How are you experiencing changes in yourself physically?
- Describe changes in your self-image and the direction you are headed.
- Describe changes in your relationships.
- How has the meaning of your work changed?
- What special difficulties are you experiencing in your present stage of development?
- What observations strike you as you look at the past development and current life stage issues?
- How are these issues contributing to your current stress?

*Adapted from the text, *Kicking Your Stress Habits*, by Donald Tubesing.

APPENDIX 2

ORGANIZING YOUR TIME

Represent Your
Present Time Allotments

1. Assess how you spend your time:

   Sleeping
   At work, on the job
   On work you take home
   Shopping
   With friends
   Alone pursuing a hobby
   Reading, watching TV
   Chores at home
   With the family
   Miscellaneous activities

FOR EXAMPLE:

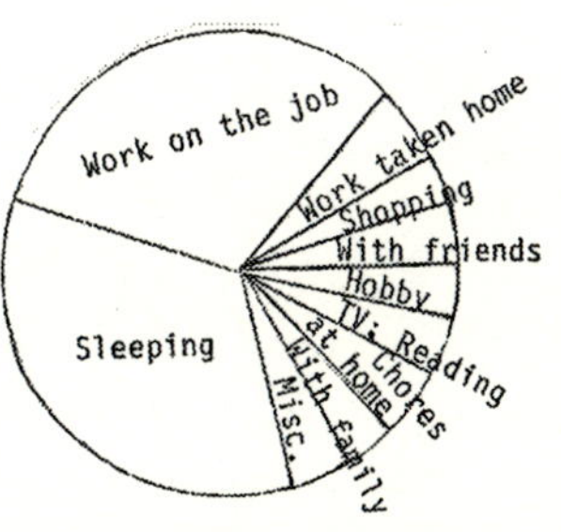

2. List the significant people in each slice.

   Is time spent on your real interests?

   List the most important people in your life. Rank according to time you invest. Do they invest the same amount in your?

3. Draw your ideal allotment of time.

4. What might you actually do to change the size of the various activity slices to make them more ideal for you?

Your Ideal Time Allotments

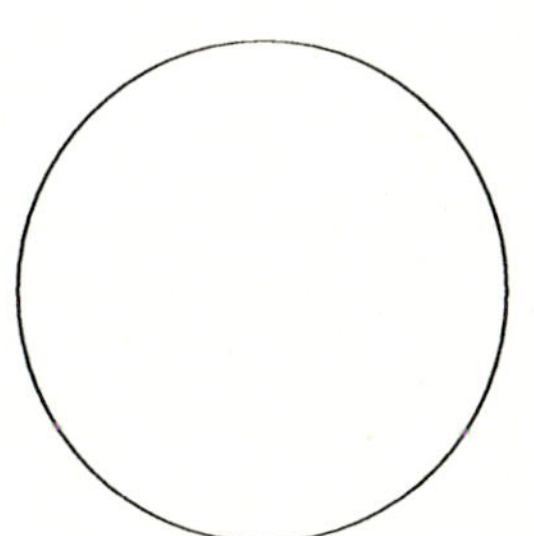

___

___

___

CHAPTER III

MAJOR HEALTH PROBLEMS

"So You Want to Live to be 90"

More people live to be 90 than ever before. But it is not automatic, since the life expectancy is 77-78 taking men and women together it is not automatic. How can one achieve that goal? Choosing ones parents and grandparents would help. The cause of variation in people is their genetic make-up, their environment, their previous medical history, their nutritional habits, mental health status and life styles. Our bodies mature between 25 and 30 years. Signs for flush of aging appear in humans and plants and other animals as soon as full maturity is achieved. Scientists do not know all the answer but they do know some. For instance, we know adding vitamins to the diet (not promiscuously) can reduce the free-radical damage. Free radicals are highly reactive destroying cells in our body. These radicals are generated as a natural part of our metabolism. They are also increased by exposure to x-ray, tobacco smoke, sunlight, ozone and auto fumes. These free radicals damage the DNA (provide the pattern for cell reproduction) that lead to disease. Besides this information, smaller amounts of food—essential components and quantities—tend to increase the years of living. NOW—TO FIND OUT where you are on the track to becoming 90 take the following questionnaire. No one needs to see this but you so be honest. Don't fudge on the life spans of your grandparents! Your weight—right! Your drinking routines. Be careful and do it correctly. Add up the pluses and the minuses and subtract or add these to the average life expectancy. Men 74, Women 78. The two blank spaces are for subtractions and additions.

HEREDITY

For each grandparent who lived past age 80, add 1 year.	_______	_______
For each grandparent who lived to 70 but not 80, add 2 year.	_______	_______
If you mother lived past 80, add 4 years.	_______	_______
If your father lived past 80, add 2 years.	_______	_______
For each grandparent, parent, or sibling who died of any type of any type of heart disease before age 50, subtract 4 years.	_______	_______
For each such relative dying of heart disease between age 50 and 60, subtract 2 years.	_______	_______
For each grandparent, parent, or sibling who died of diabetes or ulcers before age 60, subtract 3 years.	_______	_______
Women: for each sister or mother who died of breast cancer before age 60, subtract 1 year.	_______	_______
If your intelligence is superior, add two years. (IQ of 115 up)	_______	_______

HEALTH HISTORY

If your mother was younger than 18 or older than 35 at your birth, subtract 1 year.	_______	_______
If you are the first born in your family, add one year.	_______	_______
Women: If you have had no children (or plan no children) subtract 2 year.	_______	_______
If you have an annual physical exam, add 2 years.	_______	_______

CURRENT HEALTH

If your weight is 10-30 percent above ideal weight shown in standard tables, the amount you must subtract depends on your age and gender. For women: subtract 5 years if you are between 20 and 30; 4 years if you are between 30 and 50, and 2 years if you are over 50. For men: subtract 10 years if you are between 20 and 30, 4 years if you are between 30 and 45, and 2 years for any age over that.	______	______
If your weight is more than 30 percent above standard tables: Women subtract 62 years if you are between 20 and 30 years, 5 years if you are between 30 and 50, and 4 years thereafter. Men subtract 13 if you are between 20 and 30, if you are between 30 and 40, and 4 years thereafter.	______	______
If your diet is genuinely low in fat and sugar, and you never eat past the feeling of fullness, add 1 year.	______	______
If you smoke 2 or more packs a day, subtract 12 years; if you smoke 1-2 packs a day, subtract 7 years; if you smoke less than 1 pack a day, subtract 2 years.	______	______
If you never drink, neither add nor subtract; if you are a heavy drinker, subtract 8; if you are a moderate drinker, add 3; if you are a light drinker, add 12.	______	______
If you do some aerobic exercise at least 3 times a week, add 3.	______	______
If you sleep more than 10 or less than 6 hours per night, subtract 2.	______	______
If you have intimate sexual relations once or twice a week, add 2.	______	______
If you have a chronic health condition (e.g., high blood pressure, diabetes, ulcer, cancer) or are frequently ill, subtract 5.	______	______

YOUR CURRENT LIFE

If you have 4 or more years of college, add 3; if you have 1-3 years of college, add 2; if you have completed high school and gone no further, add 1; if you have less than 8th grade, subtract 2. ________ ________

________ ________

If your occupation is at a professional, technical, or managerial level, add 1 year; if you work at unskilled work, subtract 4.

If your family income is above average for your education and occupation, add 1 year; if it is below average subtract 1. ________ ________

If your job is a physically active one, add 2; if it is sedentary, subtract 2. ________ ________

If you now live in an urban area and have lived in urban areas most of your life, subtract 1; if you have spent most of your life in a rural area, add 1. ________ ________

If you are married and living with your spouse, add 1. ________ ________

If you are separated or divorced, subtract 9 if you are a man, 4 if you are a woman. ________ ________

If you are widowed, subtract 7 if you are a man, 4 if you are a woman. ________ ________

If you are a never-married woman, subtract 1 year for each decade unmarried past age 25. ________ ________

If you are a never-married man and living with family, subtract 1 year for each decade unmarried past 25; if you live alone, subtract 2 years for each decade unmarried past 25. ________ ________

If you have at least two close friends in whom you can confide, add 1. ________ ________

If your personality is noticeably aggressive and hostile and you feel regularly under time pressure, subtract 2-5 depending on how much the description fits. ________ ________

If you re a basically happy person and have a lot of fun in life, add 2 years. ________ ________

If you have had an episode of being depressed or very tense, guilty, or worried that lasted as long as a year or more, subtract 1-3 depending on how severe the depression was.	_______	_______
If you take a lot of risks, or live in a high crime neighborhood, subtract 2 years; if you use seat belts regularly, and generally avoid risks, add 1 year.	_______	_______
TOTAL	_______	_______

SOURCE: Adapted from Woodruff-Pak, 1988, pp. 145-154.

The standard deviation here would probably be in the range of 4 or 5 years below or above the projected life span.

I had several people fill this survey out and score it. This small sample indicated a variance of a few years either way. It does, however, touch on salient features that impact on longevity: Those reaching sixty-five can count on living to 81 as men and 84 for women. So, the first step is to get to 65!

Everyone is familiar with early childhood diseases such as chicken pox, measles and mumps but what types of physical strain should one be alert to in middle life? Certain ailments and stress factors do occur more often this time of life to millions of Americans. What are they? What are the symptoms and causes? How can they be prevented and what effect do they have on our bodies' systems and longevity?

Physical age represents the functional condition of one's body and its symptoms indicators. There may be a marked variation between one's chronological age and one's physiological age. Chronological age becomes a progressively poorer indication or measure of the body's capacities as one grows older as the effects of environment play a larger role.

HEREDITY AND ENVIRONMENTAL FACTORS

The influence of heredity, environment on the aging process are so intertwined, it is impossible for scientists to say with certainty where one begins and the other ends. Functional stress will affect each individual differently during the late thirties and into the 40's and 50's since no two humans exactly duplicate each others heredity, environment or experience.

Many long-lived peoples come from mountainous regions like those reported from these republics of Georgia where many are reported to live beyond 100. The oxygen-poor and pollution-free environment would be a tonic to their cardiovascular systems. Blood vessels that feed the heart widen and become more efficient. Another factor may be their isolation—that they are separated from the pressures and worries of civilization. The most important factor, however, is thought to be their life-styles, which focus on vigorous, physically demanding work. A caution suggested by research into these claims note that many of these people overstate their age due to the great veneration given to old people.

Inherited factors undoubtedly play some role for the long-lived. Part of this for them may be due to special groups inbreeding, thereby reducing the amount of dilution of genes from outsiders. However, geneticists believe interbreeding is better than in breeding for racial health. The food that all these long-lived people east is a common link also. Wasting food is unthinkable, as they never eat more than their bodies require; they strictly avoid excess fats and animal protein and intake ample vitamins, minerals and fiber in their foods. There are other groups whose patterns are like the Georgians and thereby receive benefits from these practices. The western civilization has a different culture making it difficult to duplicate an isolated and protected people.

The purpose of this chapter is to provide information on major and minor health problems and preventive medicine. Everyone eventually will face some of the circumstances noted in the following pages or if not personally some family or relative will.

MAJOR PROBLEMS

HEALTH PROBLEMS
LIFE CHANGES AND DISEASES THAT MOST OFTEN OCCUR DURING THE MID YEARS OF LIFE AND THEIR PROGNOSIS

Some knowledge of the physical changes and difficulties that become prominent by the late 30's and into the 40's and 50's are presented here. Knowledge of these problems will help us in the future by knowing the general circumstances of these situations. The categories discussed are: Heart and circulation, cancers, bone, diabetes, weight problems and associated lesser problems and preventive medicine.

Heart (Circulatory Problem)

Diseases affecting the heart and circulatory systems are the major cause of death in this country. Presently, 50 million have high blood pressure or hypertension and under control only one-third of them! It is during the middle years that many of these diseases appear. Four major types which affect adults over 40 are (1) coronary heart disease, (2) high blood pressure—hypertension, (3) hemorrhage or blood clotting in the heart, and (4) heart failure. Heart failure—this results when the heart muscle begins to weaken and the pump (heart) does not work efficiently. The result is the accumulation of fluid in the body leading to swollen legs, weight gain and shortness of breath (accumulation of fluid in the lungs). The most common cause, however, is many years of inadequately controlled hypertension. This can develop as a complication of a coronary thrombosis, drug induced heart disease (alcoholism) or simple wearing out of the heart muscle. Most cases can be controlled by the proper use of medicines.

Coronary heart disease involves two principal kinds—disease of the coronary arteries (Arteriosclerosis) or "hardening of the arteries," and coronary thrombosis. In the first of these diseases, the arteries are hardened affecting the blood supply to the heart by narrowing the tubes and creating an unsmooth lining in the artery. This has the effect of tending to allow settlement of blood in the grooves and the forming of clots. The smaller the artery the more pressure required to pump blood to the body. A major symptom here is pain over the heart, sometimes brief; (as in angina) other evidence of trouble is dizziness, nausea, fatigue and irregular heartbeat. Failure of the heart to receive enough oxygen creates the pain. Drugs may be prescribed by the physician such as nitroglycerin to bring relief to pain and increase the flow of blood through the arteries. Early diagnosis is important in heart problems; the treatment usually includes rest, diet, medication and possibly surgery which is increasingly commonplace in certain situations—by-pass, valve replacement and heart transplant.

In coronary thrombosis, a blood clot forms within a coronary artery cutting off the entire supply of blood to a section of the heart. This block (occlusion) may cause injury or destroy part of the heart muscle. The heart attack that occurs causes severe and prolonged pain. Hospitalization is essential to affect therapy, providing oxygen, good nursing, anti-blood clotting medicines and a controlled environment. An illustration of this type of heart problem follows:

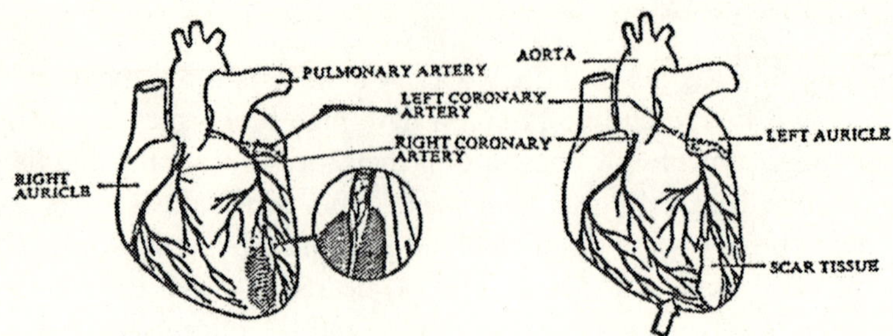

<u>Coronary Thrombosis</u>: At time of attack. The flow of blood through part of the left coronary artery is blocked (shown in inset), cutting off the circulation in the shaded area.

<u>Recovery from attack</u>: Scar tissue has built up. Blood vessels of the right coronary artery (indicated by arrow) now supply the affected area. Collateral circulation has developed.

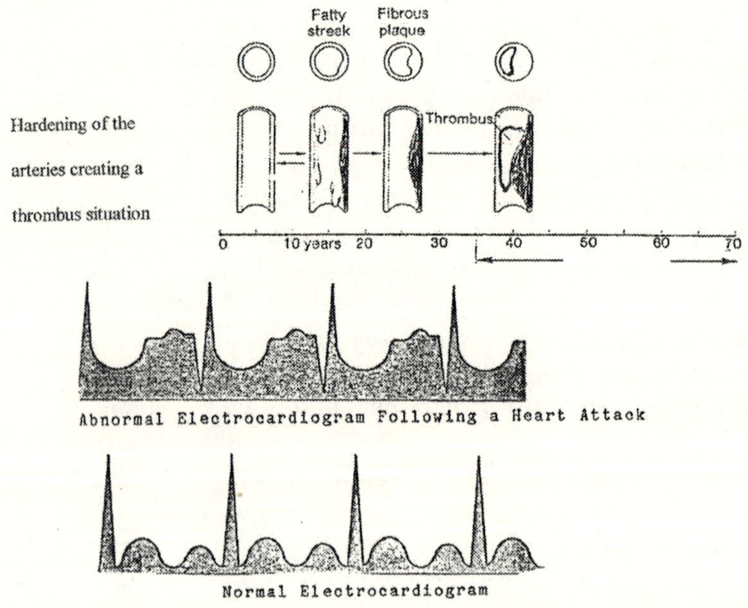

In reality, thrombosis is often superimposed on coronary plaques and most patients have a combination of both.

Hypertension or high blood pressure affects some 50 million Americans, including more than one-third of the adult population 50 and over. Worldwide a billion people have hypertension. Nearly half of the people with hypertension are undetected and of those who have been diagnosed, half of these remain untreated. The effect of high blood pressure is seen on the heart, brain, and kidneys. However, it is usual to have no symptoms at all. The symptoms may include headaches now and then, fatigue, insomnia, dizziness and excessive flushing.

Generally high blood pressure creates symptoms only after it has produced disease in some organ like the heart or kidney. Four categories are recognizable; essential hypertension, secondary hypertension, malignant hypertension and borderline hypertension. In the essential hypertension (1st stage), the most common (about 85%) the blood pressure is over 150/95, the 150 represents the systolic (the pumping pressure) inside the blood vessels and 95 represents the diastolic (the relaxed or resting) pressure between heartbeats. The tension with this type may be that the heart is pumping too much blood or that the arteries are too small to handle adequate supplies of blood. Secondary hypertension (stage two) is attributed to specific organic causes such as hardening of the arteries, kidney disease or blockage to kidney blood flow. Malignant hypertension is a situation where blood pressure sometimes jumps as high as 200/115 or higher very rapidly and damages body organs within hours or days. This type is less frequently seen. In borderline hypertension, the blood pressure intermittently rises above the normal levels for each given age group or sex—primary and secondary problems usually in these people in time. Incidentally, the word malignant does not refer to a "growth" or tumor but the severity of the pressure problem. African-Americans and men generally over 40 and men and women with a family history of high blood pressure, emotional behavior and obesity, etc., problems run greater risks of having high blood pressure than others.

New standards for blood pressure puts 45 million Americans whose blood pressure is 120-139 millimeters of mercury—the systolic—the top number in a reading (pressure in the arteries when the heart is contracting) or 80-89 diastolic (the bottom number is the pressure when the heart is at rest between beats) at risk. The new guidelines provided by the National Heart, Lung and Blood Institute (2003) are the Federal Standards for blood pressure. These standards are given on the Web site of the Journal of the American Medical Association (www.jama.com). The blood pressure categories are as follows.

New federal guidelines say blood pressure levels once thought normal actually are high enough to signal "prehypertension."

Pressure Systolic	**Normal** Less than 120	**Pre-hypertension** 120-139	**Stage one hypertension** 140-159	**Stage two hypertension** More than 160
Diastolic	Less than 80	80-89	90-99	More than 100
Treatment (Otherwise Healthy)	None	None	Diuretics for most, possibly other drugs	Two-drug combo, usually one is a diuretic
With other diseases*	None	Medically treat Diseases	Multiple medications	Multiple medications

*Previous heart attack, diabetes, kidney disease or certain other diseases
SOURCE: National Heart, Lung and Blood Institute, 2004 AP/VP

People with readings in this range (139 over 89 called high normal) do not have high blood pressure and do not need to take medication. But the new guidelines advise doctors that such people are likely to develop high blood pressure, and should be advised to try to lower their pressure by losing excess weight, exercising more, quitting smoking, cutting back on salt, having no more than one or two alcoholic drinks a day, and eating more fruits, vegetables and low-fat dairy products.

The risk of heart disease and stroke starts to rise at readings as low as 115/75, and doubles for each increase of 20/10 millimeters of mercury. The report urges doctors and patients to take high blood pressure more seriously and treat it more aggressively, often with more than one drug. High blood pressure greatly increases the risk of heart disease, stroke and kidney failure. Heart disease, which kills more than 700,000 Americans a year, is the nation's leading cause of death.

People whose reading is normal at age 55 have a 90% chance of eventually developing high blood pressure though fortunately diet and exercise can change those prospects. The National Health Institute is suggesting 30 minutes of exercise 4 or 5 times a week (split in two sessions if necessary of walking or aerobics, also weight lifting, tennis, jogging, swimming, etc.). Some authorities suggest 30-45 minutes of vigorous exercise seven days per week. More for weight loss. Remember hypertension has no symptoms until the pressure has damaged the arteries and cause them to stiffen which increases the pressure more.

Physicians often prescribe counseling for the patient and his family to help them with the fears imposed by the disease. Such things as sex and most normal living activities are not foreclosed upon by the disease. This is important to understand.

Medical science is not agreed on the cause; suspected is an inherited trait, emotional high strung individuals, so-called type A personality persons, body chemistry, trace metals such as cadmium, smoking, diet (high-fat, high salt food) tending to accelerate atherosclerosis, the tonic effects of renin (a protein secreted by the kidney) on blood vessels, and the mosaic hypothesis, involving a combination of causes. The method of treatment has usually consisted of drugs, diet, exercise, change of occupation sometimes, and rest. Surgery is rarely ever used as treatment. Long term drugs are the mainstay of treatment including diuretics for reducing fluids, vasodilators for relaxing blood vessels and drugs blocking the nerve conduction to blood vessels and specific types of drugs include hiazide diuretics, diazoside, guanethidine, reserpine, alpha blockers, methyldopa, hydrazaline, pargyline, furosemide (Lasix) and others. The best treatment comes form early discovery but, even so, if found in the 20 to 30 year old group the prognosis for success is hampered and seems to foreshadow problems for the middlescent years. One positive note—hypertensives have much less cancer than usual according to some researchers. This may be due to the chemical changes affected in the general adaptation syndrome functioning. The psychological effects of a heart attack can be devastating.

Stroke is common in middle age. The cause of this sickness is blockage in a brain artery or hemorrhage of a brain artery by rupture causing bleeding in surrounding brain tissue. A clot sometimes happens suddenly that may involve days of being dizzy, stumbling around, clumsy movement or the mouth ultimately being drawn to one side or difficulty talking. If the hemorrhage is large, often death occurs quickly. Sometimes a surgeon can remove the clot that causes the stroke. The damage to the brain usually causes the body or some parts to be paralyzed. Stroke occurs when normal circulation of the blood through the brain is cut off. Deprived of oxygen, brain cells die and fail to exercise control over parts of the body they normally direct. Damage of this type to one side of the brain usually results in the loss of control of muscles, etc., on the opposite side of the body. Usually rehabilitation methods can re-teach a person to use affected muscles, limbs and speech apparatus again. In some instances the effect of the stroke clears up without leaving apparent damage.

Small strokes or TIA's (Transient Ischemic Attack) occurs when the blood is cut-off in a small vessel (capillary) in the brain resulting in numbness in the hands, legs, face, lips or garbled speech which usually lasts a brief period or possibly an hour or so. It leaves no mark or little effect. These attacks may be the precursor of a large and more devastating one. To counter this, Coumadin (Warfarin) is often prescribed (Aggrenox or Plavix) for heart patients to thin the blood securing smooth passage through the blood vessels. In many, attention is also given to cholesterol levels, sugar control, diet in general and exercise.

Physicians will check to see if other conditions can mimic the TIA such as low blood sugar, low blood pressure, brain tumor, irregular heart rhythm and labyrinthitis (viral infection of the inner ear). Risk factors of having strokes may reduce their chances by knowing what they are and reducing them.

Risk	Lowering Risk
High blood pressure disregarded	Check blood pressure regularly once a year or more suggested by the doctor. Physical exam each year for adult. Diastolic blood pressure should be reduced.
Atrial fibrillation—erratic heart beat may result in small clots that might go to the brain.	Warfarin or aspirin can greatly decrease the risk of stroke.
Atherosclerosis and high cholesterol levels	Cholesterol level should be in line with new guidelines, eat low fat foods & diet, exercise regularly—take such medicine as Lipacore for rapid reduction.
Stroke risk is high after several months of a TIA	The precursor of the TIA, its signs and help can be given by your doctor.
People with heart problems should not smoke making proneness to clotting greater.	Give up smoking and take aspirin or anticoagulate.
Diabetes increases risk of cardiovascular disease and stroke	Taking insulin or other medicine. Tailor diet through an M.D. preferably an Endocrinologist.
Obesity even 25% overweight increases risk of serious problems.	Exercise and diet as suggested by a doctor.
A mechanical heart valve requiring thin blood by Warfarin, etc.	Physicians or a lab will assist you with regular check ups and levels of medicine.
Check vitamins and minerals particularly Vitamin E level in the diet	Take Vitamin E and other minerals to help avoid strokes.

Intravenous use of thrombolytic drugs to break up clots if given within 3 hours of having a transient ischemic stroke (TIA). The risk of dying following an attack in the period following up to 6 months but lower your risk of dying or being dependently impaired over the next six months. Most physicians recommend the drug be used to prevent long-term risks. Stroke rehabilitation specialists can assist the impaired victim adjust and recapture movement use of hand, speech, walking, etc. Most of these stroke patients are moved to short-term nursing homes then hopefully home care where independence can be established and family can help with the importance of exercise and care.

It should be mentioned that the human heart is the toughest organ in the body. The advice from physicians used to be to forestall a vigorous experience like tennis and running after 35 years of age. This advice today does not hold unless the heart has already been severely damaged or unless the activity is considerably beyond accustomed levels.

The American Heart Association claims that the best exercises are rhythmic, repetitive and involving motion, particularly of the legs. British medical studies show that men engaging frequently in vigorous activity had a lower incidence of coronary heart disease than men who did not. By vigorous we mean swimming, keep-fit exercises, jogging, running, brisk walking, cycling, tennis, climbing any stairs, and really heavy work in garden or home. Exercise should be engaged in at least four to five times a week, not irregularly and not excessive after years of lay-off or by those with high blood pressure and heavy smokers. Exercise should begin at low levels and build up slowly. People in this category should consult their physician. Exercise can aid in burning calories and help your heart and arteries have better ability to survive if a coronary artery becomes blocked. Exercise may help keep blood pressure under control, also diabetes. When you are physically fit, your heart rate is likely to become slower. You are likely to sleep better. It may slow down changes that occur with aging—stiffness, arthritis, and loss of muscle tone.

To summarize what can help prevent heart disease follows closely to those factors that cut the risk of having a stroke.

1. No smoking
2. Reduce high blood pressure
3. Reduce high cholesterol
4. Exercise—vigorously and regularly

5. Cut your weight drastically if obese (20% or greater overweight). Diet.
6. Reduce high stress
7. Be watchful for signs of problems such as family history and genetics.
8. Cut excess alcohol consumption to one or two drinks.

CANCER

Cancer (Neoplasms)

The second leading cause of death in the United States is cancer. Cancer is among the causes of death of those 65 and older, but among 45 to 64 years it is the number one killer. It is estimated that one of every four persons will get some form of cancer. It is not contagious even its terminal form. However, the AIDS virus (Autoimmune Deficiency Syndrome) which can cause a form of cancer is highly contagious through blood and semen contact. A final cure has remained elusive, but much is known and new drugs that help slow its effect or cure are improving the fight against AIDS.

Nonetheless millions of Americans have survived cancer. The incidence of cancer is high among the middlescent. Cancer is a malignant tumor—a shapeless mass of cells which keeps on growing without order. Cancer is a disease of the cells (cytology) rather than organs, which are frequently its target. Normally the nature adult body reproduces only those cells that are needed for repair of injured tissue. In cancer, there is an irregular multiplication of cells in one or more parts of the body. A lump or mass of tissue called a tumor may be benign (harmless) or malignant. A benign tumor may need to be removed because of its size or that it is potential to become malignant in the future. Cancer is greatly feared because it gives little advance warning; the warning signals emphasized by the American Cancer Association are easily confused with minor or other problems, leaving one in a quandary and fearful but more importantly its causes and cures are unknown. The types of cancer are divided into two groups: sarcomas—those which usually affect the bones and muscles, and carcinomas—make up the largest group involving the breast, stomach, lungs, womb, skin, and tongue.

Hodgkin's Disease (usually found in the young) is classified as a cancer as is Leukemia, a form of cancer where immature white blood corpuscles multiply in overwhelming numbers. These cells are produced in the bone marrow. They are longer lived than the normal white blood cells and accumulate in the marrow and various organs until they prevent enough cells to function. There are four major types of leukemia—acute lymphocytic (ALL), acute granulocytic, chronic granulocytic and chronic lymphocytic. In the acute forms malignant cells quickly take over the bone marrow making the progression of the disease rapid. The symptoms are fever, aching joints, swollen lymph glands and if you have flu that will not go away. Tests given show the types of problem through determining white and red blood cell count numbers, platelets and the presence of immature blast cells. Treatment depends on general health and how one would respond to chemotherapy and radiation therapy. Almost all ALL's and AGL's get chemotherapy. ALL is a curable cancer whereas AGL is curable in 20% to 30% of the cases. This disease is mainly an adult disease—for every child there are 15 adults with leukemia. Bone marrow transplants get cured about 80% if the patients are in their first remission from chemotherapy. People with CGL live on average 3 to 4 years after diagnosis whereas around 6 to 7 for CLL types.

There are also precancerous, and abnormal pap smears (which are in themselves harmless but affect changes in the tissues of the body). These are important to watch as they have a tendency to become cancerous—some moles, any chronically irritated spot on the skin, polyps (as found in the large intestines), some forms of lymph gland tumors and thickened white patched sores in the mouth or on the tongue (called leukoplakia). Of the four persons cancer strikes, two can be saved by treatment. Of six in twenty-four persons that are afflicted, two will survive, one will die who could have been saved by early diagnosis, three more will die of types of cancer future research must control. Even so, the chances of having immunity (protection) to cancer right now are 350 to 1, according to a recent Science Digest article. If you are under 35 and are a non-smoker, the odds are 650 to 1. Science views immunity from body sources, as for example that found in the thymus gland through the secretion of thymosin (an endocrine gland found in the upper chest) as one of the keys to survival during the middle years. Cancer is increasingly not so much a disease but an alteration in the biochemical signals to our genes. In well individuals, development of cancer may be the momentary lapse in health or an ongoing exposure to carcinogens—coal, tars, x-rays, radio active substances, as well as dust, tobacco, smoke and chemical articles, etc.

The most common forms of cancer in middle-aged women is breast cancer; however, the leading cause of cancer deaths in women is lung cancer due to smoking. An estimated one in nine life time risk that women will develop breast cancer. Breast and uterine cancer can be cured if discovered early, which proves the need for vigilance in testing and examination. But the outlook for lung and throat cancer is lethal in most instances with the five-year survival rate being only 10% or less. Besides this, smokers generally are more likely to have all kinds of neoplasms—esophagus, bladder, kidney, stomach, prostate, and pancreas (as well as heart disease and emphysema). In women, smoking causes menopause to occur earlier, it also predisposes them to osteoporosis, heart problems, and other maladies. The leading cause of cancer deaths in both men and women is lung cancer (32 of a 100 in men, 25 of 100 in women). After lung cancer, the following toll of kinds of cancer list breast 17%, colon/rectum 10%, Leukemia 8%, ovary 6%, pancreas 5%, uterus/cervix 5% and kidney 3%.

Colon and rectal cancers (the danger signals are alteration of bowel movement habits and rectal bleeding) can be cured in 70% of the cases but usually only half of this percent are cured because of late attention to the problem. The most obvious kind of skin cancer could be cured in 95% of the cases; it is discovered by a simple biopsy and is usually seen as a sore that does not heal. Over exposure to sun is an important precipitating factor in skin cancer. Middle-aged people should shield themselves from the sun with sunscreen cream, hats, etc., and limit time in the sun. Prostate cancer occurs mainly in men over 60; urinalysis aids in detection, the danger signal is urinary difficulty. Though second deadliest in men it is very slow in development. In stomach cancers indigestion is the prime symptom; fortunately this disease has declined greatly in the past several decades.

The seven warning signals of cancer, though well known, are emphasized here. With early detection, the chances of recovery are significantly improved. Here are the warning signs:

1. Unusual bleeding or discharge
2. A lump or thickening in the breast
3. A sore that doesn't heal
4. Persistent change in bowel or bladder habits
5. Hoarseness or cough that is persistent
6. Persistent indigestion or difficulty in swallowing
7. Change in a wart or mole

One should see a doctor if any of these signals persist for several weeks, for diagnosis and for reassurance.

PROBLEMS WITH THE BREAST

Infections of the breast are most common in women who are breast-feeding. Otherwise breast infections can occur in women who have had surgery on the breasts, particularly when lymph glands have been removed, or in women with compromised immune systems due to chemotherapy or diseases such as AIDS. Healthy women may also develop breast infections. Mastitis and abscesses are two kinds of breast infection. Mastitis is an inflammation of the breast tissue usually due to milk ducts that are blocked and bacteria grows. The bacteria are in the mouth or skin of the newborn baby. Abscesses are uncommon is an infection (bacterial) that produced a cyst filled with pus due generally to untreated Mastitis in the early breast feeding period. Symptoms of Mastitis are fever and fatigue, breast swelling, redness and heat sensation. Also, breast appears red and swollen in the area of the areola. Antibiotics are used to combat both problems. A physician may drain the abscess to relieve much of the pain. Compresses to the same areas, warmth helps free blocked milk ducts. It is not necessary to stop breast-feeding with either infection but it is necessary to have the milk flowing.

Breast Cancer

Breast cancer is the most common cancer in women. It begins in one spot and grows. It can spread (metastasize) to other body parts via the lymphatic system and the blood stream leading to illness and perhaps death. Earlier detection of cancerous tumors by self-examination and mammograms is the best protection against breast cancer. For those over 40, having a daughter—close kin—or mother who have breast cancer, began menstruating at 12 or younger, or starting menopause at age 55 or older, have not carried a pregnancy to term, using hormone replacement therapy for 10 years or longer, been exposed to radiation or had breast cancer before are at greater risks than those not included here. In pre-menopausal women, high levels of an insulin-like growth factor called IGF-1 may indicate increased risk of breast cancer.

The most common outward sign of breast cancer is a hard lump in the breast that is usually not moveable and may or may not be painful. The skin over the lump may look dimpled (like the skin of an orange) or indented in areas where the cancer has spread. The nipple may be inverted (turn inward) or leak dark fluid. Any lumps you feel under your arm may be cancer that has spread from breast tissue to the lymph glands under your arm. Some cancers are undetectable. Any suspicious Pap smear should be repeated to rule out error and followed up by colposcopy. It is important that women learn to examine their breasts (many middlescent women regularly monitor themselves for other reasons) on a regular monthly basis. Assistance can be readily found in the physician's office (either women or men) and no woman or man should fail, however shy, prudent or painful (rectal examination is painful and for some women the uterus examination is also) to receive some sort of medical attention in this regard. It is recommended that a mammogram should be taken annually after age 40!

	STAGES OF BREAST CANCER	SURVIVAL: 5 YEARS AFTER DIAGNOSIS
I	Cancer is less than 1 inch (2 centimeters [cm]) and has not spread outside the breast.	95%
II	Cancer is 1 to 2 inches (2 to 5 cm) <u>or</u> cancer is smaller than 1 inch (2 cm) but has spread to lymph glands under the arm <u>or</u> cancer is larger than 2 inches (5 cm) but has not spread to lymph glands under the arm.	80%
III	A Cancer is larger than 2 inches (5 cm) and has spread to the lymph glands under the arm <u>or</u> cancer is smaller than 2 inches (5 cm), has spread to the lymph glands under the arm, and the lymph glands have grown together or attached themselves to other structures.	50%
III	B Cancer has spread to tissues near the breast (such as the chest wall, including the ribs and the muscles) <u>or</u> cancer has spread to lymph glands inside the chest wall along the breastbone.	50%
IV	Cancer has spread to other parts of the body (most often the bones, lungs, liver, or brain) <u>or</u> cancer has spread to the skin or lymph glands inside the neck near the collarbone.	10%

BREAST CANCER TREATMENT

All kinds of breast cancer can be treated, usually starting with surgery to remove the tumor and part or all of the breast. There are additional treatments that may be used individually or in combination, depending on the extent of your cancer and other factors such as your overall health, gone through menopause, and response to hormones.

TREATMENT OPTIONS	DESCRIPTION
Surgery	Surgery involves removing the tumor (lumpectomy) or removing the tumor and part or all of the breast tissue (mastectomy).
Radiation therapy	Radiation is used after surgery to kill any remaining cancer cells.
Chemotherapy	Chemotherapy is the administration of anticancer drugs. It can be used with surgery and/or radiation to eradicate cancer cells and prevent them from spreading or to relieve pain and discomfort if the cancer is incurable. Drugs may be taken as tablets, liquids, injections, injections, or intravenous infusions.
Hormone therapy	Hormone therapy is used to treat cancer that grows in response to hormones. Tamoxifen and raloxifene are medications taken (either by themselves or with chemotherapy) to fight tumors that are responsive to estrogen. Hormone therapy has been used most often in women over the age of 50 (although research shows that hormone therapy can be effective in women of all ages).
Biological therapy	Biological therapy is experimental therapy that uses the body's immune system to boost specific types of white blood cells that fight cancer.
Bone marrow transplant	Higher does of chemotherapy are better at eliminating cancer cells but usually destroy bone marrow, the site where blood cells are produced. Bone marrow transplantation is an experimental approach that replaces destroyed bone marrow after high-dose chemotherapy.

Frequently in treating breast cancer, chemotherapy, surgery and radiation are utilized. Specific types of drugs for the various cancer stages are seen below. The findings here are adapted from the 2002 San Antonio Breast Cancer Symposium are adapted sources of the data that follows:

AC

Adriamycin and Cytoxan

Side effects include nausea/vomiting, diarrhea, hair loss, mouth sores, reduced WBC, and, in some cases, heart problems with higher doses of Adriamycin.

CMF

Cytoxan, methotrexate, and 5-FU (given every three weeks for four to six cycles)

Side effects include nausea/loss of appetite, diarrhea, metallic taste in the mouth, mouth sores, infertility, and lowering of white blood cell (WBC) count.

FAC/CAF or FEC

5-FU, Adriamycin, and Cytoxan (oral or I.V.)

Side effects include nausea/vomiting, diarrhea, hair loss, mouth sores, reduced WBC, and, in some instances, heart damage with higher doses of Adriamycin.

Ellence® (epirubicin) is sometimes substituted for Adriamycin in order to lessen the possibility for heart damage, although high doses of epirubicin can also cause heart damage.

Taxol

Can be used following AC or FAC for adjuvant treatment.

Side effects are seen as reduced WBC, nausea/vomiting, diarrhea, hair loss, muscle/joint aches, nerve damage, and allergic reactions.

Taxotere

Can follow or be combined with AC for adjuvant/neoadjuvant treatment (TAC).

Common side effects include reduced WBC with the possibility for infection, mouth sores, allergic reactions, fatigue, and diarrhea.

Middle Stages of Breast Cancer

As women are being diagnosed with stage III breast cancer, researchers are weighing new approaches and new drugs to further improve standard treatment.

‣ **Dose-Dense Therapy**: William Gradishar, MD, of the Northwestern School of Medicine, says that he is offering patients the option of **dose-dense therapy** after findings reported at the 2002 San Antonio Breast Cancer Symposium.

This new schedule uses the same dose of drugs as customarily given, but drugs are administered every two weeks instead of every three weeks. Results from the study found that the women who received the dose-dense treatment lived longer without their cancer coming back than women who received the traditional schedule. Trial investigators say further research is needed. To help women who receive dose-dense treatment recover faster, they are given shots of **Neupogen®** (filgrastim) or **Neulasta™** (pegfilgrastim), which boost the growth of white blood cells that fight infection.

‣ **Molecular Profiling:** A new technology that may allow physicians to look at **gene expression** in breast tumors.

"If we can identify the fingerprint of a tumor and determine characteristics of one tumor compared to another, it will help us determine who will benefit from specific therapy," Dr. Gradishar explains. "At this time, we don't know what the information means in terms of clinical decision-making, but we have the ability to collect the information from the tumor samples we are banking. In the near future, clinical trials will integrate this technology and ultimately provide clinicians with a tool to more rationally select treatment."

‣ PET Scanning: Further diagnostic information could also help the decision-making process. Elisa R. Port, MD, Memorial Sloan-Kettering Cancer Center, New York, is now studying 100 patients with stage IIB or IIIA breast cancer to gauge a possible role for **PET (positron emission tomography) scans.**

Advanced Breast Cancer

Some physicians treat advanced breast cancer patients with single chemotherapy agents, combination groups are also useful in some cases. The first treatment, in some cases, is a regimen containing Adriamycin or Ellence, known collectively as anthracyclines; treatment with Taxol or Taxotere is also common. Some common combination regimens are listed below:

- **AC: Adriamycin and Cytoxan**
- **Carboplatin, Herceptin, and Taxol or Taxotere**
- **Ellence and Taxotere**
- **FAC: 5-FU, Adriamycin, and Cytoxan (oral or I.V.)**
- **FEC: 5-FU, Ellence, and Cytoxan**
- **Herceptin with Taxol or Taxotere**
- **Xeloda and Taxotere**

For women a special word should be said about taking the PAP test for with its widespread use (more than 85% American women by the end of 1985 had one Pap smear) the ability to save most sufferers of cervical cancer is at hand. Of the various Pap classifications (I-V) I and II are negative while III is labeled suspicious, classes IV and V are positive. Some papers reports use the term dysplasia, to describe pre-malignant changes. Such a report indicates the need for further evaluation by a specialist as does the labels class III, IV, and V. Also women who at their first checkup reported gynecological complaints (bleeding, irregular bleeding, spotting, or discharge) were found to develop cancer three times more often than those with no complaints. The incidences of uterine cancer grow markedly after thirty-five.

(For recent updates, see Appendix 2.)

OVARIAN CANCER

No treatment can be affected that cures cancer for sure (no fruit juice cure or drugs, clinics or fortune teller) so do not treat yourself or take the claims of advertised cures or take the word of friends who attempt it for you. Physicians may make misjudgments but they are usually corrected before the final resolution of treatment is made—radiologists, blood analysis personnel, specialists are all usually involved in the diagnosis and subsequent therapy.

Ovarian Cancer

STAGE	LOCATION OF SPREAD	SURVIVAL 5 YEARS AFTER DIAGNOSIS
IA	Cancer is confined to the ovary and no tumor remains after surgery.	After surgery-95%
IB	Cancer is confined to the ovary but some tumor remains after surgery or tumor cells appear to be malignant.	After surgery plus chemotherapy and radiation therapy-80%
II	Cancer is confined to the pelvis.	After surgery-70%
III	Cancer has spread to the abdomen.	Following surgery plus chemotherapy-15% to 20%
IV	Cancer has spread outside the abdomen	After chemotherapy and (in some cases) surgery-1% to 5%

Cervical Cancer

STAGE	LOCATION OF SPREAD	SURVIVAL 5 YEARS AFTER DIAGNOSIS
I	Cancer is confined to inside the cervix.	
IA	Cancer has gone beyond the first outer layer of cells of the cervix and measure no more than 5 millimeters (mm), with the affected area smaller than 7 mm.	A simple hysterectomy is given (removing only the uterus)-99%
IB	Cancer has spread deeper than 5 mm or broader than 7 mm but is inside the tissues of the cervix.	Radical hysterectomy or radiation therapy-85% if the cancer doesn't spread to the lymph glands and 50% if the cancer spread to the lymph glands; chemotherapy improves survival
II	Cancer has moved to nearby organs.	
IIA	Cancer has spread to the upper two thirds of the vagina.	Following radical hysterectomy or radiation therapy-85% if the cancer spread is to the lymph glands; adding chemotherapy aids survival.
IIB	Cancer has spread to the tissue around the cervix or uterus but not to the pelvis.	After radiation therapy-5% to 60%; adding chemotherapy improves survival.

III	Cancer has spread to the walls of the pelvis, the lower third of the vagina, or the ureters (connecting the kidney to the bladder).	After radiation therapy-30% to 35%; chemotherapy improves survival.
IV	Cancer has spread to distant organs	
IVA	Cancer has spread to organs nearer to the cervix, as the bladder and rectum.	With radiation therapy or more surgery-10% to 15%; adding chemotherapy increases survival rates.
IVB	Cancer has spread to more organs such as the lungs.	Following chemotherapy or radiation therapy—less than 10% (death can come within 1 year)

Menopause

In the life of women, prior to menopause, the menstrual cycle sets the rhythm of daily activities. It influences her work life, her entertainment, her mood sometimes and colors many other things such as sex, etc. Beginning with onset of menopause (the average American woman begins at age 48-51) may begin for many at 45 and extending to 60, the ovaries secrete fewer hormones, gradually ceasing altogether. Menopause is defined as 12 months in succession with out a period. The climacteric (from the Greek meaning rung in a ladder which relates to a stage in development) is the period encompassing menopause and the average time in 5 years from the time ovaries start to decrease follicle development (estrogen is produced in the ovary follicle) to the time a woman has passed through menopause and her body has adjusted to the change in hormones. The circulating levels of estrogen and progesterone hormones dwindle and the body registers this fact. The menstrual flow diminishes becoming of less duration, lighter in color and the periods come further apart until it's over. For many women this is all there is, but for others irregular periods of heavy bleeding accompanies the menstruation. It can lead, if prolonged, to anemia. This is not normal, although irregularity is characteristic of menopause. Heavy bleeding carries the threat of uterine cancer or provides evidence to the physician to investigate of samples of tissue from the lining of the uterus gained by D & C surgical procedure (dilation and curettage) and from which one of the diagnosis can be fibroid tumor (non-cancerous) as seen in the illustration shown later. Sometimes a tumor, polyp or cyst can be removed without taking out the uterus. The decision to remove the uterus, etc., should be made in consultation with the gynecologists and your personal physician.

There are both male and female hormones in the woman's body. The female predominate prior to menopause—the female hormones maintain femininity and the ability to become pregnant. During the first half of the menstrual cycle estrogen predominates, causing growth of uterine lining tissue and preparing the ovary to ovulate and to release progesterone for the second part of the cycle. Male hormones—androgen and testosterone, the former is produced mainly in the adrenal gland found above the upper pole of the kidneys. The androgens are less influential in women prior to menopause but tend to become more prominent afterwards since the estrogen produced from the fatty tissues is not as strong as that produced in the ovaries during the child-bearing years. Testosterone produced by the testicles helps sperm mature, also, promotes the growth of male features in childhood. This is dealt with in depth later in the chapter.

Hormone Replacement Therapy

In past years HRT (hormone replacement therapy) was used to relieve the symptoms of menopause. It was learned that HRT has major long-term benefits however it carried some risks.

Women's Health Initiative

One large study of the risks and benefits involved the Women's Health Initiative (WHI) is a set of clinical trials, including two estrogen-progestin trials, in healthy postmenopausal women ages 50 to 79, which was scheduled to be completed in 2005. However, one of the trials (continuous, combined estrogen-progestin versus placebo in over 16,000 women) was discontinued early because of an increased risk of breast cancer, coronary heart disease (CHD), stroke, and venous thromboemblosim over an average follow-up of 5.2 years. Although significant benefits were also seen (reduction in risk of fractures and colon cancer), there was concern that the risks of combined estrogen-progestin outweighed the benefits for many women.

The Women's Health Initiative found unopposed estrogen versus placebo trail in women who had under gone a hysterectomy (and therefore did not require a progestin) has not been discontinued, since no unfavorable nor favorable risk-benefit profile has been observed and data are available, we recommend caution in the long-term use of estrogen alone.

The specific effects of combined continuous estrogen-progestin (estrogen 0.625 mg with medroxyprogesterone acetate 2.5 mg per day) were as follows:

Coronary heart disease—The rate of coronary events increased with combined estrogen-progestin therapy (39 versus 33 per 10,000 person years, hazard ration [HR] 1.24, nominal 95 percent CI 1.00 to 1.54). Most of the excess was in nonfatal myocardial infarction (MI), with no differences in revascularization procedures, angina, or congestive heart failure seen. The difference in coronary events developed soon after randomization with a trend towards a decline in excess risk in years two through five. There were no other predictors of risk with the possible exception of women with high LDL. Although the combined HRT arm was discontinued early, the authors calculated that it was unlikely that a beneficial effect of HRT on CHD would have been seen in subsequent years.

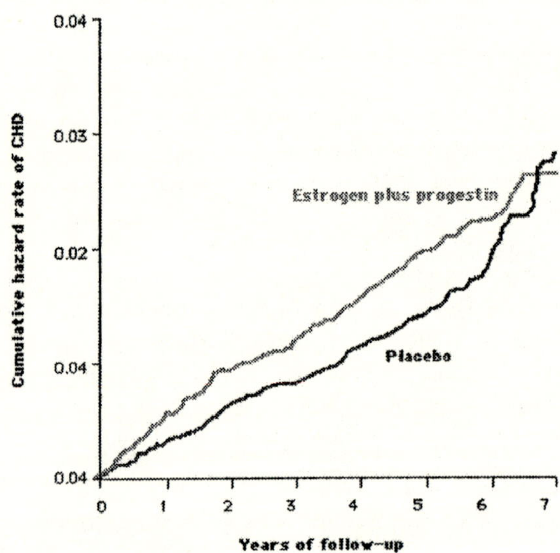

Kaplan-Meier estimates of cumulative hazard rates of CHD In the Women's Health Initiative, combined estrogen-progestin therapy was associated with a significant increase in coronary events. CHD included nonfatal myocardial infarction and death due to CHD. The overall hazard ratio for CHD was 1.24 (nominal 95 percent confidence interval, 1.00 to 1.54). Data from Manson, JE, Hsia, J, Johnson, KC, et al. Estrogen plus progestin and the risk of coronary heart disease. N Engl J Med 2003; 3499:523.

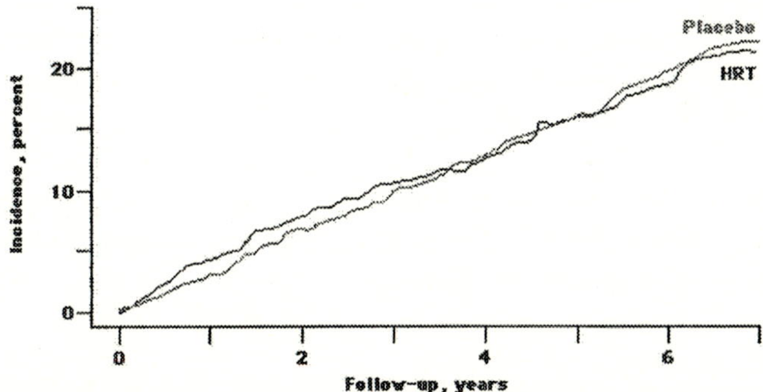

Estrogen therapy not beneficial for secondary prevention of coronary heart disease Data from the HERS-II trial on the incidence of coronary heart disease events (death or nonfatal myocardial infarction) in 2763 postmenopausal women with a prior history of myocardial infarction or interventional procedure who were treated with combined hormone.

Source: From Estrogen plus Progestin and the Risk of Coronary Heart Disease by Manson, Hsia, Johnson, Rossouw, Assaf, Lasser, Trevisan, Black, Heckbert. Printed by permission of Massachusetts Medical Society.

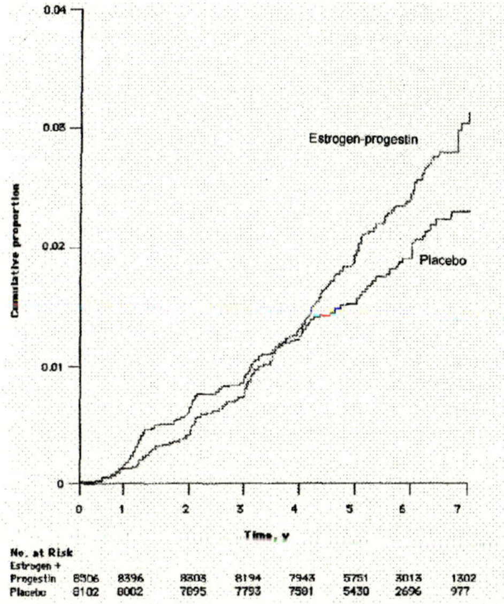

HRT increases invasive breast cancer In the Women's Health Initiative, combined estrogen-progestin replacement therapy (red) was associated with a significant increase in invasive breast cancer (HR 1.24 unadjusted 95 percent CI 1.01 to 1.543) when compared with placebo (green). Data from Chlebowski, RT, Hendrix, SL, Langer, RD, et al. Risks and benefits of estrogen and progestin in healthy postmenopausal women: principal results from the Women's Health Initiative randomized controlled trial. JAMA 2003; 289:3243-53.

The Kaplan-Meier figure clearly shows the combined estrogen-progestin hormones should increase in coronary heart disease over a six-year plus (6.8) period. Those women on placebo (typically a sugar pill—non-medicine) fared as well taking no hormone pills.

In HERS II Trials (done with a number of patients) estrogen therapy in 2,762 women who were post-menopausal and had a history of myocardial infarction was not reduced with the hormone. Here again those on the placebo did just as well as those on hormone therapy.

Stroke—In the WHI, a 31 percent increase in stroke risk was seen with combined estrogen-progestin use compared with placebo (intention-to-treat hazard ratio 1.31, 95 percent CI 1.02 to 1.68). The hazard ratios for ischemic and hemorrhagic stroke were 1.44 (95 percent CI 1.09 to 1.90), and 0.82 ((95 percent CI 0.43 to 1.56), respectively. Excess risk was seen in all age groups, and was independent of other known risk factors for stroke. The Kaplan-Meier study was part of the Women's Health Initiative investigation.

Venous thromboembolism—The rate of venous thromboembolism (increased clotting) with HRT (34 versus 16 per 10,000 person-years, HR 2.11, unadjusted 95 percent CI 1.58 to 2.82). The increase in risk was similar for both deep vein thrombosis and pulmonary embolism and was also seen in the HERS trials.

Breast cancer—The risk of invasive breast cancer was significantly increased with combined hormone replacement at an average follow-up of 5.6 years (HR 1.24, unadjusted 95 percent CI (1.01 to 1.54). Although it has been suggested that breast cancer in women taking estrogen has a relatively good prognosis, this was not the case in the WHI.

Osteoporotic fracture—The risk of osteoporotic fracture was reduced at the hip (5 fewer hip fractures per 10,000 person-years, HR 0.66, unadjusted 95 percent CI 0.45 to 0.98; and HR 0.77, 95 percent CI 0.69 to 0.86, respectively).

Colorectal cancer—The risk of colorectal cancer was reduced (6 fewer colorectal cancers per 10,000 person-years, HR 0.63, unadjusted 95 percent CI 0.43 to 0.92). This benefit is consistent with other studies (see following figures).

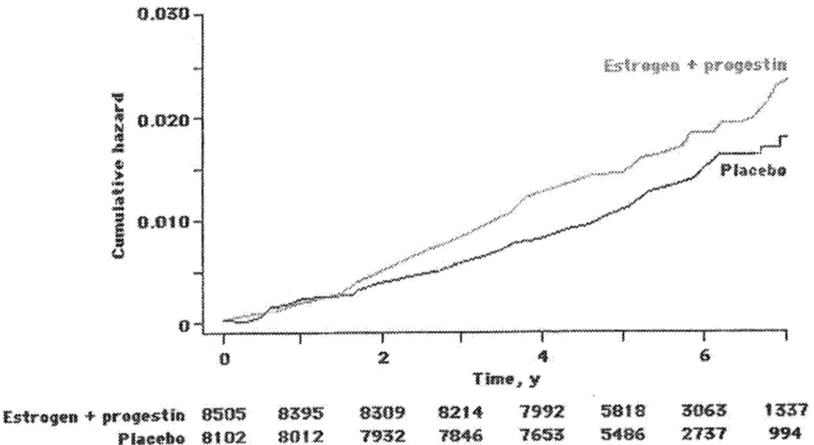

Kaplan-Meier estimates of cumulative hazard rates of stroke in the Women's Health Initiative, combined estrogen-progestin therapy was associated with a significant increase in stroke when compared with placebo. The intention-to-treat hazard ration was 1.31, 95 percent CI 1.02 to 1.68. 95 of 100 means if repeated with the same variable the (called 5% level) conclusions would be the same at the 1% level of confidence then 99 of 100 in the situation CI = Confidence Interval. Data from Wassertheil-Smoller, S, Hendrix, S, Limacher, M, et al. Effect of Estrogen Plus Progestin on Stroke in Postmenopausal Women: The Women's Health Initiative: A Randomized Trial. JAMA (Journal of the American Medical Association) 2003; 289:2673. *Copyright* © (2003), American Medical Association. All rights reserved.

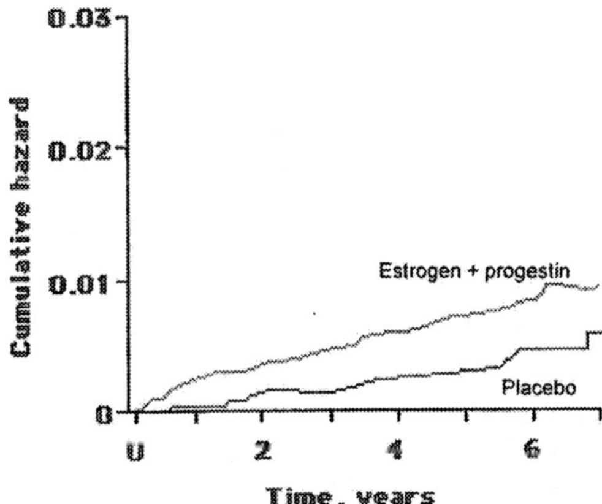

HRT increases pulmonary embolism in the Women's Health Initiative, combined estrogen-progestin replacement therapy was associated with a significant increase in pulmonary embolism (8 more pulmonary emboli per 10,000 person years, HR 2.13, unadjusted 95 percent CI 1.39 to 3.25). (Data from Risks and benefits of estrogen and progestin in healthy postmenopausal women: principal results from the Women's Health Initiative randomized controlled trial. JAMA 2002; 288:321. *Copyright* © (2002), American Medical Association. All rights reserved.

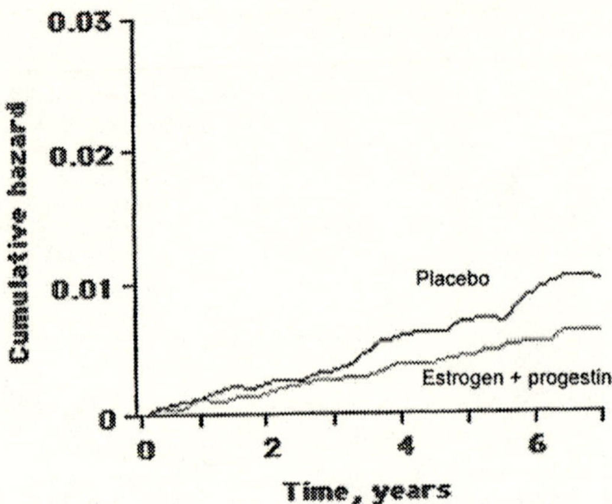

HRT reduces colorectal cancer in the Women's Health Initiative, combined estrogen-progestin replacement therapy was associated with a significant reduction in colorectal cancer (6 fewer colorectal cancers per 10,000 person-years, HR 0.63, unadjusted 95 percent CI 0.43 to 0.92). (Data from Risks and benefits of estrogen and progestin in healthy postmenopausal women: principal results from the Women's Health Initiative randomized controlled trial. JAMA 2002; 288:321.)

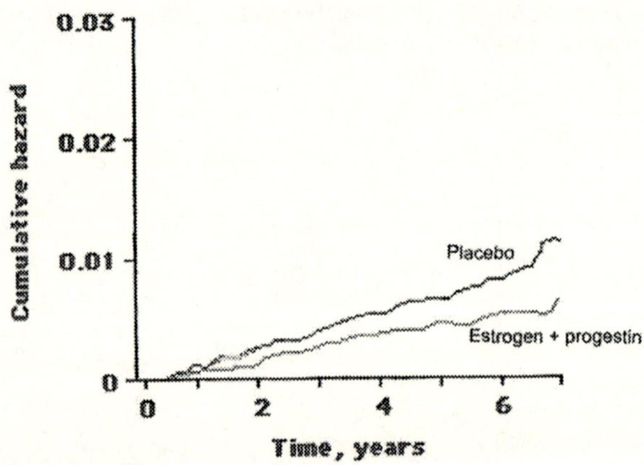

Estrogen-progestin therapy reduces hip fracture in the Women's Health Initiative, combined estrogen-progestin replacement therapy was associated with significant reduction in hip fracture (5 fewer fractures per 10,000 person-years, HR 0.7, unadjusted 95 percent CI 0.4 to 1.0). (Data from Risks and benefits of estrogen and progestin in healthy postmenopausal women: principal results from the Women's Health Initiative randomized controlled trial. JAMA 2002; 288:321.)

RISK OF ENDOMETRIAL HYPERPLASIA AND CARCINOMA

Treatment of postmenopausal women with estrogen alone increases the risk of endomentrial hyperplasia (increase size of the [cells] endometrial lining in the uterus) and carcinoma. Within one year, endometrial hyperplasia can be demonstrated in 20 to 50 percent of women receiving unopposed estrogen. Furthermore, multiple case-control and prospective studies have shown an increased incidence of endometrial carcinoma with long-term unopposed estrogen, with the relative risk ranging from 3.1 to 15.

If the absolute risk of endometrial carcinoma in postmenopausal women is about 1 in 1000, then the absolute risk in women taking unopposed estrogen increases to approximately 1 in 100. While the risk of both localized and widespread endometrial cancer is increased with long-term unopposed estrogen, the tumors that develop may be less aggressive, as survival is better in women with cancers associated with estrogen therapy.

The risk of endometrial hyperplasia and cancer with unopposed (without progestin) estrogen therapy is both duration and dose-dependent. In one study, the relative risk of endometrial cancer increased by 17 percent per year of estrogen therapy, to an odds ratio of greater than 8 after 10 years. The excess risk persisted five or more years after cessation of therapy.

In one dose-response study, lower doses of estrogen for two years did not increase the incidence of endometrial hyperplasia. When compared with no estrogen higher doses of estrogen were associated with higher rates of disease, 20% up to 50%, respectively. A low-dose (0.3 mg per day of conjugated equine estrogens) increased risk of endometrial cancer. When given for a longer period eight or more years it expanded the risk of the endometrial cancer by 9 to 10 times.

In a study by Schiff, I., Sela, H.K., Cramer, D., et al (1982) it was found that estrogen replacement elicits uterine hyperplasia rate of uterine hyperpiesia in women receiving steady or continuous cyclic estrogen replacement therapy. No difference was found between the two groups, and uterine hyperpiesia occurred in nearly one-half of the women in each group at year one.

Cognitive function and dementia—Although some epidemiologic studies suggested that estrogen may preserve cognitive function and prevent dementia, data from WHI do not support these observations. The WHI Memory Study (WHIMS) an ancillary study of the WHI, assessed annual MMSE scores in 4532 postmenopausal women who were over age 65 and free of probably dementia at baseline. After a mean follow-up of approximately four years, no significant improvement in global cognitive function was seen with combined estrogen-progestin therapy compared with placebo. However, more women in the HRT group had substantial and clinically important declines in MMSE total scores compared with placebo (6.7 versus 4.8 percent, respectively).

Although these data rule out any global cognitive benefits of combined estrogen-progestin therapy in older, non-demented postmenopausal women, the possibility of domain-specific cognitive benefits with HRT has not been ruled out.

In addition, combined estrogen-progestin therapy did not prevent all-cause dementia. After a mean follow-up of approximately four years, daily HRT with 0.625 mg of conjugated equine estrogen plus 2.5 mg of medroxyprogesterone acetate was associated with an increased risk of dementia (40 cases in 2229 women in the HRT group versus 21 of 2303 women in the placebo group; HR 2.05, 95 percent CI 1.21 to 3.48). This translates to an additional 23 cases of dementia per 10,000 women per year attributed to HRT.

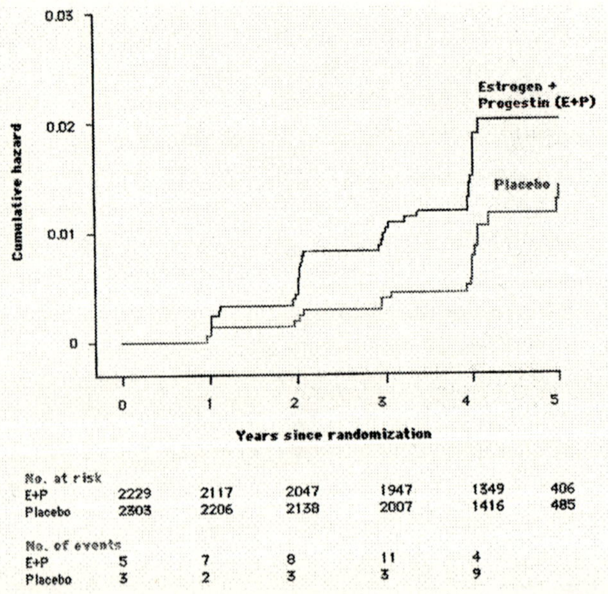

Risk of dementia with combined estrogen-progestin therapy vs placebo In the Women's Health Initiative Memory Study, after a mean follow-up of four years, HRT was associated with an increased risk of dementia (overall hazard ratio [HR] 2.05, 95 percent CI 1.21 to 3.48). Data shown only through five years of follow-up because numbers at risk are too small after this point for precise estimates. Data from Shumaker, SA, Legault, C, Thal, L, et al. Estrogen plus Progestin and the Incidence of Dementia and Mild Cognitive Impairment in Postmenopausal Women: The Women's Health Initiative Memory Study: A Randomized Controlled Trial. JAMA 2003; 289:2651-62.

The impact of unopposed estrogen use, or HRT use in younger post-menopausal (45-55 age group) women on dementia risk is not known. Current short-term (up to one year) clinical trials of oral estrogen indicate that hormone replacement therapy is not an effective treatment for Alzheimer's disease.

Other estrogen-progestin regimens that have been investigated include the following:

- Oral micronized progesterone (200 mg/day for 12 days) reduces the risk of hyperplasia to the same degree as medroxyprogesterone acetate (2.5 mg/day continuiously or 10 mg/day for 12 days.
- Medroxyprogesterone (10 mg/day) for 14 days every three months may be associated with higher rates of endometrial hyperplasia and cannot be recommended.
- There was no increase in endometrial cancer risk in the WHI in women receiving combined estrogen-progestin therapy compared with placebo (HR 0.83, 95 percent CI 0.47 to 1.47).

Medical researchers analyzing the results of data from Women's Health Initiative, HERS Trials, etc., make several recommendations for diagnosis and treatment. The doses and types of estrogen and progestin preparations that are recommended and the diagnosis and treatment of established endometrial hyperplasia are described in detail elsewhere.

For patient monitoring the following is recommended:

- Pretreatment biopsy to rule out atypical endometrail hyperplasia or carcinoma should be performed in any woman with a history of irregular bleeding or previous long-term exposure to unopposed estrogen.
- Regular monitoring for bleeding during therapy, keeping in mind that the majority of women who receive continuous estrogen-progestin therapy will have irregular uterine bleeding during the first three months of therapy, but after six months over 75 percent should have amenorrhea (abnormal discharge of menstrual substance). The prevalence of bleeding is related to the number of years since

menopause. Those women who were more than three years postmenopausal were less likely to have any bleeding during the first year of continuous therapy, as compared with women who were less than two years postmenopausl (65 versus 78 percent); the former are more likely to have had endometrial atrophy when therapy is begun.

- Women who have uterine bleeding after a period of amenorrhea should have endometrial monitoring to look for evidence of intrauterine pathology (e.g., hyperplasia, carcinoma, fibroids, polyps). Monitoring should also be performed in women with bleeding that is refractory to hormonal manipulation (such as an increase in progestin dose). In the latter case, if a biopsy is not diagnostic, consideration should be given to assessing the uterine cavity with ultrasound or hysteroscopy.

Endometrial monitoring may involve transvaginal ultrasonography or endometrial biopsy. An endometrial double layer thickness of less than 5 mm by transvaginal ultrasound is sufficient to rule out endometrial cancer in women taking continuous estrogen-progestin therapy (negative predictive value 99 percent). However, approximately one-half of women will have an endometrial thickness greater than 5 mm, which is an indication for endometrial biopsy. Thus, depending upon patient preference and the skill of the sonographer, transvaginal ultrasound may be offered first to women who require endometrial monitoring, with the understanding that a substantial number will also require endometrial biopsy.

Because estrogen stimulates the proliferation of endometrial tissue, estrogen therapy is considered to be contraindicated in women with a history of endometrial cancer, even with concurrent progestrone administration. However, two retrospective analyses found that disease-free survival in women with stage I endometrial carcinoma was no worse in women who took estrogen after surgical cure of their cancer. Therefore, some clinicians do not automatically withhold estrogen from women with low-risk endometrial carcinoma who appear to be cured. However, these women must be informed about the uncertain safety of estrogen.

Summary

It should be emphasized that the absolute risk of an adverse event (breast cancer or cardiovascular complication) occurring in an individual on the estrogen-progestin regimen in the WHI was extremely low (19 additional events per year per 10,000 women with HRT [Hormone Replacement Therapy] compared to placebo). Recommendations for HRT use were presented earlier.

HRT (Hormone Replacement)

With variable dosage shows from medical research benefits in certain situations (age, prior problems, healthcare) are relative to the following:

1. Depression
2. Falls
3. Reducing osteoporosis
4. Preserving the thickness and collagen of the skin
5. Teeth
6. Brain
7. Lower risk of Type II diabetes
8. Lower risk of cataract formation (Framington Heart Study)
9. Quality of life

Estrogen has a variable effect on quality of life in postmenopausal women, depending on the women's age and the presence of symptoms and/or comorbid conditions. In postmenopausal women with vasomotor flushes, estrogen is thought to improve quality of life by eliminating nocturnal hot flushes, and restoring more normal sleep.

HRT increases the risks of the following:

1. Gallbladder disease
2. Bronchospasm
3. Ovarian cancer
4. Systemic lupus erythematosis
5. Raynaud's phenomenon
6. Uterine leiomyomos
7. Epilepsy
8. Dry eye syndrome

In an ongoing study of the Women's Health Initiative (involving thousands of women), it was found that the development of cardiovascular and breast cancer was extremely low though increased compared to overall hormone users.

Protective effect of progestins—Among women treated with estrogen, the excess risk of endometrial hyperplasia and carcinoma can be largely abolished by concurrent therapy with a progestin given in either a cyclic or continuous regimen. In the PEPI trial, for example, combined estrogen-progestin therapy led to marked reductions in the incidence of simple (0.8 versus 27.7 percent), complex (0.8 versus 23.7 percent), and atypical hyperplastic (zero versus 11.8 percent) endometrial lesions.

In the PEPI trial and in a review from the Cochrane Database, cyclic progestin (when given at least 12 days per month) was an effective as continuous low-dose progestin. Shorter duration progestin therapy (<10 to 12 days) may be less protective.

The most commonly used combined continuous estrogen-progestin regimen in the United States is low-dose medroxyprogesterone (2.5 or 5 mg daily) given each day with estrogen (conjugated estrogens 0.625 or its equivalent). This regimen is associated with a low risk of endometrial hyperplasia, and has the added advantage of inducing amenorrhea in 60 to 75 percent of women after more than six months of treatment.

Use of HRT is a serious matter. It is, therefore, extremely important that you get the best medical attention possible. You need to have a physician who understands women's problems and has definitive knowledge of the use of hormone replacement—diagnostic, treatment and follow-up. The Women's Health Initiative designed to settle the question of whether long term hormone therapy could prevent heart disease and other degenerative conditions in healthy postmenopausal women. Women who had a uterus were placed on a specific combination HT pill (Prempro) or placebo. Women who no longer had a uterus were given one particular estrogen pill (Premarin) or placebo. These pills were used because physicians prescribed these HT formulations most often. In 2002 WHI reported the results of Prempro trials. Like most studies before this cohort studies, the HT users had reduced rates of colorectal cancer, hip fractures and spinal fractures and increased rates of invasive breast cancer and blood clots in the veins mainly those traveling to the lungs.

The WHI Prempro Trials found the opposite of many cohort studies for the risks for heart attacks and strokes increased in the first two years of the study and breast cancer thereafter. Because of these risks WHI concludes long term risks of Prempro out weighed the benefits. Sixteen thousand women were told to stop taking the medicine and suggested six million women on this medicine reconsider it's use with their doctors.

This followed a report for women to understand Prempro did little to improve health or cognitive and didn't relieve menopausal symptoms. It also doubled the risk of dementia for women over sixty-five. The risks of taking Prempro clearly over balanced the gains. The risks were not large but significant leading to more strokes and heart attacks. Some argued those included too many older people, the average age was 63 and many women were in their early fifties a time when the typical menopause begins (51 years) in the U.S. Actually 5,000 with over thirty percent were younger than 60. The results were not statistically different of the older women. To decide if age matters in the use of HT would require a tremendously large sample many times the use of the WHI one which was 16,000 and the outlay in size of money gigantic. Small cohort studies are under way using randomized and control study of HT use in younger women. These new studies focus on markers of atherosclerosis such as thickness of the arterial walls of the main arteries.

Harvard investigation raises the question of whether or not the estrogen and progesterone/progestin preparations other than Prempro and Premarin been used could result in the difference. But some argue the earlier HT studies showing earlier good effects of the hormone on heart attack and strokes were based upon Prempro and Premarin. It should be noted that different forms of estrogen have different effects on tissues, such as the lining of blood vessels in the breast. Prempro uses a synthetic form of progesterone that is different from that made from a woman's ovaries. HT is taken by most women in pill form then absorbed in the intestine on their way to the liver in much lower concentrations goes through the blood to reach the rest of the body, this is different from what happens normally. The estrogen and progesterone go immediately to all parts of the body by passing the liver. High amounts of estrogen going through the liver causes the liver to make increased amounts of certain molecules that promote atherosclerosis for this reason even before the results of WHI were known doctors were using the estrogen skin patch rather than the estrogen containing pill to reduce blood clots.

The use of HRT is relative to heart disease, osteoporosis, bladder infection and urinary incontinence. Some options to the use of drugs as ways to reduce the risk of health problems follow below.

Problem	Suggestions
Vaginal dryness	▪ Put estrogen ointments and creams into your vagina. ▪ Wear a soft estrogen-containing ring in your vagina. ▪ Use water-based lubricants during intercourse. ▪ Remain sexually active, which helps preserve the elasticity of the vaginal wall. ▪ Do Kegel exercises regularly.
Lessened sex drive	▪ Use testosterone in pills, in cream applied to the vulva, or under the skin.
Hot flashes and night sweats	▪ Dress in layers and clothes that you can remove during a hot flash. ▪ Avoid alcohol and caffeine-containing drinks and food. ▪ Add soy ingredients to your diet. ▪ Doctors may suggest you should take clonidine, a medicine that is not a hormone but can reduce the strength of hot flashes.

D & C (DILATATION AND CURETTAGE)

The uterine lining is scraped to isolate the cause of frequent periods, to terminate a pregnancy, to treat an incomplete abortion or miscarriage.

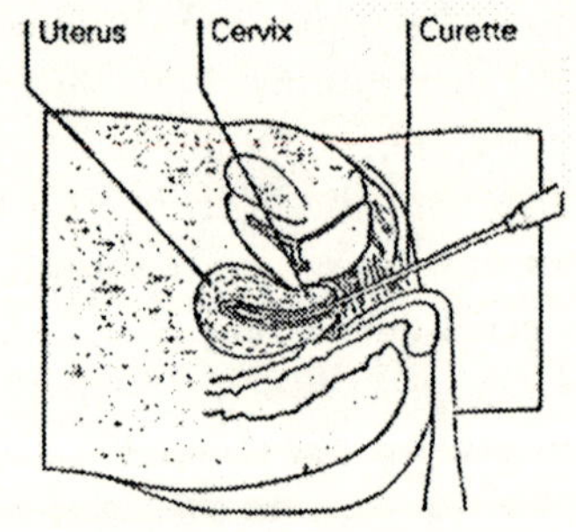

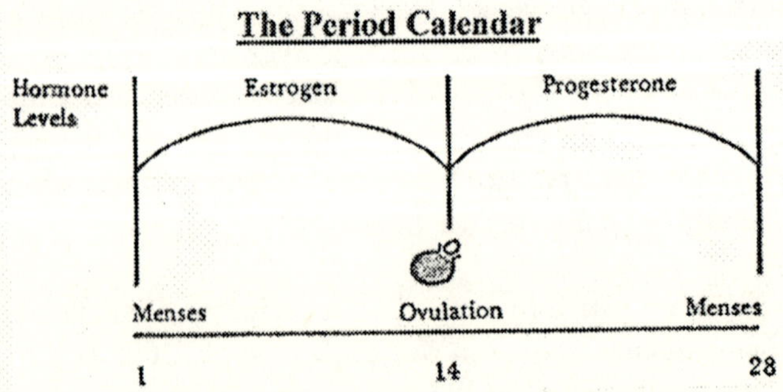

The ovaries and gonad glands give trim hips, drive, cause hair to grow in unlikely spots and provide sexual urge. Their levels of flow are not lessened by menopause. The loss of estrogen means unfortunately decreased immunity to diseases that plague men (hardening of the arteries) but fortunately offset by increased sexual vigor. All women continue to secrete some estrogen, its just so low that its influence is minimal.

Menopause—Scenario

Women experience menopause in different ways. Your body is influenced by your general health, nutrition, stress level, exercise routine, heredity, and life style.

The following chart lists the most common symptoms. Most women do not experience all of them and many women experience only a few.

WHEN	SYMPTOM	DESCRIPTION
Menopause beginning	Irregular periods	Menstrual cycle shortens and is irregular, you may still be fertile.
Menopause	Hot flashes	Dramatic changes in body temperature that could begin several years before periods stop.
	Insomnia/night sweats	Sleep problems, possibly caused by nighttime hot flashes.
Post-Menopause	Vaginal dryness; urinary irritation or incontinence	Thinning of the vaginal wall and bladder, along with decreased vaginal secretions, can cause vaginal dryness, pain during intercourse, also risk of vaginal or urinary tract infections, and urinary incontinence.
	Sexual problems	Loss of libido due to low testosterone (produced by the ovary before menopause) levels but can result in vaginal irritation because of vaginal dryness.
	Mood changes	Irritability, anxiety, stress, and depression are not caused by lower estrogen levels, but may occur as a result of disturbed sleep.
Long-term	Bone loss	Bones become more porous, with risk of breaking a bone.
	Heart disease	Blood vessels are less flexible and cholesterol levels rise, causing the risk of having a heart attack.

Oral contraceptives influence hormone levels. Most birth control pills contain estrogen and progesterone hormones, producing even hormone flows during the month in eliminating the trough at 14 days that come with ovulation. These pills also control menstrual flow, which can be sped by stopping the pills a few days early or put off by taking the pills a few extra days at the end of the month. The difficulty with the pill is for a few women it has ulterior effect, their contraception problems can be solved by other methods. The medical profession has not in the past prescribed the use of hormones for cosmetic purposes, to delay softening of bones, preserve breast fullness, youthful feminine tissues, to combat masculinizing facial hair, loss of hair, etc. This however is changing at the present time. Estrogens are used (Premarin, Ethinyl Estradiol or Menest) for prevention and treatment of vascular instability (hot flushes, flashes, vaginal dryness and osteoporosis). Artificial progestational agents may be prescribed like diethylstilbestrol or sometimes Provera tablets. Some of these hormones have been linked to vaginal and breast cancers and the decision to use them should be a matter of serious thought in consultation with your doctor. Birth control pills are not prescribed after 35 because of the high incidence of cardiovascular and thrombotic problems associated with their use after this age. However, the woman who is still ovulating can get pregnant, and contraception is a major concern (especially now that the IUD is not being advised by some physicians). Most IUD's are not off the market. A new IUD, ParaGard, is marketed primarily to doctors. ParaGard is aimed at only women who have no history of pelvic inflammatory disease, are involved in stable mutually monograms relationships and have had at least one child. This IUD (Model T380A) is marketed by Gynophorma of Somerville, New Jersey. The manufacturers claim it is safe. For those over 35 who do not wish to bear children, sterilization is a safe option and either the man or woman can undertake the operation.

It is true, according to the physicians to whom I talked, that the menopausal woman is frequently emotionally upset and given to crying spells. It may be a depressing time for many women because the ovaries no longer supply the body with enough estrogen and progesterone. These hormones along with some other (thyroxine, adrenalin, etc.) and along with the nervous system, influence behavior. The hormone upheaval upsets body control with flushes of heat causing sweating without apparent reason and feeling of suffocation. They sometimes occur during eating, sleeping or exercise. The problem here lies with a hormone (gonadotropin) released by the pituitary (master gland) which serves to control and adjust body level of estrogen and progesterone. At menopause the ovaries secrete less and less of these female hormones so in order to counteract this the pituitary gland pours more hormones into the system with the resultant effect of creating the "hot flash." The pituitary levels of FSH and LH (gonadotropic hormones) remain high for life but at menopause the temperature control is upset affecting some women. Replacement therapy (by tablet or injection) of the missing hormones can be used but should be attempted only with your physician's guidance. For the woman with a normal menopause, the ovarian function diminishes gradually and the symptoms mentioned above are few and spread over two or three years and sometimes longer.

A hysterectomy is sometimes given to correct a uterine fibroid tumor. The tumor when it occurs usually begins early in the life of a young woman and by the later thirties or forties has become a problem that is large enough to be removed. Dilation and curettage (D&C) is a way to diagnose and control causes of abnormal bleeding, i.e., post menopausal bleeding. Surgery for fibroids is the more common way to treat them. In many instances, if the woman is through childbearing and the fibroids are getting larger, the surgeon will do a vaginal hysterectomy. Brigham & Women's Hospital, Boston, is trying a non-invasive method without surgery. The ovaries are often removed (called oophorectomy) in conjunction with a hysterectomy and sometimes the fallopian tubes are removed (called a bilateral salpingectomy). In a D and C performed under anesthesia, the cervix is widened and the uterus lining is scraped to get a sample of cells. This is the third most frequently performed operation in the United States and it is simple. It has been claimed that a sizable number of these operations mentioned above are not needed. Even though much is probably done for preventive measures, second opinions should be obtained. If abnormalities exist suggesting removal of the womb, then losing the uterus or fallopian tubes will cause few menopausal symptoms but the ovaries lost will create some difficulties as outlined above.

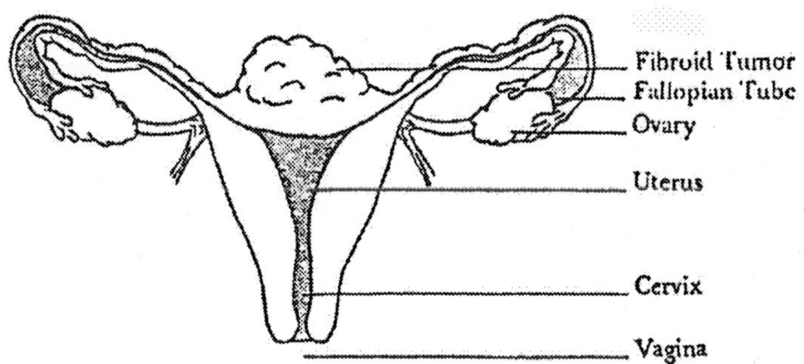

Summary on Hormone Therapy

The WHI studies have caused many women to ask whether they should use HT at all, even for short-term symptom relief as they begin to experience menopausal onset.

If your menopausal symptoms are severe, HT is an option that can help, but there are others. If you take HT, you need to estimate the risks and if you're willing to accept them. Only you can gauge the value of the risk however your doctor can help you understand it.

Hormone therapy (HT) remains the most effective treatment for hot flashes and vaginal dryness, two of the most disruptive menopausal symptoms. HT does not always work, and often causes more symptoms (vaginal discharge, uterine bleeding, breast discomfort) than it relieves. Other remedies are less effective than HT, but carry fewer risks. Neurontin (an epilepsy treatment) and certain antidepressants and blood pressure medications can help relieve hot flashes. Soy products (foods) relieve symptoms partially but soy in pill form does not. Lifestyle change is definitely an approach worth trying. Exercise and relaxation techniques can help control hot flashes. Some women get relief by avoiding caffeine, spicy foods, and other "triggers."

Does HT make sense? The average women using combined HT lowers the risk of osteoporosis and colorectal cancer but increases the risk of breast cancer, blood clots, heart disease, and stroke. (Stroke is the main hazard of estrogen alone.)

If age, family history, or lifestyle makes you especially vulnerable to breast cancer or cardiovascular disease, then HT will carry higher-than-average risks. But HT will pose fewer hazards if you start out at low risk for these conditions—younger, good life styles, nonsmoker or drinker, diabetes, obesity, late menopause.

Everyone should try nonhormonal/strategies first. Kegel exercise, vaginal cream, avoid alcohol, have sex. They're safer than HT and many women find them effective. If that doesn't work, and you want to consider HT look at the risks associated with taking Prempro. Most women will not develop breast cancer or cardiovascular disease during any five-year period, whether they take HT or not.

If you take HT, take the lowest effective does for the shortest possible time. Half the standard does is often enough. If you experience substantial improvement on HT, stick with the regimen for 6 to 12 months, then gradually taper off (cut dosage to every other day then cut doses in half the second week on alternate days then stop). If your symptoms return with a vengeance try another 6 to 12 months of treatment. But if they return in a milder form, try managing them with lifestyle changes or nonhormonal medications. If vaginal dryness if your primary complaint, an estrogen cream or ring may relieve it without affecting the other parts of your body.

If your symptoms persist after two years of hormone therapy, you should carefully reevaluate the dangers, for they increase over time. Your doctor can assist you with a decision on this matter.

Prostate Problems

The enlargement of the prostate gland in males can cause an obstruction to the flow of urine by pressing against the urethral canal. One of every 3 men has an enlarged prostate gland but symptoms are not serious enough to warrant an operation. The waste accumulates in the bladder and finally backs up into the kidney where infections can generate very easily. Cancer of the prostate is a serious problem among men and the danger increases with age especially in the over 60 age group. Earlier problems with a non-cancerous enlargement of the prostate places the man at greater risk of developing prostate cancer. Prostate disease symptoms include difficulties in urinating, loss of force in the stream of urine and getting up at night to urinate (nocturia). A regular yearly prostate examination is important to detect early problems and increase the chance for a positive outcome. Surgery is the typical way of taking care of this problem.

Prostate Stages

Stage T1 is the first stage identified by being confined to the prostate and is too small to be felt by the doctor during a manual rectal examination or to be observed by transrectal ultrasound. Stage T2 the cancer is still located to the prostate but can be felt by the physician during a rectal examination. In Stage T3 the cancer invades most of the gland and bursts through the prostate capsule. In the first stage—M the cancer cells have metastasized (spread). The Gleason Tumor grading is based upon the appearance of the cancer. Examination of the cells under a microscope then if they differentiate from grade from 1 to 5 (the most malignant). Grade 2, 3, and 4 lie between the extreme. Cells vary in appearance from a single biopsy pathologists score the two most representative regions separately then add them to arrive at a single Gleason score 1, 2, 3 or 4 have the scores of 5, 6 7 carry an intermediate prognosis.

Treatment

Stage T1 and T2 and have low Gleason scores indicate slow growing cancer will be observed to discover need for treatment. In older men the treatment may be more damaging than the disease and if they have a life expectancy of 10 years or less may be left with the disease. The best men for radiation therapy especially older men who may not tolerate surgery is external radiation the standard method—rays are aimed straight at the prostate tumor and sometimes nearby lymph nodes from a machine five times a week for 7 weeks. Side effects in this procedure are diarrhea, rectal bleeding, impotence and rarely incontinence. Breahy therapy, a recent technique delivers radiation by seeds or pellets of radioactive material put into the prostate gland through a needle. Ultrasound is used by the doctor to see the location of the cancer. There are few side effects to this method though it is less well tested.

Surgery (radical called prostetatectomy)

The gland is removed and sometimes the lymph glands in the pelvis through an incision in the abdomen. Type T1 and T3 under 70 years of age are the best subjects for this surgery.

Androgen Deprivation Therapy

Prostate cells are stimulated by androgen testosterone (male hormone) and other hormones. When removed slow the growth of cancer. This is the best treatment for men whose cancer has spread beyond the prostate gland and into the lymph nodes and other organs (Stage M). It is viewed as an adjunct to radiation for men in Stage T3 though it cannot cure the cancer itself. New approaches are cryosurgery, which applies cold to destroy cancer cells. It is accomplished by using a general anesthesia, takes 12 hours and requires a hospital stay of 1 or 2 days. Some advocates believe it is less likely to cause undesirable side effects. This approach does protect potency and spares urinary incontinence. It may it has been found to bring short-term soreness, scrotum swelling and painful urination also some 5 to 20% have blockage of the urethra.

Women may have need of the following tests:

CA-125 (Cancer Antigen 125) Test

Where there is a strong family history of ovarian cancer. This simple blood test is a screen for elevated levels of CA-125, a protein produced by cancer cells. This test is given to women who have completed menopause as the test is less accurate before menopause.

Cervical Biopsy

Removal is made of a piece of tissue from the cervix for analysis under a microscope. A punch biopsy used collects a small circle of tissue. This can be performed in a doctor's office without anesthesia. Cramping and spotting may occur following this procedure. A core biopsy is used for diagnosis and treatment in a hospital using anesthesia. Core section is removed from the cervical opening and closed by stitches and by applying heat (cautery).

Colposcopy

The use of a small binocular magnifying glass that reveals cell changes that might indicate a tendency to development cancer. This approach helps identify the best site for a biopsy. Does not usually require anesthesia.

Endometrial Biopsy

A sample of tissue is removed from the lining of the uterus. A plunger is inserted and pulled back, some small pieces of the endometrial tissue is sucked inside the catheter. The biopsy is performed in the doctor's office or nurses causing some discomfort and produces spotting a day or two afterwards.

FSH and LH Blood Tests

These tests measure the level of follicle-stimulating hormones (FSH) and luteinizing hormones in your blood. These two hormones help determine the cause of abnormal menstrual cycles, lack of ovulation and infertility also may determine onset of menopause.

Hysteroscopy

This is a thin wand inserted through the vagina and cervical canal to the inside of the uterus. A light source to show the uterus along with a device that sprays carbon dioxide or a saline solution to inflate the uterus to keep the wall of the organ from touching a scalpel, laser or scissors can be inserted into the hysteroscopy to perform the surgery. This procedure is usually formed on an outpatient basis.

Mammogram

This procedure that takes about fifteen minutes is an x-ray of the breasts. With the breasts exposed one stands before a machine with a camera positioned above the breasts. A technologist positions the breasts on the lower of two compression plates and slowly brings the top plate down to flatten your breast. Side and front views of the breast are made and then repeat the procedure of the other side. Another view may be required particularly if the woman has had implants.

Pap Smear

This test makes it possible for the doctor to recognize and treat abnormal cells in the cervix before they become malignant. A speculum is inserted in the vagina to bring the cervix into view. A spatula is brushed along the outer surface of the cervix. A small brush is put into the cervical opening and moved around to collect cells from inside the cervical canal. The cells are placed on a glass slide, which is sent to a lab for analysis. This procedure is painless.

Breast, Pelvic and Vaginal Ultrasound

The use of ultrasound is painless and used to see the internal reproduction organs and breast. A cool gel is spread on the skin and then a transducer moves over the area that's being inspected. The vaginal ultrasound uses a wand-shaped transducer (about the diameter of a tampon) which is inserted into the vagina to get a close look at the uterus and ovaries.

Testing for Fungi

Vaginal infection with yeast or with Trichomonas (parasitic) can be recognized by examining vagina secretions under a microscope.

Lung Cancer

Lung cancer is the leading cause of death due to cancer in both men and women in the United States. Eighty-five percent of lung cancer is caused by cigarette smoke. The risk of cancer increases with more smoking. Cigar and pipe smokers and not as much risk as cigarette smokers but greater by far than non-smokers. Other risks beyond smoking is asbestos, radon, uranium, also chronic infections such as Tuberculosis increase likelihood of cancer. Once diagnosis of cancer is determined 85% die within five years. Most lung cancer is not discovered until it has spread. Lung cancer is preventable by first stopping smoking, live in a smoke-free environment, check for radon in your home and if you work where industrial dust and fumes exist follow all the safety rules and wear protective clothing.

The types of lung cancer are:

(1) Squamous Cell Carcinoma—This type of lung cancer comprises 30-35% of all lung cancers. It originates on the surface of the lining of the larger airways (bronchioles) and is usually found in the center part of the lungs. They are slow growing but metastasize quickly to lymph glands near the lungs and other organs.

(2) Adenocarcinoma—Represents 35-40% of being cancer patients. Often originates in the smaller airways and is found in the periphery of the lungs. It sometimes spreads too the lymph glands where it started and then spreads to other organs.

(3) Large Cell Carcinoma—Causes 10-20% of all lung cancers. These cancers often spread inside the lungs before going to other parts of the body.

(4) Small Cell Carcinoma—Sometimes known as oak cell carcinoma represents 20 to 30%. It is usually found in large airways and most of the time spreads to other organs. It is likely than any other cancer of the lungs to spread to other organs and the effected cells are more apt to respond to chemotherapy though unfortunately it is temporary.

Emphysema and (COPD) Chronic Bronchitis Chronic Obstructive Pulmonary Disease

Another common disease afflicting the middle age population is emphysema. Its victim is most commonly men over 40. Women and young people may also suffer from this respiratory ailment sometimes as an after effect of infections. Unfortunately, since women are increasingly taking up smoking, and smoking has been identified as the major cause of obstructive pulmonary disease they are highly vulnerable. Physicians estimate that there are 5 million Americans with emphysema or bronchitis. Bronchitis is hard to distinguish from emphysema but is marked by excessive mucus in the lungs and air passages. Emphysema progressively cuts off the exchange of oxygen for carbon dioxide by killing air cells little by little, making the chest muscles work harder to try to make up the deficiency. Without oxygen the muscles do not function properly. Thus the disease has a cyclical effect. The symptoms are shortness of breath, a difficulty in breathing or a winded feeling. Chronic bronchitis has the same symptoms.

Our breathing apparatus is constructed in the form of a bush with branches, positioned upside down in the chest. The main tube, the "windpipe" or trachea, is the trunk of the bush; it leads air from the nose and mouth down into the chest. There the trunk divides into two chief branches, the bronchi (a single one is a bronchus). These go right and left into the two tissue sacs that are the lungs. Within the lungs each bronchus branches out as smaller and ever more numerous bronchi. The smaller of these are bronchioles.

Each bronchiole ends in a tiny structure that looks much like a cauliflower, made up of very small air sacs, or alveoli. There are estimated to be 750,000,000 of them. The alveoli are the destination of the indrawn air, and it is in them that the work of the lungs is done. Small blood vessels near the surface take the oxygen into the blood cells by osmosis. If inhaling of air and exhaling through the bronchi is not coordinated so air gets smoothly in and out, air is strapped in the bronchiole eventually breaking down the alveolar walls. What follows is the increasing inability to get oxygen in the body.

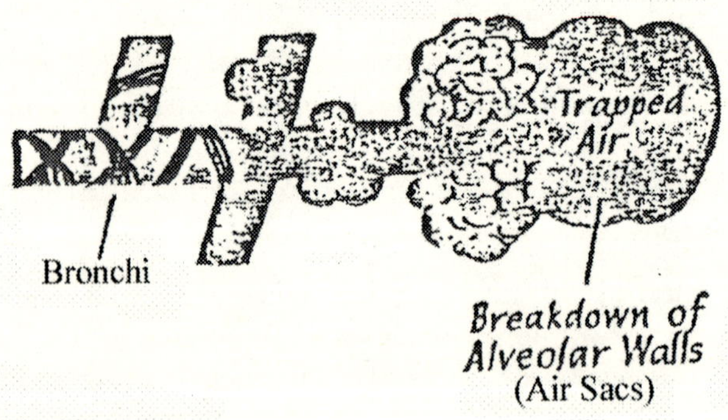

The exact causes of emphysema are not known. It is thought that it may result from the accumulated effect of all the lung ailments we have managed to live through as well as the polluted air we have breathed. Cigarette smoking is the most important cause. An inborn tendency making one more susceptible for damage if discovered may help to determine those who are most likely to contract the disease. Environmental pollutants, like excessive acids and corrosive materials in smoke, asbestos fibers from the brake lining of cars, excessive dust and particles in the atmosphere are suspect when we are constantly breathing this type of air. My mother died of this disease after a fifteen-year bout. She never smoked but did live in an industrial town where the air was polluted. At times she was also under considerable stress.

Suggestions for prevention are: prompt attention to infections of the eye, ear, nose, throat and chest, no smoking and try to escape air pollution. Early detection is most important since doctors are unable to reverse the damage already caused.

Best Medical Care

The rule based on evidence from the American Journal of Medicine, Journal of Urology and Northwestern Medical School states that those hospitals that do procedures in greater numbers such as coronary bypass, angioplasty, carotid (endutectomy), pediatric heart surgery, prostate surgery, abdominal aortic aneurysm repair, mastectomy, major liver surgery and pancreatic cancer surgery provide less risk of death.

Beyond this to get the best care one has to be aggressive. Insurance companies cover but they sometimes "cut deals" to cut costs (discount/with certain hospitals when they agree to send the patient to specific hospitals). You may have to fight by enlisting the aid of medical staff in the hospital where you want to be treated is important, also your local doctor can look into top hospitals who have physician to physician referral lines or your physician might help you find a specialist at Mayo Clinic, Johns Hopkins, or UCLA Medical Center, Los Angeles. You can get information on choosing the right care—quality care through the Web page www.healthfinder.org or call 1-800-624-8773. The latter provides information on how to get managed care to work on your behalf.

The U.S. News & World Report often provides a list of hospitals that gives the best expertise in a number of specialties based upon reputation, mortality ratio, COTH (Council of Teaching Hospitals), technology services, discharges and RNs to beds. In most instances they list 50 medical hospitals or centers. Cancer list includes these as the top 5.

<u>Cancer (Top 5)</u>
1. University of Texas, M. D. Anderson Center, Houston
2. Memorial Sloan-Kettering Cancer Center, New York
3. Johns Hopkins Hospital, Baltimore
4. Mayo Clinic, Rochester, Minnesota
5. Duke University Medical Center, Durham, NC

<u>Heart (Top 5)</u>
1. Cleveland Clinic, Cleveland, Ohio
2. Mayo Clinic, Rochester, Minnesota
3. Massachusetts General Hospital, Boston
4. Johns Hopkins Hospital, Baltimore
5. Duke University Medical Center, Durham

<u>Hormonal Disorder (Top 5)</u>
1. Mayo Clinic, Rochester, Minnesota
2. Massachusetts General Hospital, Boston
3. Johns Hopkins Hospital, Baltimore
4. Brigham & Women's Hospital, Boston
5. University of California, San Francisco Medical Center

<u>Respiratory Disorder (Top 5)</u>
1. National Jewish Center, Denver
2. Mayo Clinic, Rochester, Minnesota
3. Johns Hopkins Hospital, Baltimore
4. Barnes-Jewish Hospital, St. Louis
5. University Hospital, Denver

<u>Eye, Nose and Throat (Top 5)</u>
1. Johns Hopkins Hospital, Baltimore
2. University of Iowa Hospital & Clinics, Iowa City
3. Massachusetts Eye and Ear Infirmary, Boston
4. University of Pittsburgh Medical Center
5. Mayo Clinic, Rochester, Minnesota

<u>Rheumatology (Top 5)</u>
1. Mayo Clinic, Rochester, Minnesota
2. Johns Hopkins Hospital, Baltimore
3. Hospital for Special Surgery, New York
4. Brigham & Women's Hospital, Boston
5. University of Alabama, Birmingham

<u>Neurology & Neurosurgery (Top 5)</u>
1. Mayo Clinic, Rochester, Minnesota
2. Massachusetts General Hospital, Boston
3. Johns Hopkins, Baltimore
4. New York Presbyterian Hospital
5. University of California San Francisco Medical Center

<u>Kidney Disease (Top 5)</u>
1. Brigham & Women's Hospital, Boston
2. Massachusetts General Hospital, Boston
3. Cleveland Clinic
4. University Hospital, Denver
5. Mayo Clinic, Rochester, Minnesota

It continues with Urology (Johns Hopkins), Eyes (Johns Hopkins), Psychiatry (Massachusetts General Hospital, Boston), Rehabilitation (Rehabilitation Institute of Chicago), Digestive Disorders (Mayo Clinic, Rochester, Minnesota), Geriatrics (UCLA Medical Center, Los Angeles).

There are many fine hospitals besides these probably hundreds. Many of these centers offer trials or protocols for the purpose of research and study of disease. This is usually handled on an outpatient basis although some bring you into the hospital, clinic or center for a week or so each year for complete check-ups, etc. There are usually no costs associated with these arrangements. Your physician can locate one of the places for you. Typically documentation is required which the physician can assist you, also inservices, may be over the phone. These trials frequently provide funds for travel, food, lodging for a night or two awaiting admission and provide medicine incident to your malady. Kinds of trials are varied but include diabetes, neurological illnesses, cancer, AIDS, and other problems. For example, Bristol-Myers Squibb sponsors clinical study if you are a Type II diabetic (uncontrolled through a medicine), call 1-877-897-2025. The National Institute of Health, Bethesda, MD, U.S. government controlled, offers this number to find out about trials through the patient recruitment line and Public Liaison Office, 1-800-411-1222, http//www.cc.nih.gov.

Angioplasties

Is a procedure used with heart attack victims a snake, thin tubes tipped by plastic balloons into the blocked arteries and then inflate them restoring blood flow. Over a million persons in the U.S. suffer heart attack could be aided by use of angioplasties procedure. Most heart attacks are treated by drugs primarily.

Most heart attacks are treated only with clot-busting drugs, which can be given anywhere. Most hospitals cannot do quick artery-clearing angioplasties, and doctors are reluctant to postpone treatment while patients are moved to hospitals that can. A Danish study published in Summer 2003 New England Journal of Medicine concludes that a transfer to an angioplasty center cuts the risk of death and major complications by about 40 percent. Comparing 1,129 patients with major heart attacks, 14 percent either died or suffered another heart attack or disabling stroke when treated with drugs alone during the month-long study. Only 8 percent died when transferred to another hospital for angioplasty. Nearly all were transferred within two hours.

The question of transfers potentially affects hundreds of thousands of patients. In the United States, heart attacks kill about 460,000 yearly, according to the National Institutes of Health.

The attacks occur when clogged and clotted arteries crimp the stream of blood to heart muscle. Several factors have limited angioplasties, though. They require sophisticated surgical backup in case something goes wrong. Clot dissolving drugs like TPA can be given by emergency room doctors. Several studies have suggested that the benefits of angioplasties might outweigh delays for hospital transfer. The Danish study helps settle the question, some doctors said. In the nationalized Danish health system the researchers took special precautions that ordinary hospitals might not take. Potential transfers were whisked past emergency rooms straight to a cardiac care team.

Overweight

Overweight and obesity while not defined as a disease is a major cause of physical problems in middle age. Estimates indicate about 50 million persons in this country are 10% or more overweight. Another 5 million are at least 20% overweight. The main cause is over-eating and under-exercising with metabolic disorders accounting for only one or two out of every 100 overweight persons.

The causes for over-eating are varied ranging from (1) family habits, (2) economic and cultural factors, (3) pregnancy, to (4) psychological factors including tension, anxiety, depression and frustration. Studies have shown 9 out of 10 persons over-eat when they are nervous, worried, or idle. The side effects of overweight range from heart disease and hypertension to hardening of the arteries; from diabetes to osteoarthritis (breakdown of the lower spine, hips and knees).

If a middle-aged person is 10 pounds overweight the danger of death is increased by 8%; a 20 pounds it rises 18%; at 30 pounds to 28%, and at 50 pounds 56%. Hypertension, circulation problems and diabetes are all possibilities for those exceeding 20 pounds. Prevention is the best approach to obesity. Treatment, of course, is to follow medical advice to reducing safely. For those slightly over the norm a routine of daily vigorous exercise should be initiated (running, tennis, swimming, weight lifting, brisk walking exercise routines, body bends, etc.). Sharply curtailing fats, starches and sugars in our food selection is indicated. It is not recommended that you diet by using patent medicines, pills or any other kind of drug on your own. Smoking is a dangerous and unreliable substitute for long-term weight reduction. A general estimate of your weight class follows; how does your weight fit? A discussion of food and the balanced diet is death with under preventive medicine.

*DESIRABLE BODY WEIGHTS: MEN** Ages 30–60

Height		Small	Medium	Large
Feet	*Inches*	Frame	Frame	Frame
5	2	128-134	131-141	138-150
5	3	130-136	133-1143	140-153
5	4	132-138	135-145	142-156
5	5	134-140	137-148	144-160
5	6	136-142	139-151	146-164
5	7	138-145	142-154	149-168
5	8	140-148	145-157	152-172
5	9	142-151	148-160	155-176
5	10	144-154	151-163	158-180
5	11	146-157	154-166	161-184
6	0	149-160	157-170	164-188
6	1	152-164	160-174	168-192
6	2	155-168	164-178	172-197
6	3	158-172	167-182	176-202
6	4	162-176	171-187	181-207

*Weights at ages 30-60 based on lowest mortality. Weight in pounds according to frame (in indoor clothing weighing 5 lbs. for men; shoes with 1" heels).

*DESIRABLE BODY WEIGHTS: WOMEN** AGES 30–60

Height		Small Frame	Medium Frame	Large Frame
Feet	*Inches*			
4	10	102-111	109-121	118-131
4	11	103-113	111-123	120-134
5	0	104-115	113-126	122-137
5	1	106-118	115-129	125-140
5	2	108-121	118-132	128-143
5	3	111-124	121-135	131-147
5	4	114-127	124-138	134-151
5	5	117-130	127-141	137-155
5	6	120-133	130-144	140-159
5	7	123-136	133-147	143-163
5	8	126-136	136-150	146-167
5	9	129-142	139-153	149-170
5	10	132-145	142-156	152-173
5	11	135-148	145-159	155-176
6	0	138-151	148-162	158-179

*Weights at ages 30-60 based on lowest mortality. Weight in pounds according to frame (in indoor clothing weighing 3 lbs. for women; shoes with 1" heels).

These tables are derived from the Metropolitan Life Insurance Company studies and represent the range of weights for heights, which parallel the lowest mortality rates.

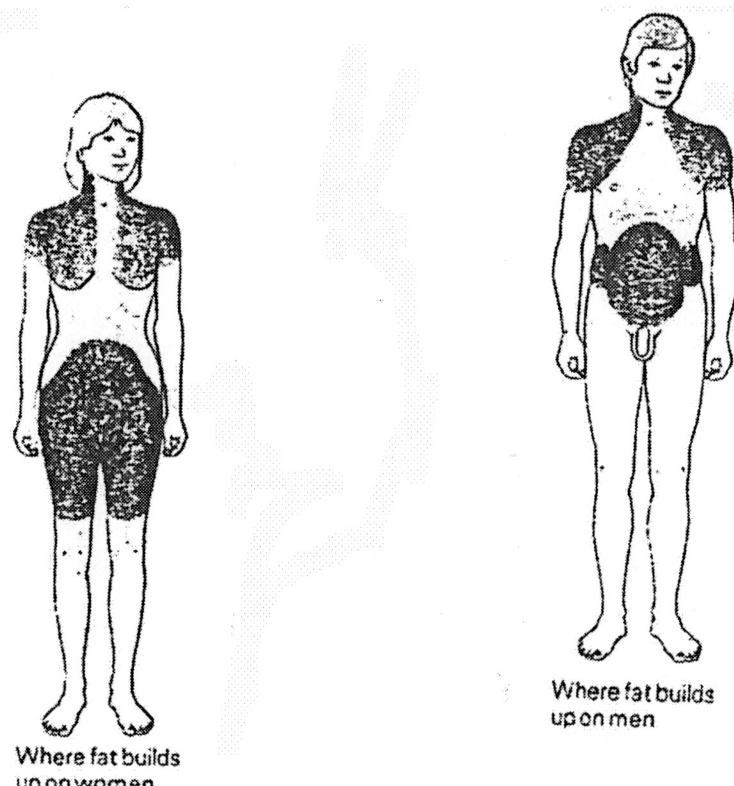

Another slightly different view of weight is the use of the Body Mass Index (BMI). Using the following scale of weight and height check where they intersect on a 90° angle (down and across). That gives you a general estimate of your BMI. This index is based upon mortality hence should be considered trustworthy.

Your Body Mass Index (BMI)
To estimate body mass index (BMI), identify your weight (to the nearest 10 pounds) in columns across the top. Then go down the column until you come to the row that represents your height. Inside the square where your weight and height intersect is a number that estimates your BMI. If you weight 170 pounds and are 5'8" your BMI is 26. You are overweight slightly, of course, muscle weighs more than fat and you may be healthy with this BMI.

BMI INTERPRETATION

Underweight	Under 18.5
Normal	18.5-24
Overweight	25-29
Obese	30 and over

	WEIGHT															
HEIGHT	100	110	120	130	140	150	160	170	180	190	200	210	220	230	240	250
5'0"	20	21	23	25	27	29	31	33	35	37	39	41	43	45	47	49
5'1"	19	21	23	25	26	28	30	32	34	36	38	40	42	43	45	47
5'2"	18	20	22	24	26	27	29	31	33	35	37	38	40	42	44	46
5'3"	18	19	21	23	25	27	28	30	32	34	35	37	39	41	43	44
5'4"	17	19	21	22	24	26	27	29	31	33	34	36	38	39	41	43
5'5"	17	18	20	22	23	25	27	28	30	32	33	35	37	38	40	42
5'6"	16	18	19	21	23	24	26	27	29	31	32	34	36	37	39	40
5'7"	16	17	19	20	22	23	25	27	28	30	31	33	34	36	38	39
5'8"	15	17	18	20	21	23	24	26	27	29	30	32	33	35	36	38
5'9"	15	16	18	19	21	22	24	25	27	28	30	31	32	34	35	37
5'10"	14	16	17	19	20	22	23	24	26	27	29	30	32	33	34	36
5'11"	14	15	17	18	20	21	22	24	25	26	28	29	31	32	33	35
6'0"	14	15	16	18	19	20	22	23	24	26	27	28	30	31	33	34
6'1"	13	15	16	17	18	20	21	22	24	25	26	28	29	30	32	33
6'2"	13	14	15	17	18	19	21	22	23	24	26	27	28	30	31	32
6'3"	12	14	15	16	17	19	20	21	22	24	25	26	27	29	30	31
6'4"	12	13	15	16	17	18	19	21	22	23	24	26	27	28	29	30

Problems associated with being overweight are legion such as, those overweight by 40% are twice as likely to die prematurely as those of normal weight; raises the rate of getting Type II diabetes and heart problems—high blood pressure, stroke and certain kinds of cancer. In men overweight prostate cancer is a threat, in women breast and uterine cancer. Both women and men are likely to develop colon and rectal cancer, also gallbladder diseases and gallstones, osteoarthritis and gout. In addition there are also psychological and emotional maladies in a culture that equates slimness with attractiveness. Those obese persons may run up against bias and job discrimination. Treatment for overweight usually involves diet, exercise, behavior modification, perhaps medicine, and in a few cases surgery. The overweight and obese must eat fewer calories than they burn: exercise can reduce weight also provides the strengthening of the heart:

(1) Better cholesterol level LDL (harmful type) can be reduced while the HDL is increased.

(2) Stronger lungs help to use oxygen more effectively and ups the breathing capacity.

(3) Makes for strengthened bones and muscles particularly for women at menopause and afterwards when lowering levels of estrogen can contribute to osteoporosis.

(4) Lower blood pressure thereby reduces risks for stroke and heart disease.

(5) Provides protection against cancer B reduces time passage of waste through the colon and may help against breast cancer and endometrial (abdomen) cancer.

(6) Protection against diabetes—and reduces the long term risks and associated problems of neuropathy, eye and kidney failure.

(7) Reduces appetite—true some exercise increases the desire for food but sustained regular exercise at a sustained clip takes away appetite in the long run—it also reduces sugar (glucose) levels and weight and makes for better circulation.

The material that follows paraphrases an article by Dr. Jim Carraway, M.D. of the Eastern Virginia Medical School in Norfolk, Virginia on Living Long and Well.

BMI's of 49 (100 lbs. overweight) or over if Type II diabetic are candidates of Bariatric Surgery. The removal of fat may not reduce blood sugar level. After this surgery you would be eating less of everything so for improved control one would have to work closely with a physician on nuroeducation. It becomes obvious that we can be in control of our life, our health, and our longevity. The question is how can we live long and well? The answer is by learning everything we can about what makes us better. This process of self-education is not an easy one. However, a continual, systematic approach with a high awareness level of new information is the best way to gain the proper knowledge about health and longevity. How do you get the information to follow this pathway?

In the Harvard Women's Study of 16,000 nurses over 20 years, four major factors which helped determine wellness and longevity included maintaining a good body weight, not smoking, exercising, and take a multivitamin if 40 or older. It seems clear from the many studies which have been done that a multivitamin with additional vitamin C, vitamin E, and omega-3's (fish oil or flaxseed oil) is essential. These can improve health and can reduce the risk of cardiovascular disease, neurological problems, and even cancer. For our plastic surgery patients, we recommend the following minimum supplements:

- multivitamin with minerals
- 1000 mg vitamin C
- 400 units vitamin E
- Ca/Mg/Zn tablet B 1000g/550 mg/50 mg (for ages 45 years and older)
- Fish oil capsule 2-4/day

Exercise is another major area of importance in our lives. Because many of us are sedentary, we need to increase our activity level by exercise. According to Patrick Quillen, author of *Beating Cancer With Nutrition*, thirty minutes of exercise every other day cuts the risk of breast cancer by 75%. Exercise also helps maintain the proper acid-alkaline balance in your body, which enhances the enzymatic reactions, brain function, and cardiovascular function. It is ideal to burn about 2,000 calories by aerobic exercise weekly. According to Dr. Vince Giampapa in *Principles and Practice of Anti-Aging Medicine*, burn more than 2,000 calories per week and it causes excess free-radical and cortisol production, both of which accelerate aging rather than slowing it.

Supplements are an important consideration, and you should constantly expand your knowledge of traditional supplements, which have been around for a long time, as well as some of the newer supplements. As you consider adding supplements to your diet, think of them as a kind of life insurance.

Reducing "white" carbohydrates (bread-potatoes-pastry) in our diet is another key factor in improving our health. One of the reasons that good diets such as The Zone Diet emphasize elimination of white carbohydrates is because they have little nutritional value and provide empty calories. If you eat fruits, vegetables, nuts, grains, beans, meat, seafood, eggs, olives, and other nutrient dense foods, you will, for the most part, get a complete spectrum and amounts of vitamins and minerals.

<u>A Healthy Diet</u>

(1) Eat a variety of foods to get energy, vitamins, protein, minerals and fiber.

(2) Keep a healthy weight. *Look at the charts presented in this section.*

(3) Use a diet of low saturated, trans-unsaturated fats, and cholesterol.

(4) Choose a diet with plenty of vegetables and fruits that provide complex carbohydrates, minerals, vitamins, and fiber.

(5) Use a small amount of sugar.

(6) Use salt (sodium) sparingly.

(7) Drink alcoholic drinks limited to 1 or 2 drinks that amount has a salutary effect on atherosclerosis (hardening of the arteries). No alcohol if pregnant.

(8) Eat no more than 4 ounces of lean meat—poultry with the skin off (one or no more than twice a week). Including fish several times a week is a good antioxidant.

(9) Check your glucose every day with a meter that gives a cumulation mean (average) of daily takings over several months. This will be fairly similar to the AIC tests taken by our physician.

One should eat at least as much vegetables and fruits as the grain, bread, pasta basically carbohydrates, carrots, beets, corn, potatoes have considerable amounts of carbohydrates in them for those turn quickly into sugar. The 50% to 60% of a daily diet (recommended by some diets) is too much carbohydrates (sugar to add to your diet). Wheat bread is better than white. Eat no sugared cereals but choose from 100% wheat from those with low sugar (seen on the nutrition facts found on the boxes and packages) and saturated fats. One should also take if 40 to 45 years or older, multivitamins, many studies show the importance of the following multivitamin should have additional Vitamin C.

The U.S. Department of Agriculture's pyramid, which had not been updated since 1992 (Diabetes Management, 2003) until now, provides a new one discussed here. (1) The old guide had several problems it treated all fats as equally bad, though science now distinguishes between healthful fats 1 P monounsaturated, Omega-3 fatty acids and damaging fats such as <u>Trans</u> fats and saturated fats. (2) The old pyramid showed all dairy products as equally beneficial and did not recommend the necessity to choose low fats or non-fat products. (3) The old guide strongly emphasized breads and cereals which provides many carbohydrates but fewer nutrients. Whole grain is now recommended whenever possible but the printed boxes of cereal or bread wrapper fats to suggest whole grain. (4) Critics said of the guide that the USDA was overly influenced by the meat, wheat and dairy industries.

A new guide calls the Healthy Eating Pyramid developed by nutrition experts Drs. Willett and Stampfer and promoted by the School of Public Health at Harvard suggests the alterations—whole-grain foods are at the base of the guide but white bread, white rice, pasts and potatoes are at they tip of the pyramid and use sparingly like sugar, red meat is also relegated to the tip category for limited use. The generic protein group of nuts and legumes (peas and beans) by eating 1-3 times a day and fish, poultry or eggs be eaten 0-2 times a day. Vegetables and fruits are to be eaten in abundance 2-3 times a day de-emphasizing dairy products. Dairy products are calcium supplements only 1-2 times a day. They also suggest a daily multivitamin for meat and alcohol in moderation (1-3 a day) unless not indicated. The American Diabetes Association suggesting 50-60% of one's daily food should come from carbohydrates seems off the mark for remember many vegetables, a different category as function basically as simple sugar in the white calories (grain group) like potatoes, corn, also beets and carrots are loaded with carbohydrates. The author suggests we up the use of vegetables and fruits and eat fish once or twice a week limited the diet to good fats and oils.

Control of sugar (glucose levels) is essential for handling diabetes and for closing on future troubles. Taking one's own sugar with the use of a lancet is easier once it seems. Now on new machines as much blood is needed even the forearm can be used by a Free Style machine (also keeps record for several months) and others. This must be done daily, may be several time to keep track of the sugar to have adjust to food amounts, exercise and dosage. An endocrinologist (MD) is the best source of regulation. Your insulin or tablets although most doctors in general practice can help plan a regime for you. Below is the target for glucose levels that are appropriate (this is known as the A_{1C} test. Levels above 7 means your diabetes is out of control. Taking your glucose level means that you will be confronted with coming to grips with diet, exercise and style of living. It should be remembered that with calcium and Vitamin D weight loss is promoted by increasing the intake of these. Vitamin D also helps with muscle strength, fall prevention and osteoporosis.

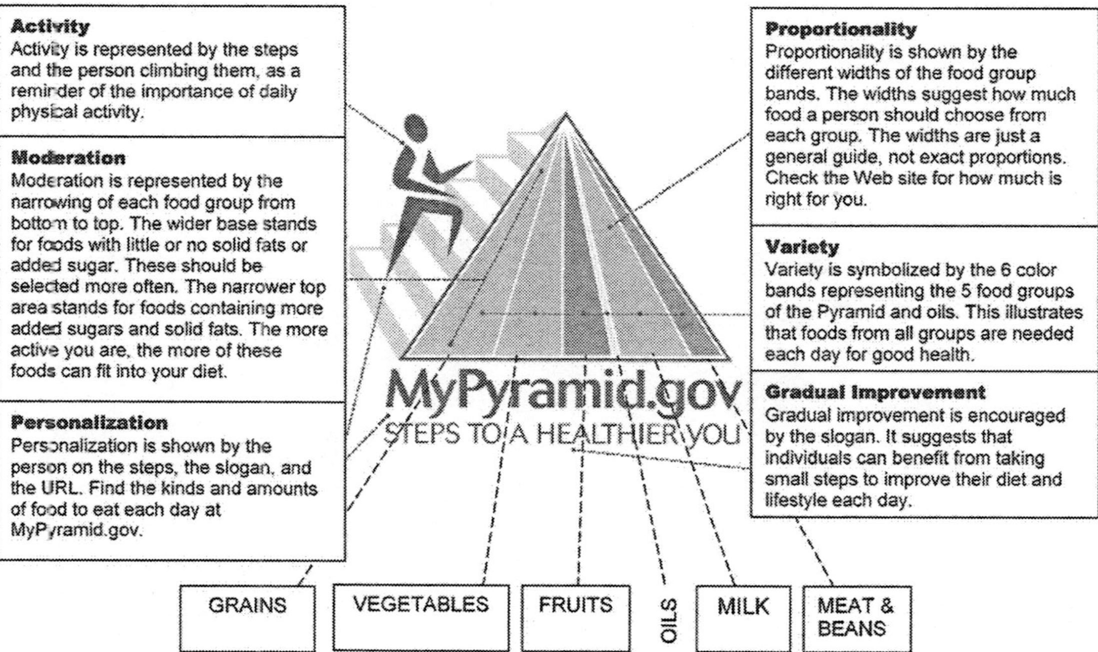
Anatomy of MyPyramid
Activity
Activity is represented by the steps and the person climbing them, as a reminder of the importance of daily physical activity.
Moderation
Moderation is represented by the narrowing of each food group from bottom to top. The wider base stands for foods with little or no solid fats or added sugar. These should be selected more often. The narrower top area stands for foods containing more added sugars and solid fats. The more active you are, the more of these foods can fit into your diet.
Personalization
Personalization is shown by the person on the steps, the slogan, and the URL. Find the kinds and amounts of food to eat each day at MyPyramid.gov.
Proportionality
Proportionality is shown by the different widths of the food group bands. The widths suggest how much food a person should choose from each group. The widths are just a general guide, not exact proportions. Check the Web site for how much is right for you.
Variety
Variety is symbolized by the 6 color bands representing the 5 food groups of the Pyramid and oils. This illustrates that foods from all groups are needed each day for good health.
Gradual Improvement
Gradual improvement is encouraged by the slogan. It suggests that individuals can benefit from taking small steps to improve their diet and lifestyle each day.
MyPyramid.gov
STEPS TO A HEALTHIER YOU
GRAINS
VEGETABLES
FRUITS
OILS
MILK
MEAT & BEANS

An A_{1C} test reveals how much sugar (glucose) is attached to the hemoglobin in your red blood cells. The longer the glucose level remains high, the more glucose attaches to the hemoglobin and other substances. This high blood glucose raises the risk of complications (cataracts, hardening of the arteries, heart problems, stroke and kidney diseases).

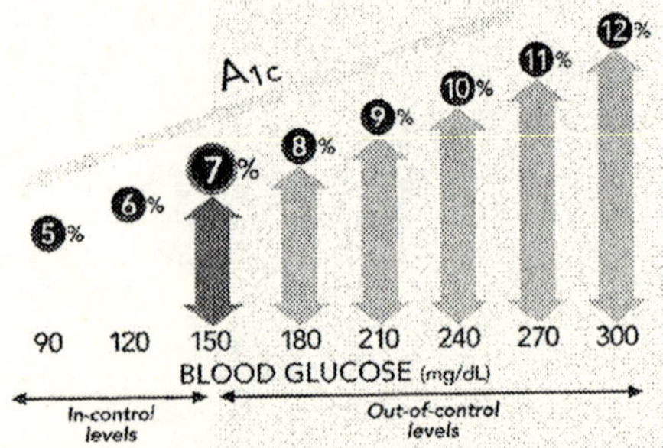

A fasting blood glucose test shows how you're doing during that period of the day. An A_{1C} test shows where your blood sugar level has been over the past two months.

Food Choices and Helping Sizes

FOOD GROUP	ONE SERVICE SIZE
Grain	1 slice bread; 2 cup cooked cereal, rice or pasta; 1 ounce ready-to-eat cereal
Vegetable	1 cup raw, leafy vegetables; 2 cup other vegetables (cooked or raw); 3/4 cup vegetable juice
Fruit	1 medium apple, banana, or orange; 2 cup chopped, cooked, or canned fruit; 3/4 cup fruit juice
Meat	2-3 ounces cooked lean meat, poultry, or fish (1 egg or 2 tablespoons peanut butter counts as 1 ounce of meat); 2 cup cooked dry beans
Dairy	1 cup milk or yogurt; 12 ounces cheese; 2 ounces processed cheese

Eating according to the 2005 USDA Food Guide MyPyramid may take some adjustment. Think of grains, fruits, and vegetables as a primary portion of your diet and be cautious of hidden fats in meat and dairy products. The servings listed are smaller therefore better than the average American helping and will help maintain the best weight and food balance. Eating less is better.

Types of Fat

Different kinds of dietary fats are shown below. Some are better for your health than others. Fats you eat should be in the main food categories.

DIETARY FAT	USED FOR	INGREDIENTS	
Polyunsaturated fat	Needed by the body to help form the membranes covering every cell	Natural vegetable oils; soft (tub) margarine	**GENERALLY GOOD FOR YOU**
Monounsaturated fat	Needed by the body to help form the membranes covering every cell	Natural vegetable oils; soft (tub margarine	
Omega-3	Protective against coronary heart disease.	Fish and marine foods	
Saturated fat	Raises blood cholesterol and increased heart disease if eaten in large quantities	Animal fats (fatty meats, butter, whole milk, chicken skin)	
Cholesterol	Plax accumulates on carotid arteries cause strokes if excessive	Animal fats	
Transunsaturated fat	A type of unsaturated fat that has recently been found to be probably harmful	Animal fats; stick (hard) margarine	**WORKS AGAINST YOU**

Fats and Oils Comparison

Oils contain different amounts of the types of fats. Oils and fats that are high in monounsaturated fat (such as olive and canola oils) or polyunsaturated fat (such as safflower oil). Use saturated fats (such as butter) only in moderation. These fats have a positive effect on you. The fats and oils good for you are at the top of those listed toward the bottom are contraindicated.

OIL OR FAT	% SATURATED FAT	% MONO-UNSATURATED FAT	% POLY-UNSATURATED FAT
Olive oil	14	70	11
Canola oil	6	62	31
Sunflower oil	13	32	50
Peanut oil	20	45	35
Soybean oil	15	43	38
Safflower oil	10	20	66
Corn oil	13	24	59
Soft (tub)margarine	14	32	31
Chicken fat	30	45	21
Lard	39	45	21
Butter	62	29	4
Coconut oil	87	6	2

Vitamins and Minerals

One should eat a variety of foods, i.e., whole grains, vegetables (green and yellow), fruits, (2 to 3 ounces per meal) of lean meats, skinless poultry, or fish.

VITAMIN OR MINERAL	FOOD	RESULTS FROM EATING THESE FOODS
Fat dissolvable vitamins		
Vitamin A	Milk with Vitamin A and eggs; cheeses; liver; fish oil (lower fat)	Helps eyes stay healthy; essential for development, growth of cells in organs, skin, and hair; works as an antioxidant (protecting cells)
Vitamin D	Milk with Vitamin D	Assists in absorption of calcium; and forms bones and teeth; also nervous system and muscles
Vitamin E	Nuts; seeds; wheat germ; leafy green vegetables and vegetable oil	Serves as an antioxidant (protects cells); contributes to the formation of blood cells
Vitamin K	Spinach; greens; collards; broccoli; milk; eggs; cereals	Essential for making proteins that brings about blood clotting

Water-dissolvable vitamins		
Vitamin B_1 (thiamin)	Pork; legumes; seeds; nuts; grains; cereals	Converts food into energy; essential for the function of muscles and nervous system.
Vitamin B_2 (riboflavin)	Milk; yogurt; meats; leafy green vegetables; whole-grain breads and cereals	Helps convert food into energy; aids in the formation of red blood cells; essential for the body's use of some hormones
Vitamin B_3 (niacin)	Meats; fish; legumes; nuts; whole-grain and enriched breads and cereals	Helps convert food into energy; aids in the formation of red blood cells; essential for the body's use of some hormones
Vitamin B_6 (pyridoxine)	Chicken; fish; eggs; brown rice; whole-wheat products	Needed for formation of red blood cells; helps the body make proteins; assists in fighting infection; may reduce risk of atherosclerosis
Vitamin B_{12}	Meats; fish; poultry; eggs; milk	Makes red blood cells; support nervous system; may reduce risk of atherosclerosis
Vitamin C	Citrus fruits; vegetables; fortified cereals	Acts as an antioxidant (protects cells from damage); necessary for healthy skin; regulates metabolism during stress or illness
Folic acid (folate)	Fortified cereals; dark green vegetables; fruits; beans; yeast breads; wheat germ	Makes new body cells; before pregnancy and in first 3 months of pregnancy aids in preventing birth defects; helps red blood cell formation
Minerals		
Calcium	Milk and dairy products; green leafy vegetables; tofu; sardines and salmon with bones; calcium-fortified orange juice	Necessary for formation and maintenance of bones and teeth; contraction of muscles (including the heart muscle); aids normal nerve function; aids blood clotting; may reduce risk of colon cancer
Chromium	Brewer's yeast; calf's liver; American cheese; wheat germ	Makes fat into energy
Copper	Shellfish; nuts; seeds; legumes; liver; whole grains	Needed in the formation of skin and connective tissue; also for many chemical reactions related to energy; essential for heart function
Iron, Calcium Phosphorus, Potassium	Food sources: milk, liver, dried prunes, raisins, apricots, whole grain, ripe fruit, nuts, leafy greens	Iron important in hemoglobin making. Calcium needed for building bones. Phosphorus metabolizes fats and carbohydrates to generate energy. Potassium and sodium—needed for healthy nerves and muscles
Selenium	Seafood; kidney; liver; cereals; and grains	Serves as an antioxidant protecting cells from damage; essential for healthy heart muscle
Sodium	Table salt; vegetables; many prepared foods	Holds fluids in body; helps nerve transmission, muscle contraction and helps control rhythm of the heart muscle
Zinc	Meats; poultry; oysters; eggs; beans; nuts; milk; yogurt; whole-grain cereals	Helps in sperm production; needed for growth and production of energy; helps immune function and blood clotting

Diabetes

The likelihood of becoming diabetic increases with age. Millions of Americans who have diabetes don't know it—although it is one of the most common diseases affecting an estimated 25 million people. Diabetes is fairly easy to detect and if found in early stages, can be controlled but that requires understanding the problem and willing to follow a regimen. With the growing universal problem with overweight (one of two in the adult population) it is crucial that we take note of it. The body handles sugar less well as one gets older.

Diabetes is a condition in which the body can no longer make use of sugar in a normal way. Glucose accumulates in the blood (high blood sugar) making the kidneys work overtime to expel this wasted sugar from the body. Long time inability to handle sugar leads to destruction of renal tissue (kidneys); it can lead to heart attacks and contributes to retinopathy, neuropathy, nephropathy bacterial infections and atherosclerosis. Symptoms include: excessive thirst, excessive urination, hunger, loss of weight, easy tiring, slow healing of cuts and bruises, changes in vision, intense itching, pain in fingers and toes and drowsiness.

Hyperglycemics (diabetics) typically are treated with diet (low carbohydrates, high mineral-vegetable food) calorie reducing diet programs (typically 1800-2500 calories per day depending upon the person). Accompanying this is the use of insulin particularly for those diabetes prone to ketosis (a poisonous substance where the body uses fat for a substitute for glucose to provide energy) and had its onset in youth (Type I diabetes). For the older diabetic who are ketoacidotic, weight reduction (also for Type II—adult onset) exercise, both very important, and insulin are used when patients cannot control their weight or diet. Insulin should be used for all Type I (Insulin Dependent Mellitus) persons, for those actively ill, the pregnant, those under stress from surgery infection or use of cortisone-like drugs and the symptomatically diabetic with fasting hyperglycemia of over 300 mg per dl. Medicine for increasing production of insulin by the pancreas are the Sulfonylureas Glipizide and Glimperide are about 65% effective with Type II diabetes. Biguanides reduces and releases glucose from the liver and improve the tissues sensitivity to insulin. Metformin should not be used by most people who drink heavily and have heart, kidney, liver and congestive heart failure. Sometimes an oral agent (Ortinase, Tolinase, Diabinese) or Glucotrol on the local market Formantin and Glipizide a drug on the foreign market are used typically for those over 50 (sometimes among younger adults when sugar levels are being controlled in conjunction with diet and/or exercise). Those otherwise healthy, free of all allergies to sulfonamide preparations (enhancing the insulin receptors or their affinity for insulin) and those who have an interest in using oral agents rather than insulin. This is allowable within acceptable risks. We would stress and reiterate the following concerning Diabetes. Type I Diabetes must be treated with insulin and typically both a fast acting, mealtime insulin and long acting basal insulin are used. Pills, in general, are ineffective. Type II Diabetes has more treatment options. Sometimes weight loss via diet and exercise cures or controls it. When medication is needed there are several choices. Sulfonylureas—Modern, commonly used agents include glipizide, glyburide Glimperide and the closely related agents repaglenide and nateglinide all these stimulate increased insulin production. Older agents in this group are Diabenase, Tolinase, Tolbutanide, Biguanides—only metfornum is available. It mainly reduces the liver's overproduction leads of glucose which often to high fasting blood sugar Thiazolide medicines Rosiglitazone and P10—gletazone enhance muscle and fat's sensitivity to insulin.

The incretins are a new class of agent which enhance insulin's action exenatide and others. Insulin is necessary for most Type II Diabetics after about 10 years since decline in insulin production inevitably occurs. Some will become Type I over time with complete dependence on insulin. The AMA Drug Evaluation continuing since the 2005 Edition has stated insulin is preferred over oral agents. They report "insulin may be safer with respect to mortality caused by cardiovascular disorders." Actually, stress related or unmasked diabetes mellitus, will as some drugs, such as corticosteroid, precipitate awareness and help the situation. For some, an increased incidence of yeast infection, for example vaginitis in women, heralds onset of diabetes. Also the repeated occurrence of rhino infections for no apparent reason. Stress, it should be noted, is not the basis of most middle age diabetic onset but is some times associated with it.

The use of sugar of various kinds (lactose, milk, fructose—fruit, galactose—milk component, sucrose—any sugar) relate in some way to hyperglycemia and hypoglycemia (hyper-over hypo-under). The former, too much sugar in the blood; the latter, too little. As a method of handling the high and low sugar problems, diet for weight reduction is a prime importance. Typically for the low sugar blood problems, a diet of high-protein and low carbohydrate is indicated with complex sugars some fruit (like dates or raisins) plus frequent feedings five to six times a day to maintain an adequate blood sugar level. Mealtime schedules must be strictly maintained for these people. For a suggestive diet plan, ask your physician or request literature on this form your public health agency.

Sugar's importance and relation to stress is a complicated one but, simply put, it affects the use and control of adrenaline, which serves the ability of the body to react and adjust to stress. Those who are the most likely candidates for diabetes include, people with diabetic relatives, people over forty, and overweight, and women over men. It is important to know that:

1. Diabetes is hereditary (that is a genetic predisposition; it increases with age; environment is important particularly stress and the social environment. People with a family history of diabetes need to be alert especially as they get older for elevated sugar levels.
2. Note this fact that due to obesity and sedentariness Type II now exceeds Type I in adolescents. This is scary!
3. Obesity is a tremendous risk factor non-Insulin Dependent Diabetes mellitus because the body loses its sensitivity to insulin with increased fat. Eighty percent of adult (middleagers) diabetics are obese or have a history of overweight.
4. The timing of meals for the insulin dependent diabetic is critical.
5. For Type I diabetes knowledge of Ketoacidosis is critical. The lack of insulin results in high sugar and acid levels. The symptoms are weakness, confused state, tired, fast breathing, immediate treatment is required with intravenous fluids and insulin.
6. Monitoring one's sugar blood level is crucial. Every diabetic should get a meter (i.e., Cone Touch) and check the sugar level once or several times a day. If a reading is high then adjust your eating pattern, exercise, life style and insulin or other medicines on the advice of your physician.
7. Oral agents are usually used only on a short-term basis, that is when someone is being started on a weight-reduction program until the time when diet and exercise can control the sugar level. For long-term control they are not efficient enough to control the disease.
8. Over weight persons who gain year to year by the middle years can expect some problems relative to sugar levels.

Treatment includes proper diet, insulin and exercise. There is a high tolerance in the body for glucose where exercise is taken regularly and vigorously. Care should not be sporadic and left to chance and it must be done in coordination with other remedies. With today's treatment methods, diabetes may be controlled and the diabetic may lead a normal life but it continues to be the fifth leading cause of death by disease. For uncontrolled diabetes, one can forecast eye problems leading to blindness and kidney problems leading to kidney failure and hardening of the arteries and other problems. Therefore it is important to recognize its symptoms early and seek medical treatment.

DIABETES-ITS ORIGIN

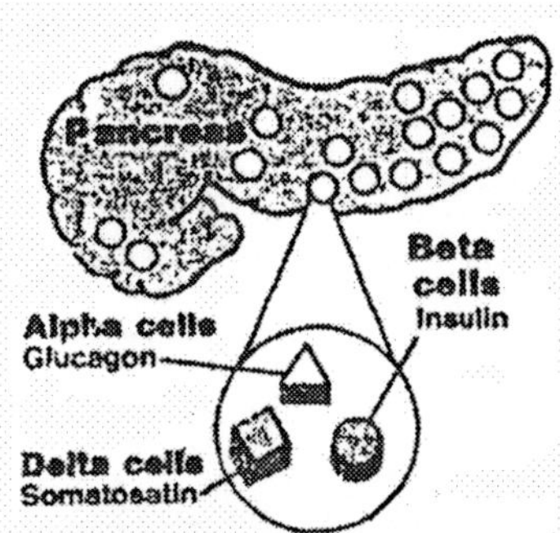

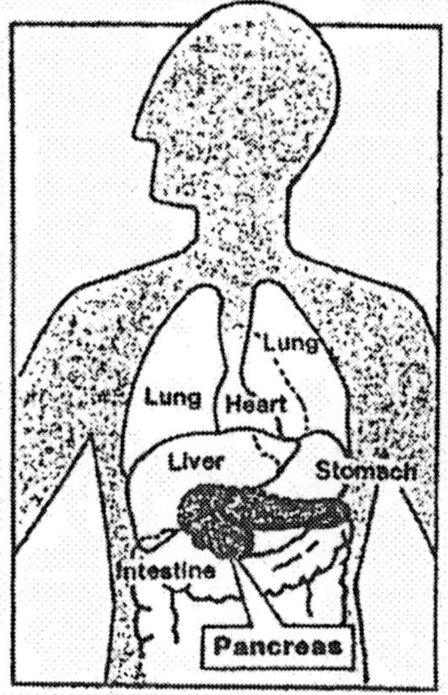

TYPE 1

Insulin-dependent diabetes begins in children or young adults. None of the insulin-producing cells functions properly. Daily insulin injections are necessary for the diabetic to stay alive.

TYPE 2

Non-insulin dependent diabetes has its onset in adults when some insulin-producing cells stop functioning. This type of diabetes can be controlled with diet and oral medication. About 90 percent of all diabetes are type 2.

TYPE A 2

Middle age diabetics who no longer produce insulin—requires daily insulin injections.

Appendices

APPENDIX 1

Common Vaginal Infections: Symptoms and Treatments

This chart lists the common vaginal infections, their causes and symptoms and tells how they are treated.

INFECTION	CAUSED BY	SYMPTOMS	TREATMENT OPTIONS
Vaginosis	Bacteria	Genital itching or burning; gray vaginal discharge with an unusual fishy odor that may be especially noticeable after intercourse	Antibiotics in tablet form taken by mouth or as a cream inserted into the vagina; sexual partner should be treated also
Candida	Yeast-like fungi	Intense burning and genital itching; clumped, white, cottage cheese-like discharge; possible pain during sexual intercourse	Prescription or over-the-counter antifungal cream or suppositories inserted into the vagina soothe the burning and itching for some women; antifungal tablet taken in one dose by mouth
Trichomonas	Protozoa, which are single-celled organisms that are sexually transmitted	Genital itching and burning; possible frothy, gray-green discharge with an unusual odor	Antibiotic in table form taken by mouth; sexual partner should be treated also

APPENDIX 2

COMBO TREATMENT REDUCES RECURRENCE OF EARLY DISEASE

The National Cancer Institute released the results of two large clinical trials showing that a monoclonal antibody, trastuzumab (Herceptin), given with chemotherapy reduced recurrence of breast cancer in women with HER-2 positive invasive disease by more than 50 percent.

Dr. Edith Perez of the Mayo Clinic, who chaired one of the studies—the North Central Cancer Treatment Group (NCCTG) trial. "These data confirm that we now have a very potent weapon against the recurrence of cancer cells that overexpress HER-2, which tend to grow fast and are generally more likely to recur."

Perez, an internationally known breast cancer researcher and co-director of the Multidisciplinary Breast Clinic at Mayo Clinic in Jacksonville, started work on the study seven years ago.

Past research had indicated that trastuzumab added to chemotherapy slowed tumor growth in patients with advanced or metastatic breast cancer. It seemed logical Perez says, to wonder whether the monoclonal antibody might stop the cancer from recurring. Even so, the dramatic results astounded her.

About 25-30 percent of breast cancers overexpress HER-2. These tumors tend to grow faster and are generally more likely to come back than tumors that do not overproduce HER-2. Trastuzumab is a monoclonal antibody designed specifically to attack the oeverexpressed protein. Monoclonal antibodies are used for other types of tumors, such as lymphoma, but this is the first one targeting breast cancer.

Perez says that women who have been diagnosed with early stage invasive breast cancer should be sure that their physicians have their tumors sent to appropriate laboratories to be tested for HER-2. Although it's been the standard at Mayo for several years, it's not being done everywhere. She also advises women to discuss the findings of these studies with their physicians and ask if there is other research being done from which they might benefit.

Moving forward, researchers will focus on finding other ways of attacking HER-2. They'll also be looking for other proteins and genes that may be important in breast cancer growth so they, too, can be targeted. Research continues hoping for a cure in our lifetime.

For more information: Multidisciplinary Breast Clinic, (904) 953-0707, www.mayoclinic.org/trastuzumab/

Adapted from Check Up Mayo Clinic, June, 2005, Vol. 12, No. 2, Jacksonville, FL

CHAPTER IV

MINOR HEALTH PROBLEMS

"Be Alert For The Little Things"

Diseases of the Eye

The two most common eye ailments occurring during the middle years are cataracts and glaucoma. There are no symptoms, vision stays normal and there is no pain. Detection is found by the use of the "air puff" test or other tests used to measure eye pressure in an eye examination. But, this test alone cannot detect glaucoma. Glaucoma is found most often during an eye examination through dilated pupils. This means drops are put into the eyes during the exam to enlarge the pupils. This allows the eye care professional to see more of the inside of the eye to check for signs of glaucoma. Both can lead to blindness, which is the ultimate symptom of these diseases. Two other common problems lie with Diabetic Retinopathy and Macular Degeneration. More people fear these diseases, according to a recent Gallup Poll, than any other excepting AIDS and cancer. Cataracts, which may occur from thirty-five onward, are opaque spots which form on the lens of the eye. The lens becomes milky and cloudy not allowing the light to pass through to form a clear image in order to focus on the retina. This impairment affects the picture carried by the optic nerve to the brain. The cause of cataracts besides age related changes include heredity, eye injury, and some medicines like corticosteroids, health problems and diabetes mellitus.

Cataract Surgery

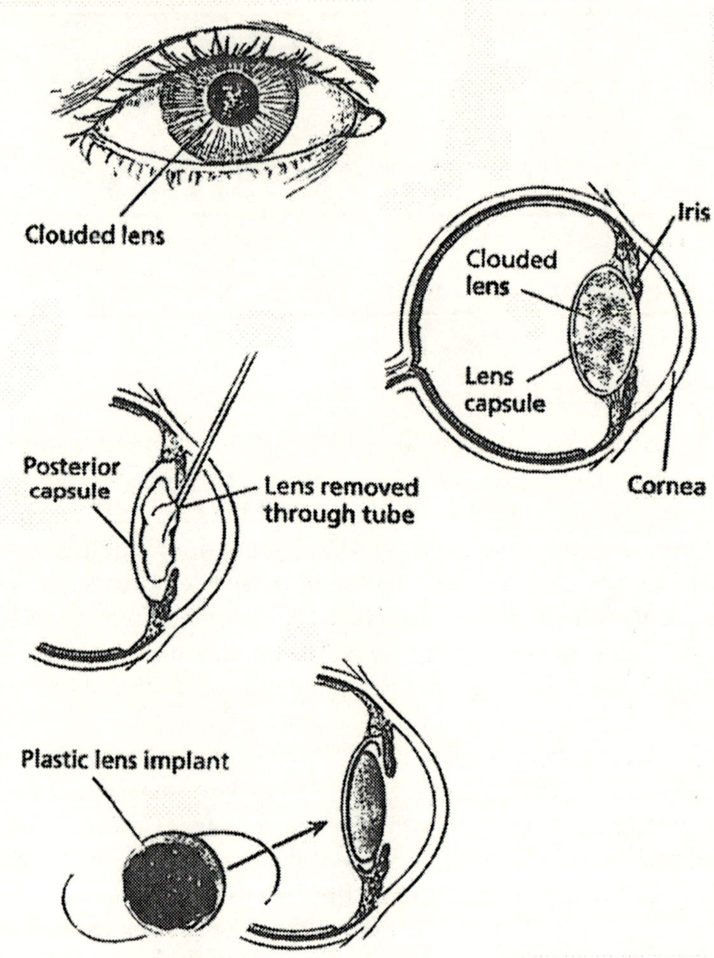

The only effective cure involves removing the clouded lens and replacing it with a plastic implant. Diagnosis of cataracts doesn't mean immediate surgery, if the vision is only slightly blurred. A correction to the prescription of their glasses and better lighting may be sufficient to help. Some medicines that dilate the pupils help some people. Some people delay surgery for years. Risks for cataracts involve smoking, drinking alcohol in excess, exposure to ultraviolet radiation, have diabetes at an early age and have used corticosteroid for a long time. By the time people are 75, 45% will need surgery. Only 2 of 100 from 45-54 and 5 of 100 55-64. Surgery is painless and is done on an outpatient basis and the operation requires an hour or slightly less and most are effective.

In glaucoma (hypertension of the eye) extreme internal pressure is exerted within the eyeball causing it to harden. In acute cases considerable pain is noted along with dimming of the vision. The most damaging type of glaucoma doesn't cause pain, but injures the vision silently and very slowly. Sometimes an indication of this disease is accompanied by the appearance of colored rings and halos about bright objects, or vision remains good centrally but dims on the periphery. Half of all blindness comes from this disease and it seems particularly to affect women in the middlescence years. There are now non-painful tests for glaucoma. If diagnosed early vision can be almost always be spared.

Eye problems are serious and should not be left unattended. Those twenty-five years of age should see an eye specialist at least every two to three years. Those over fifty should see an ophthalmologist (eye physician) once a year. Eye injuries should be treated promptly, one should avoid, glare; using lighting along with television viewing and do not try to treat infections of the eye yourself. Most of these minor infections like pink eye (conjunctivitis) can be cleared up by using ophthalmic ointment containing antibiotics. Boric acid is not as good as it used to be thought for eyewash. No wash should be used frequently unless professionally advised. One should rinse eyes every morning to rid eye of the granules (sleepers) which cut the eyelids and tend over time to have them turn in to the eyeball. Eye drops such as Refresh have been found to be effective.

In Glaucoma there is usually an increased pressure in the aqueous humor (the fluid that fills the chambers of the eyes). This pressure causes damage to the optic nerve. Aqueous humor is always being produced and excess fluid is always being eliminated through the canal of Schlemm to keep a good balance of pressure in the eye. If the drainage system becomes blocked and pressure rises, pressure in the blood supply of the optic nerve increases. If it continues the nerve fibers that carry optical messages die and vision begins to fade. Vision loss might also occur by the blocking of very small blood vessels that feed the retina and optic nerves. Nerve fibers on the outer edge are affected first, so vision loss begins with peripheral vision and gradually closes until the cells supplying central vision are killed. The damage done is not reversible so early identification is important. Glaucoma does run in families. Those most likely to get glaucoma: Blacks over age 40; everyone over age 62 especially Mexican Americans; people with a family history of glaucoma.

Glaucoma

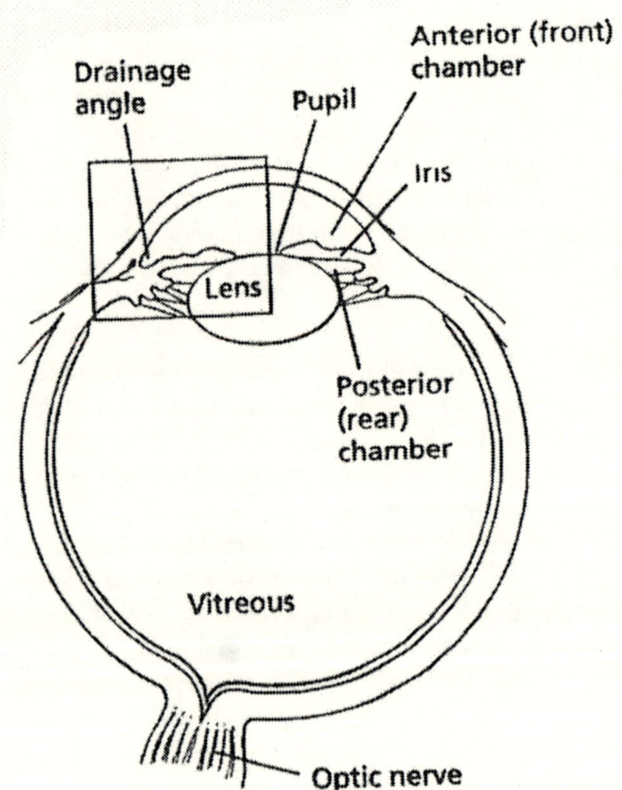

Most Glaucoma is open-angle type (90% of cases) sometimes called simple or chronic Glaucoma. The angle in the front chamber of the eye remains open, yet the aqueous humor drains out too slowly leading to a backup but a gradual but persistent rise in pressure. Closed-angle Glaucoma is known by a rapid rise in eye pressure over hours as the drainage angle suddenly becomes blocked preventing the outflow of fluid.

Most ophthalmologists start with medicine that is the lowest Glaucoma medicine to reduce the side effects. This requires people taking these medicines to see their physician once every three months.

The usual drugs used for amelioration are Timbolol and betaxolol hydrochloride, which reduces the amount of aqueous humor. This may be accompanied by burning, itching eyes and may have the effect of slowing heartbeat, cause depression and fatigue. Another drug Pilocarpine and echothiophate iodide that constricts the pupils to widen the drainage angle. This drug use may cause blurred vision, aching brow, and tearing.

Latanoprost is a drug that reduces pressure and dilates the pupil temporarily and has similar effects like other drugs but may cause aching muscles and chest pain. Brimonidine tartrate another drug that is used for treatment reducing pressure by decreasing the fluid production but carries with it burning eyes, blurred vision and generally may cause fatigue and dry mouth. Epinephrine, dipivefrin, and epinephyl borate reduces pressure and creates dilation. This use by by-products of irritated eye and may generally increase heartbeat, sweating and high blood pressure. Other drugs used by physicians are Dorzolomide hydrochloride and Apraclonidine hydrochloride. Both reduce pressure and fluid production. Your doctor will carefully monitor your medication.

Diabetic Retinopathy

This condition involves deterioration of the blood vessels of the retina in people with diabetic mellitus. It usually occurs in both eyes. The longer one has diabetes the greater the risk. The symptoms though limited at first reaching an advanced stage without notice can be observed by an ophthalmologist. A dilated fundus examination involves placing eye drops in the eye in order to dilate (widen) the pupils and your retina as seen through an ophthalmoscope. Sometimes a fluorescein agniography is performed. In this case a dye is injected into the vein in your arm, the dye travels through the blood vessels to the retina and photographs are taken to determine whether or not the vessels are leaking. In case of leaking blood vessels and enlargement of the macula, laser surgery is used. The laser is focused on the damaged retina to close the ruptured vessels. This procedure is done in a doctor's office. Where new and fragile vessels have developed, the use of laser surgery is utilized. The beam is spread on the damaged retina creating scars that stop the growth of blood vessels and protect the retina to the back of the eye. A local anesthesia is used and procedure is performed in an office.

Another circumstance exists where the vision from bleeding occurs. Freezing therapy is indicated. This shrinks new blood vessels until blood settles then laser surgery is used. It is sometimes performed in an operating room requiring a local anesthesia. Advanced proliferative retinopthy removes the vitreous gel and replaces it with a clear solution. This operation is performed under a powerful microscope in an office or operating room using local anesthesia. In the case of retinal detachment repair surgery is performed re-attaching the retina to the back of the eye. This repair work is done in an operating room.

Macular Degeneration (ARMD)

Generally age related, ARMD is the leading cause of blindness in people over 60. The problem is the macula, the area on the retina responsible for sharp, central vision when it deteriorates gradually causing blurred vision making reading difficult and finally leaving a blind spot in the center area of vision. Risk factors are smoking, exposure to bright sun light and ultraviolet radiation, light colored eyes, farsightedness, hypertension, high cholesterol and coronary artery disease.

The ARMD occurs in two forms—wet and dry. The majority of people have dry or atrophic form—it may affect one eye producing a gradual distortion of vision mainly in the dry form. Blurred vision and difficulty reading or distinguishing faces are usually the first symptoms. The second is effected. One-eyed vision masks their perception of vision for they seem to have normal sight. Wet ARMD is more severe. It results when blood vessels develop in the choroid layer, the back layer of tissue under the retina and extends like tentacles toward the macular. The new vessels tend to leak fluid and blood which injures tissue and photoceptor cells. Distorted vision is a first symptom, straight lines seem wavy, colors seem faded and a blind spot may develop in the center of the focus area. People with ADMD do not go blind they retain peripheral vision. Treatment for dry macular degeneration unfortunately doesn't exist however this form of ARMD progresses very slowly and people manage well in daily chores even with central vision loss. Laser surgery is sometimes used in wet ARMD with the laser aimed at the leaking blood vessels to seal them. This procedure works better when accomplished on newly formed vessels that have not grown over the Fovea. It is not a cure but slows down the progress of the disease. It is thought diets high in vegetables and antioxidants (Vitamins C & E) slows the progress of wet ARMD.

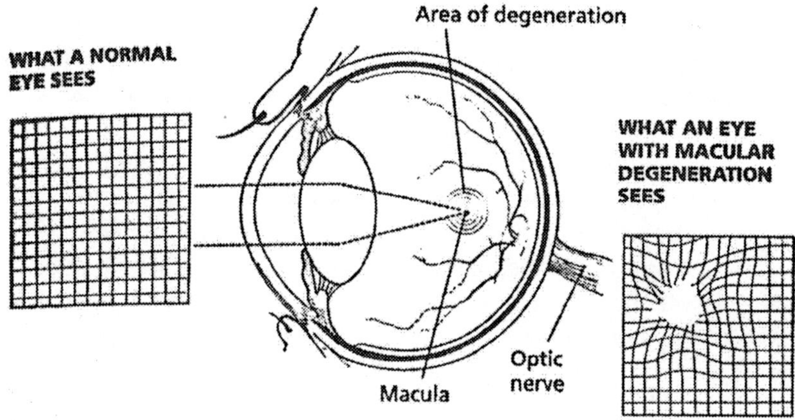

Age-Related Macular Degeneration

Detached Retina

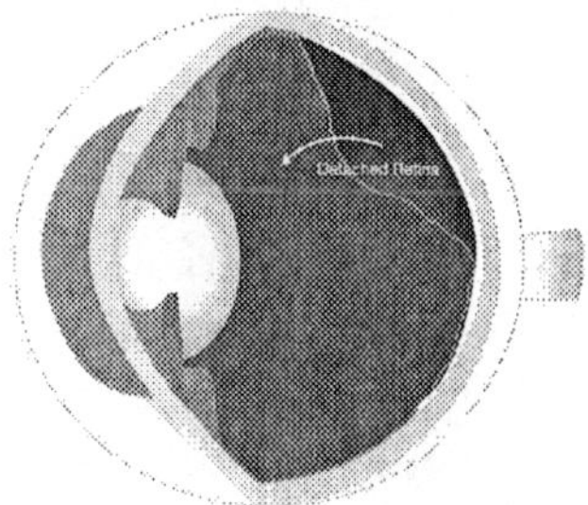

Detachment of the retina happens when the retina lifts away from the Choroid, which contains an inner layer of blood vessels. If treatment is delayed the pulling away continues until the retina hardly hangs on the cilicry body and the optic nerve. Both eyes may be affected. The separated retina is a serious situation that can lead to permanent loss of vision. Middle age and older people are most likely to be smittened. Near sightedness increases the chances of detachment. Cataract removal increases the risk of retinal separation. Notable occurences that signal detachment are flashes of light and floaters—small black bits go across the field of vision.

MINOR HEALTH PROBLEMS

Hemorrhoids

Sometimes called piles, hemorrhoids are enlarged veins situated inside or just outside the rectum. Prolapsed hemorrhoids are recognized because of the mass protruding from the anus. They can move back into the canal or you can push them back gently. Internal hemorrhoids are permanently prolapsed become inflamed and may issue a watery discharge. They cause itching, pain and sometimes bleeding. They are like varicose veins in the legs. Usually they can be controlled by medicine or surgery. There are two reasons for seeing the physician promptly if you think you have hemorrhoids. First, though rare hemorrhoids may signal something as an internal disease (a liver problem or cancer growing in the rectum or intestines). Second hemorrhoids may bleed. Bleeding from the rectum area whether from the hemorrhoids or something more serious should be investigated fully. One of the best remedies to avoid hemorrhoids is to avoid constipation—a big problem in middle age. To circumvent this one should exercise regularly, drink 6-8 glasses of water daily, eat fruits, vegetables, some chocolate, cheese and milk and complex carbohydrates such as bran. In some people one bowl of bran cereal a day may solve the problem. Secondly, bleeding hemorrhoids can cause anemia or if a clot should form in the vein it can be very painful and somewhat dangerous. Do not use advertised remedies or cures instead consult your physician. For some help in emergency, apply very cold (ice) water or witch hazel (it eases the pain) or hydrocortisone cream (controls the inflammation) on a cloth directly to the anal area, continuing for five to ten minutes until relief is obtained. Hot baths in the morning and at night often help as well as certain over the counter aids like petroleum, lidocaine. The doctor may us an anoscope, which has a light at can see any difficulty internally up in the intestine such as cancer, internal hemorrhoids. Bathing in warm water helps so does drinking 6-8 glasses of water a day and eating a lot of fruits and vegetables. Increase fiber in the diet is recommended. Bathe with unscented soap and when using the toilet, use unscented tissue. Also important is taking Kegel (see Appendix) exercises and promptly attending to the first sign of bowel movement activity.

Incontinence

This is a disorder found mainly in women involving the leaking of urine when laughing or straining. A muscle weakening or relaxing in the genital area creates this condition. Metabolic problems such as diabetes, neuropathy, damage from infections, or anatomic abnormalities may be the cause of incontinence. Sometimes this happens due to some infection. Treatment depends upon the cause and usually consists of proper exercise and in many cases surgery upon the advice of a specialist.

There are four kinds of incontinence called stress incontinence, urge, overflow and transient incontinence. Ten million people are affected with one type or the other. A majority (90%) could be helped or cured, however, only 1 in 4 seek a physician. Many people resign themselves to wearing adult diapers, many think incontinence is part of growing old or are embarrassed to acknowledge the problem.

Kinds of Incontinence

Stress—This is seen in the leaking of small amounts of urine when coughing, lifting heavy objects, sneezing, exercise or put pressure on the bladder. This is more common in women after childbirth and in men after prostate surgery. Among women whose age is under 60 this is the most common type. The Harvard Medical School and Family Guide gives the following information on types and treatment for incontinence follows:

Urge—The bladder in this case develops a spasm. A sudden contract makes the urine flow with little warning. For men and women this is the most common type.

Overflow—This can occur with women after pelvic surgery or men who have prostate enlargement. With partial blockage, the bladder cannot empty completely so urine dribbles frequently. Urological problems can cause weakening of the bladder and unsolicited urine flow.

Transient—Is caused by a temporary condition and most often in people older than 65. The causes that predominate are low estrogen levels, medicine (sedatives and channel blockers), delirium, urinary tract infection, drinking great amounts of fluids, drinking diuretic beverages as coffee or alcohol, heart failure, difficulty getting to the toilet when the urge to urinate, and fecal impact occurs.

Keep a daily log on the daily urination, the circumstances, etc., for a week. Having this information the doctor will perform a genital examination and one on other simple reflex and muscles. If your bladder is usually full it may mean you are not able to completely empty the bladder.

For stress incontinence which can be alleviated 50% to 75% of the cases by

(1) Performing exercise to strengthen the urinary sphincter.

(2) Learning biofeedback to help you contract the correct muscles.

(3) Holding weighted cones in your vagina to strengthen pelvic muscles.

(4) Wearing a tampon or pessary while you exercise to prevent leakage. They press against the vagina wall and compress the urethra.

(5) Taking drugs such as phenylpropodamine or pseudoephedrine which increase the urinary sphincter ability to contract. This helps up to 20 of every 60 women.

(6) Using a vaginal estrogen.

(7) Having collagen implants. Purified collagen from cows is injected into the urinary sphincter. The body breaks down the collagen and forms scar tissue, which in turn bolsters the muscles.

    About half of the women taking this procedure find improvement but in men, it's less successful.

(8) Having surgery to strength the pelvic muscles or to lift the bladder. Many surgeries require only a small incision in the abdomen others are done through the vagina.

Urge incontinence can be improved up to 75% in people who have it. Increasing the capacity of the bladder by learning to suppress sudden urges and prolonging the intervals between urination for 1 to 2 hours then 3 to 4 hours. Or another way is to set time schedules. Drugs can improve urge incontinence like Oxybutynin, Propantheline anti-depressants. Side effects like dry mouth are common with this drug. Overflow incontinence may improve with blockers Prazosin, Terezosin or Doxagosin if the problem is an enlarged prostate. These drugs are often used for high blood pressure, they can also help relax urethral muscles and the fibers of the prostate. Implants can be used which stimulate coordinated activity of the bladder when medicines provide no relief. The Simon Foundation for Continence provides further information about causes and treatment of incontinence (1-800-237-4666).

Preventing Incontinence by Taking Kegel Exercises

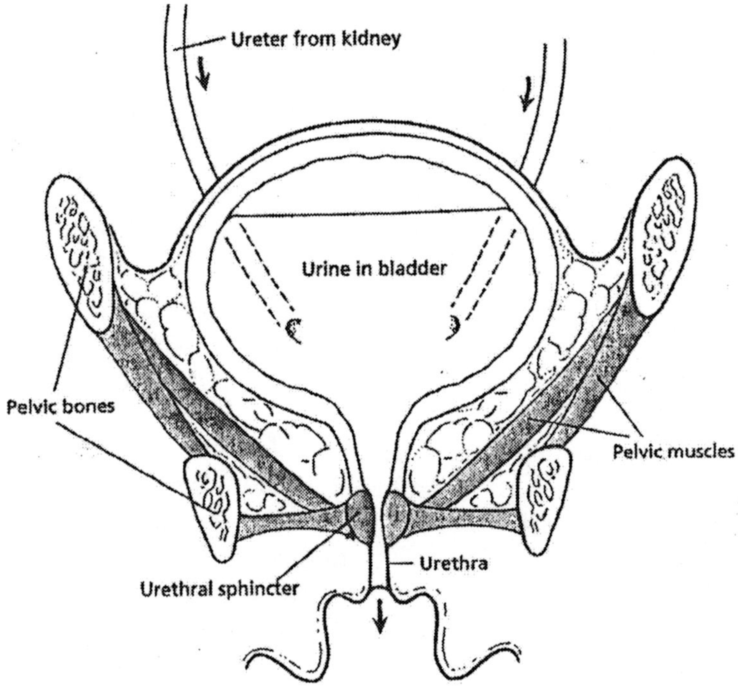

Allergies

Allergies are groups of symptoms caused by contact to substances that are usually harmless but are viewed by the immune system as being hurtful to the body. The immune system overreacts to these substances (allergens) releasing histamines, etc., that causes runny noses, itchy eyes. Allergies affect one or more systems as nose, throat, lungs, intestine, stomach and eyes, skin. Allergies run in families. But your children may not inherit your specific type but another kind.

Allergies (Reactions)

There are many kinds of allergic reactions: (1) Those caused by the digestive system by allergic foods such as chocolate, wines, cheese, tomatoes, etc.; (2) those due to contact with material or substance on plants like poison ivy, cosmetics, medicines, clothing, detergents, etc.; (3) those substances like food and medicine which cause hives and welts; (4) Eczema is another type seen in the development of rough, red patch found around the elbows and back of the knees. It is difficult to manage. Eczema is not contagious. Calamine lotion will usually relieve the itching but beware of "cures." Cortisol creams provide the best treatment. Some reactions from bee stings can be serious. Some people require shots to protect them from these effects. Wasps can create painful swelling or cause a person to become unconscious. Locally, apply a drop of diluted ammonia or vinegar will help after pulling the stinger out, with significant reactions, see a doctor immediately. The main remedy is to find the precipitating cause. For eczema and asthma consult your physician who may suggest an allergist. A guide to relief is found in the appendix.

Food Allergies

Many people are allergic to foods. Those some on those foods are intolerant to the body. Nearly everyone at some time has a food they do not digest well. A common food milk (lactose) is an intolerant food. In these cases an enzyme is lacking that is needed to digest milk sugar lactose. Food allergies are an abnormal response of the immune system as in other categories of allergies is usually causing a reaction to a small bit of food. The reaction occurs when a body manufactures antibodies causing a reaction, which includes itching, swelling of the mouth, lips, or airways, sometimes causing extreme breathing problems, itchy skin, rash, wheezing and though rare loss of consciousness. Symptoms appear in minutes up to 1 hour later after eating the offensive food. The most reliable test for the culprit is the elimination diet. In this situation all possible offending foods (dairy products, grains, caffeine, alcohol, red meat and sugar) one at a time for 2 weeks then gradually reintroducing them one at a time. Blood tests are also utilized, one kind is the radio allergo sorbent test also an assay used to indicate the presence of IgE antibodies in the blood. The foods responsible for 90% of all food allergies are: cow's milk, eggs, wheat, peanuts, soy, tree nuts, fish and shellfish. In some people kissing someone who has eaten a peanut recently may cause a severe reaction.

Treatment is solely avoidance of the offending food. Those at risk of severe reaction should carry portable injections of epinephrine for use at the first indication of an anaphylactic reaction.

Hay Fever (Rhinitis) Allergy

This allergy is triggered by pollen in spring, summer and early fall though some people have it all year round. These people may be affected by indoor allergens such as dust that harbors mites that produce irritating substances especially in warm humid weather. Molds, hair of skin cells known as dander is shed by animals. Most rhinitis allergens come from the air. At 50 years of age most allergies are less severe the symptoms are nose running, eyes become red and itchy, may produce mucus, frequent sneezing and irritated throat and skin. Treatment—some medicines like Beta blockers, oral contraception pills, and thyroid hormones can cause nasal symptoms. If allergy is suspected skin testing—scratch tests or an injection just under the skin may confirm it. Decongestant pills (non-prescription) with the medicine pseudoephedrine can also help. If you have high blood pressure, diabetes, coronary artery disease, narrow angle glaucoma or trouble urinating check with a physician about its use. Non-prescription antihistamines such as Chlospheniramine or diphenhydramine are cheap and very effective also in some people they may cause drowsiness, blurred vision, trouble urinating, etc. If these do not work your doctor will prescribe a more powerful drug that's non-sedating like Cetirezine, Lasatadine or Fexofenadine. People with liver disease should be careful with other non-sedating antihistamines Terfenadine and Astemizole can cause heart rhythm abnormalities. Nasal sprays on a short period basic may be help.

Allergies to Medicines

Some adverse reactions to medicines are caused by an allergic problem in which your body produces antibodies to a drug. The antibodies bind to the drug to rid it from the body. In this operation the clumps of antibody bound to the drug travel through our blood and can harm body tissues or interfere with normal body functions. Allergic reactions are most often outbreaks of minor problems involving the skin they may also attack cells in the kidneys, liver, joints and blood. Inform your doctor if you think you are having an abnormal reaction. The worst type of reaction comes from anaphylactic shock that lowers the blood pressure and the airways become so narrow you cannot breathe, this requires emergency treatment. Sun exposure may cause photosensitivity of a drug you are taking like antibiotics, Tetracycline, Sulfa antibodies. Alas some birth control pills have the same affect, as does NSAIDS (nonsterodol anti-inflammatory drugs). Everyone needs to ask the doctor what are the side effects to his prescribed medicine and how do they interact with my other medicines.

Eczema and Dermatitis

These allergies are forms of reactions that are interchangeable for several situations that cause inflammation of the skin. Most common ones listed here they have like caused but common symptoms, red areas of skin, red lumps, blisters itching, rash and scratching. This type is called atopic dermatitis. If one has this type of problem its likely another family member has another type of allergy. This allergy usually goes away on its own and usually is confined to one part of the body such as the hands.

Contact Dermatitis

Touching or rubbing a substance which creates a rash or is marked with blisters. Contacts may be with laundry detergents. Metal from jewelry, clothes fasteners, some rubber products (gloves or condoms), some cosmetics, plants (poison ivy) and some drugs. In rare cases a person contact with another body. The reaction usually occurs one or two days after contact.

Stasis Dermatitis

Occurs on ankles, calves and feet also in people who have varicose veins or circulatory problems. Symptoms include mild redness and swelling along with itching. It the swelling is not treated the rash will become crusted and leak fluid. Infection can occur and injury to the area can lead to ulceration. Treatment starts with wearing compression stockings.

Seborrheic Dermatitis

Typically observed at scales over red patches which most commonly appears on the scalp in the form of dandruff. It also affects the eyebrows, eyelids, ears and folds near the mouth. The cause of this condition is not known.

Perivral Dermatitis

Often confused with Rosacea the small red papulses and pustules are limited to the skin around the mouth, nose and under the eyes. Young women are the most likely to be affected. It usually clears up in 1 to 3 months with an antibody; its cause is unknown.

Treatment to these problems can be treated by the individual involved through using hydrocortisone cream and skin moisturizers. Dandruff can be treated by medicated shampoo. Antihistamine can help the itching and can be purchased across the counter.

Asthma

This disease is a disorder of the airways, inflammatory that is marked by recurring bouts of breathlessness and wheezing. The symptoms are caused when the breathing tubes of the lungs clamp down and fill with sticky mucus, making it difficult to get air in and out of the lungs. Some 5 million people in the USA, a third being children, are affected. The researchers do not fully understand the cause of asthma. Aspects of the environment especially allergies. Adults who have had Asthma as children have a 10% reduction in lung capacity.

Common causes of Asthma are as follows:

Allergens

Cockroaches, paper lice and dust mites
Feathers, molds, animal dander, saliva or pollen
Foods with sulfites—used in wine, beer, salad bars, and dried fruit
Coloring dyes.

Strenuous Exercise

Too much at one time and by cold, dry air

Polluted or Cold Air

Air pollution outdoors
Tobacco or wood smoke
Indoor polluted air as fumes from dry cleaning, new carpeting, cleaning materials
like mixing bleach and ammonia and wood finishing products.

Medicine

Aspirin and other non-steroidel and inflammatory drugs as Ibuprofen or Indomathacin, Beta blockers, cholinergic drugs used as eye drops in glaucoma or bladder contraction

Viral Respiratory Tract Infection
Flu and common cold
Occupational Substance

Metal salts, wood or vegetable dust and some solvents and plastics

Stress and Emotional Upsets

Stress worsens with the coming of impending Asthma attacks. Allergies caused by insects can be countered with ultrasonic repelling devices you can buy from Wal-Mart and other stores. Also filters are now on the market which placed in a room will rid the air of 90 percent or more of the dust and dust mites. These hold promise for the Asthma patient.

Treating Asthma involves four aspects—evaluation, medicine, environmental control, and education about the problem.

Evaluation of the Problem

Measures of lung capacity and volume are made to gauge the severity of Asthma. Many physicians like patients to monitor their lung function with a device called a peak flow meter. Inexpensive, portable it can be used at home to measure your peak expiratory flow rate, this gives you advance warning of an impending attack setting off the reminder to take medicine or see your doctor. Getting a baseline level, measures when you are feeling well and when you are under duress. Measures should be taken every day. These baselines can tell you how well you are doing. Seventy-two percent of those monitoring their Asthma as opposed to 42% who do not require days off within four months—three levels describe the peak flows—Green, 80 to 100% the ideal level—non-symptom; Yellow level, 50-80% take medicine regularly—may not have symptoms; Red levels—unacceptable, i.e., 50% less than your ideal level get help immediately (your doctor or emergency center).

Medicines

Drugs can prevent and reverse inflammation while treating narrowed airways. Medicines for long-term control help to achieve and maintain better levels of lung functions. Some anti-inflammatory medicines include: Cortisosteroids, Cromolyn, Nedocromil, Leukotriene and Antagorids, bronchodilators designed to open airways by relaxing the 8 mouth muscles are Beta-agonist, methylxanthines, and immunotherapy.

Environmental Control

Those measures that help control factors that bring on asthma attacks heretofore mentioned in this section.

Education

Learning about the nature of your problem through American Lung Association publications or other medical hard books such as *The Harvard Medical School Family Health Guide,* available now in 2005; *American Association Medical Guide,* and *The Home Medical Advisor*, 2002.

Arthritis

Some 15 to 20 million Americans seek treatment for one or more of a 100 different conditions which fall under the category of arthritis. The word means inflammation of the joint. The three major concerns of middle-age people are rheumatism, osteoarthritis and gout. There are seven main types of arthritis:

(1) Rheumatoid—the most serious affects nearly 3 million in the USA; is an inflammatory disease that damages the synovial tissue connecting bones and joints and it is chronic. Women are affected three times as often as men. However, very few are severely disabled because of it. It is not known what triggers the immune system to produce the substances that cause the inflammation which can in time all the components of the joint, the synovial tissue normally smooth, becomes grainy and rough invading the joint cavity eats into the cartilage bone, tendon areas of tissues (called pannus causing the bones to fuse). If tendons rupture, it will create floppy joints.

Treatment—Taking a part in your treatment is important—following the plan for therapy, recognizing the flare-up and drug side effects and exercising. Nonsteroidel antiflammatory drugs, like Aspirin or substitute. If this isn't effective then methotrexate or hydroxychlaroquine in large dosage can improve your situation. Some other disease changing drugs are antirheumatics—gold therapy, penticillimine and sulfacalazine. One needs to pay attention to diet, rest and exercise, protecting joints and saving energy. Diet—recommend two servings of fish per week rich in omega-3 polyunsaturated fatty acid found in salmon, mackerel and sardines—taken in capsules form is beneficial also.

Rest and Exercise—During periods of flare-ups you may need 8 to 10 hours sleep. Short naps may be needed for during hiatus periods some people will overdo their activities becoming very tired—rest is preventive. Exercise reduces pain, relieves stiffness and fatigue.

Joint Protection and Saving Energy—Overuse needs to be avoided for it increases swelling and pain. Occupational Therapists can teach you how to reserve energy and protect your joints while doing your daily chores. Rules—do not sit in one position too long, use your strongest joints and muscles, modify your home to make it easier to live in, ask for help when you need it and avoid movement that puts extra stress on your joints.

Newer drugs that hold promise are TNF blockers adding TNF blocker etanercept to methotrexate makes for great improvement and leflunomide, a drug taken by mouth. This latter drug is taken six to eight weeks to begin to work. Cognitive therapy can provide a sense of control and provide understanding thereby reducing depression and stress.

It usually occurs first between the ages of 25-45. Fever, a loss of appetite and weight loss are symptoms. One or two of the smaller joints become swollen and are acutely painful. Mental depression is common to its victims.

(2) Osteoarthritis B A degenerative joint disease less dramatic than the rheumatoid type; it affects fewer joints. Most everyone over fifty will develop this to some degree as the process begins in middle age. Frequently symptoms first appear after a joint injury or strained joint in compensating for the injured one. The distal joints (hands and feet) are the ones affected whereas in rheumatoid arthritis it is the proximal that are affected. Many people 20,000,000 perhaps have this problem. Their hips, knees and spine, for women the hands, boney joint in the tip of their fingers are affected. These are called Herberden nodes. Friction creates pain and irritation. Pain is felt directly in the joints but many radiate out from the hip, and osteoarthritis of the neck and lower back. Physicians focus on pain relief use acetaminophen or nonsteroidal anti-inflammatory drugs, protecting the joints from overuse by canes, splints and weight reduction. Exercise with physical therapy to improve muscle tone is recommended.

Sometimes surgery is necessary to relieve extremely painful or misaligned joints. Hip and knee replacement may be an option for people whose mobility is limited if they are in generally good health. Many people forget that exercise helps slow progressive degeneration. Needed is range of motion, strengthening the muscles and low impact aerobics or endurance exercise like walking, swimming or stationary bike riding. Do exercise daily after a hot bath and when your medicine is having its greatest effects. Analgesic creams containing capsaicin obtained at drug stores help some people reduce pain and tenderness. Glucosamine Chondroitin is a good over the counter joint remedy. It has been found to provide relief for pain, etc. If this is used do not touch your eyes, nose or genitals.

(3) Rheumatic fever—A generalized inflammatory disease affecting the whole body; may cause heart damage. It usually follows a streptococcus infection such as tonsillitis or scarlet fever. (This disease causes only transient arthritis in most cases and rare in itself.) This is seen mainly in children. Aspirin helps if more serious involving streptococcal antibodies to combat this is used.

(4) Gout—a situation where the uric acid accumulates in the blood attacking the small joints, especially the big toe; occurs most frequently in men. This disease is due to a deficiency of a substance needed in breakdown of certain meats and therefore a build-up of uric acid develops because of this deficiency and creates the problem. The kidney cannot handle an overload of uric acid leaving the joints vulnerable irritating the synovial tissues during pain and swelling. Drink plenty of water, less alcohol. Foods such as liver, anchovies, kidney, herring, sardines rich in protein—foods, which prevent kidney stones, should be eaten.

(5) Infectious arthritis—A joint inflammation caused by a bacterial infection; the most common of which is gonorrhea, a sexually transmitted disease. Thousands of cases each year, untreated gonorrhea can spread through the blood stream can cause infections in the joints, bones and skin. Women have no symptoms so need to be tested to ascertain this situation—in several weeks' discharge from the urethra or vagina and painful urination. Men have discharge from the urethra, which is clear or white or thick yellow or pus like. Treatment is with antibiotics, which cure the problem and keep it from spreading through the body. Sexual partners should be warned about their situation. Not common in middleage, however, it is seen as a non-GC (gonorrhea coccus) (Chlamydia) seen in young women and men or inflammatory problem in people with immune system problems, diabetics or damaged joint (Rheumatoid arthritis, Trauma).

(6) Bursitis—The inflammation of a bursa (sac) filled with fluid that lies between a muscle and bone. Pain occurs outside the elbow where the tendons are connected to the bone. The sac assists the movement of the arm. Frequently this is called tennis elbow (only 10% get Bursitis in this manner) but can also occur in the shoulders and knee by people who garden a lot, job related lifting and screw driver use or wrist overuse, the muscles of the forearm. Rest and

medical or surgical procedures can effect a cure. (Injection of cortisone frequently helps this problem.) Nonsteroidal inflammatory drugs relieve the pain. Physical therapy and shoe insoles use can improve the problem.

(7) Reiter's Syndrome—This is a non gonorrheal cause of arthritis which is most frequently due to an altered immune response to a venereal disease type organisms known as chlamydia. It has a genetic component. This syndrome affects joints, eyes and urethra (the tube that connects the bladder to the outside world). Many times antibiotics cure the disease. Some forms of Reiter's syndrome are chronic and others may be recurrent.

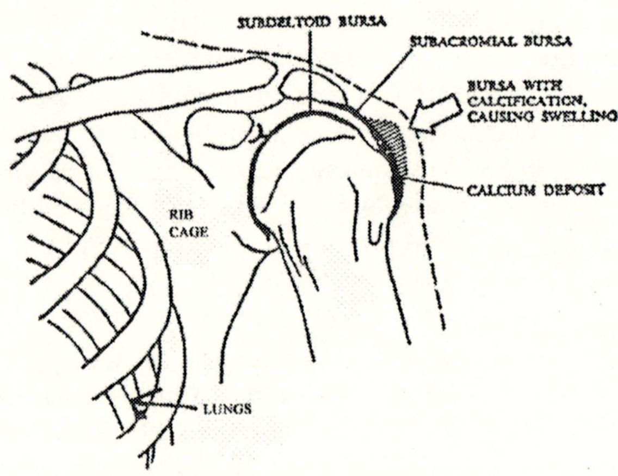

Signs and symptoms which often occur in middle-age by nearly everyone sometimes need to be recognized and treated early regarding arthritis: The symptoms include:

1. persistent pain and stiffness on arising.
2. pain and tenderness in joints.
3. swelling in joints.
4. tingling sensations in fingertips, feet, hands.
5. unexplained weight loss, fever, and weakness.

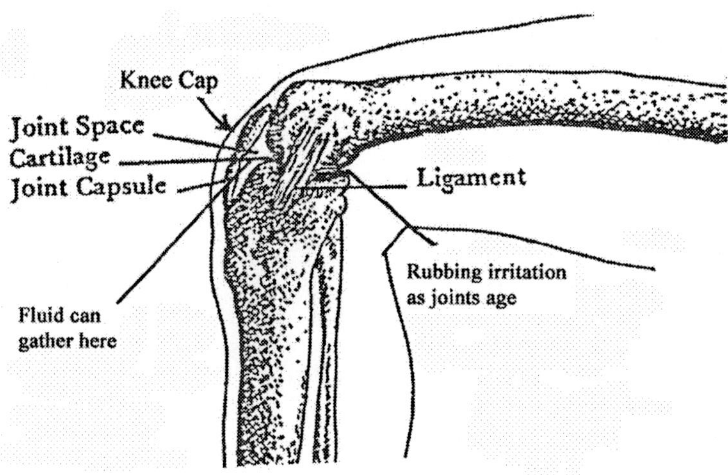

Arthritis victims are continually exploited by quacks with useless remedies, usually anti-inflammatory such as aspirin and other drug therapy. They are not only wasting money but valuable treatment time. The American public is paying over a billion dollars a year for quick relief, which doesn't occur.

Treatment includes special diets and dietary supplements, aspirin, exercises, rest, special supports, drugs and climate change. Additional advice includes guarding against cold and dampness, avoiding strain, fatigue (don't do all your house or yard work or ironing at one time). Unfortunately, there is no cure for most forms of arthritis.

Teeth Problems

Tooth decay, periodontal disease and gingivitis are common ailments during middle years. Teeth play a vital role in our nutritional health and must be free of disease to continue their proper function. More serious than decay is periodontal disease caused by plaque organisms from it-secretions of toxins damage the ligaments as a result gums become inflamed and pull away the teeth from the gums. Over time they can damage gums, the roots of the teeth and finally the bone. This infectious ailment of gums can have serious side effects such as heart disease by causing infection of the heart valves. It is an ailment of major proportions in the United States with one out of four American being seriously affected. This disease affects some ninety-percent over 50 years of age. Progressive stages and symptoms include redness and swelling, bleeding when gums are pressed, pink after brushing with toothbrush, bleeding and painful gums. Pain is killed by Aspirin, Tylenol, Acteminophen or Ibuprofen. Vitamin deficiencies, improper brushing and flossing, and malocclusion, contribute to the disease. Treatment for advanced and serious cases involve surgery.

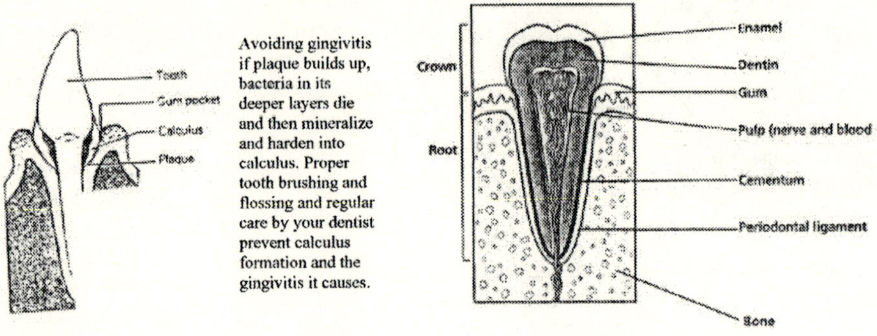

Avoiding gingivitis if plaque builds up, bacteria in its deeper layers die and then mineralize and harden into calculus. Proper tooth brushing and flossing and regular care by your dentist prevent calculus formation and the gingivitis it causes.

Prevention by proper dental care flossing and brushing regularly and professional cleaning are of single importance is the best cure. We should regularly visit our dentist thereby forestalling the unexpected and for receiving preventive maintenance. Replacing broken teeth or lost ones can easily be done to make your teeth appear normal by your dentist by capping teeth, making bridges to avoid loss of teeth, using implants and braces, crowns and partials.

Deafness and Loss of Hearing

The ability to hear begins to fade with age. By twenty-one our hearing peaks. By middlescence it is estimated that some 25 to 30 million have some degree of hearing loss. Sensitivity to high pitches is the first to go. Deafness may be caused by disorders such as vitamin deficiencies, infections, metabolic and glandular disorders, head damages, or wax build-up. Deafness also may be inherited.

Types of deafness are as follows:

(1) inherited deafness (otosclerosis) this is a common form of trouble usually beginning in younger adulthood becoming more pronounced during middle-age. One of the middle ear bones experiences abnormal growth, which prevents vibrations from activating the nerve leading to hearing. Surgery is sometimes necessary to correct this disorder of the middle ear.

(2) Catarrhal deafness is a conduction problem which sinuses, tonsils, adenoids, etc., create the inflammation of the Eustachian tube connecting the throat and the middle ear. These conditions act as sound insulation and interfere with the sound transmission through the middle ear to the inner ear where the hearing apparatus is located even though the nerve endings may be normal. Medicine to sure infection is a treatment and/or surgery.

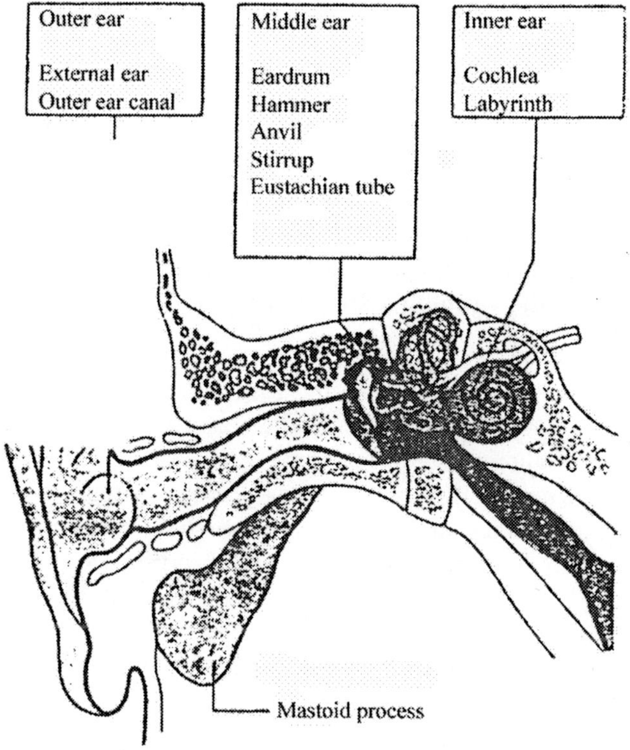

(3) Nerve Deafness is seen when sound is sent to the hearing nerve but the hearing organ has degenerated (the nerve that transmits impulses to the brain, or the brain itself).

(4) Mixed deafness may be a combination of any two types of deafness.

(5) <u>Meniere's Disease</u>

The increase in the amount of fluid in the labyrinth, the part of the ear involved in balance, causes pressure in the inner ear, which distorts and often ruptures the labyrinth wall. This disease affects one ear and about half the time the other. Symptoms include vertigo, dizziness, ringing in the ear, distortion, nausea, vomiting and pressure in the ear. This problem usually clear up on its own, when it starts lie down also cut down on fluids and salt on occurrence. See a doctor (Otolaryngologist if possible). He will effect a loss of fluid, check for infection and tumor on the auditory nerve inside the skull.

(6) Labyrinthitis

Involved with balance results from a virus that inflames the ear. Like Meniere's disease it is characterized by dizziness everything seems to be spinning. If you move your head vertigo ensures in some nausea, etc. Though very debilitating it is not a dangerous condition when cared for correctly. A quick trip to your doctor is in order. He will rule out other causes than Labyrinthitis. Rest for several days will be needed and some medicine to combat the vertigo, nausea, etc. Usually the symptoms disappear in 1 to 3 weeks.

(7) Tinnitus

This problem is a case where ringing in the ear occurs when there is no sound present. Causes include diseases of the Eustachian tube or ear or underlying disease as an allergy, high blood pressure, heart problems or anemia. Hearing loss itself may be the cause and even earwax. Injury to the head or neck and some medicines such as aspirin, non-steroidal anti-inflammatory drugs, antibodies and sedatives may also cause Tinnitis. Exercise, decreasing salt, keeping the blood pressure in the normal range and avoid loud noises. Some help is afforded by white noise tapes or steady sounds as the ticking of a clock even hearing aids to amplify environmental sounds reduces Tinnitis.

The family doctor should be consulted about hearing problems, and where a specialist is needed, he will advise. If the hearing loss is sufficient, a hearing aid, if appropriate, will be recommended. In the case of conduction problems due to infection or an inherited problem, a surgical operation may be advised. In any case people with hearing problems must help themselves by being cooperative and providing feedback to those providing the therapy. Hearing specialists are not in the business of selling aids but will recommend, if available, a hearing rehabilitation center or supplier. An adequate aid will allow one to hear sounds unheard in years through its ability to amplify. Do not consult a hearing aid company on your own without first consulting a physician for there are no miracles despite advertised claims. Companies are trying to sell their product and will, often, give you a typical sales pitch—low costs and fantastic results. Take it with a grain of salt. The cosmetically desirable small size aid may take in a smaller spectrum of sound waves. Allow your physician or audiologist to decide if a hearing aid will help you or not and abide by their advice.

Revitalization (Hormones and Replacement Therapy) for Sex Glands

Outside of recognizable disease affecting the major ductless glands (endocrine glands composed of the pituitary, sex glands [testes and ovaries] thyroid, parathyroid and adrenals are the islets of langerhans-pancreas (insulin related) the hormones secreted are sufficient to carry one to old age, 80 or more. However, by the time many women are 50 and many men are 60, there is a functional loss in gonadal hormones provided by the sex glands (testes) in men and (ovaries) in women. Though whatever the cause (usually due to the running out of eggs in women, eggs produce estrogen), the tendency exists for men and women in the latter middlescence period 55-65 for men to produce less testosterone and women less estrogen. When gonadal reproductive activity fails so does the sex steroid production. This does not mean that life is over by any means, perhaps less sex drive for men and little change of potentia in women, but for them it may be improved with the fear of pregnancy removed. Women manufacture estrogen from adipose tissue so some do not need replacement therapy. Sex activity may suffer from lack of partners, rather than desire to engage in sex. Sex hormones replacement which has been sometimes used for both sexes to improve and perhaps forestall the diminishing large supply of hormones is in a ratio of 20-1 (in milligrams) of testosterone (essentially male hormone) over estrogen (essentially a female hormone). Replacement use is under the physician's direction. Estrogen shortage can lower libido and cause vagina dryness. Recent controversy over estrogen and patches has bothered many women. Alternatives exist in locally applied creams such as Premarin, Estrace, and vaginally inserted drugs like Estring and Vagifem are helpful. Women treated in this manner will generally find there is no breast tenderness, vaginal bleeding will not occur nor will there be a lowering of the voice or excess hair growth. Most medical experts have concluded that estrogen replacement therapy (ERT) is safe when properly used. This means low doses—usually 3 milligrams or 0.625 milligrams used for two years. These doses are combined with progesterone, the other women's sex hormone. The estrogen builds up the uterine lining and the progesterone prepares the lining to be shed just like the menstrual period for the next part of the month. These kinds of uses protect from osteoporosis also helps with heart disease and reduces the risk of uterine and breast cancer. There are two types of hormone therapy:

- **Estrogen replacement therapy (ERT).** ERT is estrogen alone. Because ERT may increase the risk of cancer in the lining of the uterus, it is usually prescribed for women who have had a hysterectomy.
- **Hormone replacement therapy (HRT).** HRT combines estrogen with progestin, another female hormone. Progestin reduces the effect of estrogen on the uterine lining and protects against cancer of the uterus.

Hormone therapy reduces the discomfort of menopausal symptoms such as hot flashes and vaginal dryness. However, hormone therapy can have unpleasant side effects, including bloating, cramping, nausea, breast tenderness, and periodic vaginal bleeding.

Hormone pills are taken every day. Some forms of hormone therapy are available as skin patches. There is very little risk in taking hormone therapy for a year or less to manage symptoms of menopause. However, hormone therapy is not usually recommended for women who have had breast cancer, trouble with blood clots, liver disease, or undiagnosed uterine bleeding.

Hormone therapy though used for a long time or in increasing amounts does not protect against heart disease (Women's Health Initiative study showed this). It might help with osteoporosis. Talk to your doctor before deciding whether or not hormone therapy is a good idea for you.

Long term risks associated with progesterone use are unknown at the present time. There is some evidence of lipid metabolic effects. Men treated on this formula will not develop breasts, protein wastage nor the dangerous state of relaxed blood vessels (vasodilation). Treatment of men with this mixture has had far less beneficial results than treatment of women. Also there is only limited data to suggest that men benefit from this treatment. Estrogen prescriptions are used for three main reasons only; (1) vasodilation instability, (2) changes in vaginal mucus, (3) osteoporosis. Women with pre-existing cancers shouldn't take estrogen at all. Some decline in sexual function may occur towards the end of the middlescence period but physical causes should always be investigated, as these are frequently at fault, for example diabetes, hypertension medication, prostatic problems and fatigue. About half of the men 75 years old can achieve satisfactory intercourse.

Help is now coming to the aid of women—the problem for men it is erection in the middle years, for women it is libido or desire to have sex. Recent drugs are now on the market with others coming most of these for women. With 1.7 billion spent on Viagra in 2002 many companies are trying to reproduce the same kind of success. For men, the newest drug is Levitra being touted as more vigorous than Viagra. Sex can be had for 24 hours and is alleged to have 6 to 9 times more potency. It takes effect in 15 minutes and works for nearly 82% of men. Another drug available now called Cialis known as the weekender for it works up to 36 hours. Clinical Trials data says 64-92% of men find it effective—works in 16 minutes. Some side effects, headaches, facial flushing, upset stomach and nasal congestion. But it doesn't cause blurry vision or eye trouble experienced by some Viagra users.

Sex

Viagra heads the list, unbelievable but true. A recent study found women treated with Viagra for four weeks showed improvement in arousal, orgasm and sexual enjoyment. It may improve lubrication problems better than libido problems, which for women tend to be more about hormones and psychology than blood flow. Scientists have discovered the basic functioning of men's sexual format but they haven't as yet discovered all that's involved in women's physiology leading to a quick libido booster.

A new birth-control pill, Seasonale (Barr Pharmaceuticals) developed by Eastern Virginia Medical School in Norfolk, Virginia, in its Jones Institute for Reproductive Medicine (the nation's first vitro fertilization clinic) reduces women's menstrual periods from 13 to four per year. On the market for less than a year is showing now nearly 13,000 prescriptions a week. This medical school has become an international leader in women's health. Typically women using oral contraception follow a 28-day regimen. They take "active pills" for 21 days, then switch to placebos for a week. Stopping the hormone regimen causes "withdrawal" bleeding that resembles a period, even though ovulation hasn't occurred. In what is known as an "off-label use," doctors have advised women to delay their periods by starting a new pill pack at the end of three weeks. Because they don't skip any active pills, they forgo withdrawal bleeding that month.

Seasonale works in a similar way. Women take a pill with the same hormone level for 84 days and placebos for seven days, during which time they get their periods. The reduced frequency of periods is at the heart of Seasonale's appeal.

Androgen

Androgen is basically a male hormone but women possess some which usually helps in menopausel time with their potentia. According to Irvin Goldstein, M.D., Director of the Institute of Sexual Medicine at Boston University, estrogen imbalance isn't even half the problem. There are 10 sex steroids only three are estrogens, the other seven are androgens. Three of four women who they see in their clinic is for lack of desire have serious androgen shortages. Therapy focuses on upping female levels of Testosterone, the biggest emphasis is on DHEA, a chemical cousin of Estrogen and Testosterone. DHEA use shows large improvements in their self-evaluated sexual performance. This drug should not be taken on one's own. Side effects of Testosterone can include weight gain, clitoral enlargement and hair growth. DHEA has been linked to cancer. More research is needed such as the unsolved mystery of women's sexual functioning. It is coming!

For the upper middle age (60-70) middlescent person, use of certain drugs have a good effect upon fatigue (sometimes it is principally a psychological phenomena—boredom, lack of activity, etc.). Frequently among the overweight, the lack of thyroid hormones may cause the drowsiness—that can be remedied. For women during the menopause some estrogen used with progesterone is beneficial; it helps the body retain calcium. For older men some thyroid extract aids overcoming fatigability particularly where the basal metabolic rate is low and the cholesterol level high. The use of certain drugs as Deosxyephedrine, Neosysephrine and Benzedrine have powerful effects in counteracting undue fatigue where other methods have failed. These drugs, however, have the potential for being habit forming and should be used with caution. Iron deficiency, a common cause of lack of energy, in women and men can be treated with iron tablets. The use of these type drugs at present time, on a chronic basis, is only in documented cases of narcolepsy or cataplexy. These conditions are sleep disorders leading to fatigue. Caffeine may work as well and has less side effects but limited use is suggested for it has side effects of its own. Stimulant drugs are not given where blood pressure is chronically high, in the presence of coronary, artery disease and other vascular disease. One should remember that there are more people who complain of "being tired" who do not have enough to do than those who work very hard. Let us not lose sight of the fact that an important cause of fatigue in middlescence is depression (see Chapter II). This problem can be readily helped by medication and by becoming more involved with outside interests and less involved with one's self and therapy.

It should be emphasized that some danger lies in the administration of hormones, particularly the sex related hormones. Use of androgen for men with prostate problems is questionable and certainly the use of the "pill normally for birth control," as a tonic stimulation or replacement has some hazards for women. The fact remains, that there are no "monkey glands" or elixir which will bring the forty or fifty-year-old man back to twenty or the 35-45 year-old woman back to eighteen. Beware of quacks and promises of being made over functionally! A good face-lift may be worth it but your physician will give you the advice about the "fountain of youth." When responding to claims for "making you over" make sure you go to a medical doctor (M.D.) (Plastic Surgeon). Many bogus degree-holding people claiming to be doctors or specialists are bilking the public with degrees in everything (like N.D. Doctor of Natureopathy) to poetry. Check the licensure displayed and give the local Public Health Department a call to validate the credential and specialties claimed if there is some doubt.

Cholesterol and Fats

The accumulation of cholesterol with some mineral salts in the linings of the blood vessels leads to the condition of hardening of the arteries. We have dealt with this subject generally before but need to emphasize it again in light of the new guidelines for cholesterol levels. The body has no specific system with which to detect the cholesterol concentration in the blood in order for it to be regulated by a separate homeostatic mechanism (the ductless glands are examples of homeostatic mechanisms). We synthesize cholesterol whenever fat fragments accumulate in the blood sera (the liquid part of the blood). When by-products as triglycerides are released into the blood as fat bits (they are energy sources for cells of the body) most are lost in the kidneys, some in feces and urine. Cholesterol is formed in the liver and is not dependent on food we eat to be present. If we eliminated all cholesterol from food, our body would form enough cholesterol on its own to meet our daily needs. Two kinds of lipoproteins in the diet are high density which as a salutary effect and the low density which have a negative effect on the system and is associated with risk of heart disease. High density lipoproteins can be increased by exercise and low fat cholesterol diets using complex carbohydrates in the diet (whole grain cereals, breads, etc.). HDL is beneficial because its primary purpose is to take cholesterol from the body cells and send them to the liver where they can be removed. It is the stress response that begins the cholesterol synthesis. An accumulation amounts of cholesterol that is absorbed from cheese, eggs, fish or meats in the diet is debatable but it has some effect on the amount synthesized from sugar fats. These foods do not contain carbohydrates but do contain calories, cholesterol and saturated fat. No more than 3-ounce servings at lunch and dinner is recommended. Lean cuts are best and baking and broiling is better than frying. Fat foods, salad dressing, margarine, mayonnaise, oil, butter and cream cheese add calories one serving per meal. In any event the amount taken in has a relationship to the amount of cholesterol that shows up in the blood.

In the middlescent years many Americans are plagued with high cholesterol. Even younger adults are affected; in the autopsies of a number of American soldiers in the Korean War, massive evidence was found of high levels of cholesterol, resulting it is believed from heavy fat and carbohydrate diets of their adolescent and many young adult years. Many adults in their middle years are ladened with stress, under exercised and overfed, meaning that there are numbers of people nationwide who have arteriosclerotic vascular disease. Far too much milk products, eggs, fried foods, certain seafood, beef, butter and mayonnaise and fast foods have been consumed. Substitution of eggbeaters, imitation mayonnaise, polyunsaturated oils, low fat milk, (better still no fat), lean beef and margarine should be utilized. One should eat baked or broiled chicken, turkey and fish and less lean beef (maybe twice a week). Another excellent way of treating cholesterol is by physical fitness that helps cholesterol break down faster and in other ways not to build up in the body.

A daily cholesterol intake of less than 200 milligrams (mg) is recommended to prevent hardening of the arteries, heart attack, etc. The fat amounts should provide about one-third of the calories, they are considered the low fat foods, 30% says the American Heart Association with no more than 40% from saturated fat. A 2000-calorie diet should include no more than 67 grams of fat. Carbohydrates 83 per meal. A 1200-calorie diet, 50 grams (Bayer Aspirin Research). The following provides amounts of cholesterol and fats found in some foods.

Figuring Fat

$$\frac{\text{Grams of fat} \times 9}{\text{Calories per serving}} \times 100 = \% \text{ of calories per serving from fats}$$

Food	Portion	Milligrams of Cholesterol
Egg yolk	one medium egg	250
Egg white	one medium egg	0
Beef liver	32 oz.	438
Butter	1 tablespoon	10
Lobster	32 oz.	85
Oyster	Raw 32 oz.	50
Lard	1 tablespoon	12
Cheddar cheese	1 oz.	28
Bacon	one strip	15
Beef	32 oz.	90
Chicken	white or dark 32 oz.	80-91
Corn oil		0
Turkey	white or dark 32 oz.	77-100
Brains	raw 2 oz.	2000
Sweet breads	32 oz.	466
Milk	whole 1 cup	34
1%	1 cup	14
2%	1 cup	22
Skim		5
Ice cream	2 cup	26
Ice milk (10% fat)	2 cup	13
Yogurt, low fat	1 cup	17
Tuna (canned in oil, drained)	32 oz.	65
Shrimp (canned, drained)	32 oz.	150
American cheese	1 oz.	21
Veal	32 oz.	100
Pork	32 oz.	90
Lamb	32 oz.	98
Flounder (raw)	32 oz.	50
Mayonnaise	1 tablespoon	15
Margarine	1 tablespoon	0
Cottage cheese	32 oz.	19
(4% fat)	32 oz.	9
(1% fat)		
Chocolate milk	1 cup	32
Salmon	32 oz.	55

Most of these foods have some unsaturated fats and some saturated fats though in much smaller amounts than the cholesterol. Guidelines for cutting back on fat. (American Heart Association) There are other factors in cholesterol production, perhaps heredity, stress, exercise and maybe something else as yet unidentified. All things being equal the person who avoids cholesterol and saturated fats has an edge in the middlescent fight to escape coronary heart condition.

You should test cholesterol every three to five years, if you have high cholesterol levels more often.

	Desirable	**Borderline**	**Undesirable**
Total Cholesterol	Below 200	200-240	Above 240
HDL Cholesterol	Above 45	35-45	Below 35
LDL Cholesterol	Below 130	130-160	Above 160
Total Cholesterol/HDL	Below 4.5	4.5-5.5	Above 5.5
LDL/HDL	Below 3	3-5	Above 5

Adapted from Jerry Gordon, 2004

Reducing Your Cholesterol

The first is to eat a low-fat, low-cholesterol diet. Your total fat consumption—saturated, polyunsaturated and monounsaturated should be less than 30 percent of your daily intake of calories. Keep your cholesterol intake to fewer than 300 milligrams per day. Saturated fats contained in butter, whole milk, hydrogenated oils, chocolate, shortening, etc. should be one third of your total fat consumption. Reduce your total fat and cholesterol intake, limit your consumption of meats such as beef, pork, liver and tongue (always trim away excess fat). In addition, avoid cheese, fried foods, nuts and cream, and try to curb your intake of eggs to no ore than four per week. Try to eat meatless meals several times a week, use skim milk and include fish in your diet. Eat a variety of vegetables, pasta, grains and fruit. Check the label of the foods you buy, and restrict your choices to foods containing 3 grams of fat or less per serving. If you are overweight reduce by regular exercise, walking, swimming, aerobics, health spa exercise machines.

Carrier molecules (HDL and LDL) are made of protein and are called apoproteins. They are necessary because cholesterol and other fats (lipids) can't dissolve in water which also means they can't dissolve in blood. These apoproteins are joined with cholesterol and form a compound called lipoproteins. The density of these lipoproteins is determined by the amount of protein in the molecule. "Bad" cholesterol is the low-density lipoprotein (LDL), the major cholesterol carrier in the blood. High levels of these LDLs are associated with atherosclerosis. "Good" cholesterol is the high-density lipoprotein (HDL); a greater level of HDL—this is like a drain cleaner you pour in the sink—is thought to provide some protection against artery blockage.

A high level of LDL in the blood may mean that cell membranes in the liver have reduced the number of LDL receptors due to increased amounts of cholesterol inside the cell. Once a cell has used the cholesterol for its chemical needs and doesn't need any more, it reduces its number of LDL receptors. This enables LDL levels to accumulate in the blood. The LDLs then begin to deposit cholesterol on artery walls, forming thick plaques. In contrast, the HDLs—the "good"—act to remove this excess cholesterol and transport it to the liver for disposal. A third group of carrier molecules, a very low-density lipoportein (VLDL) are converted to LDL after delivering triglycerides to the muscles and adipose (fat) tissue. The levels of HDL, LDL and total cholesterol are all indicators for atherosclerosis and heart attack risk. People who have a cholesterol level of 275 or greater (200 or less is desirable) are at significant risk for a heart attack, despite a favorable HDL level. In addition, people who have normal cholesterol levels but low HDL levels are also at increased risk for a heart attack. Risk factors are diet, age—increase after fifty, weight, gender (men at a younger age, women after 50), genetics (some predisposed to high levels), disease (diabetics, health problems, stress and life styles). Medicines that lower cholesterol are Mevacor, Zocor, Lipitor, Cresta, Pravochol, Trica, Lopid, Wellchol.

PREVENTIVE MEDICINE

A number of things should be kept in mind about health maintenance in the middlescent years.

Balanced Diet

The foremost is eating properly. A balanced diet should consist of the following proportions in percent as calories:

Proteins (meat, fish, peanut butter, eggs, milk, nuts)	25%
Fats (butter, whole milk, oils, animal fats)	30%
Carbohydrates (breads, fruits, rice, potatoes)	45%

(check new pyramid guidelines which follows)

Along with these proportions one should include Vitamin A (spinach, carrots, squash, peaches, apricots, margarine and beef liver); Vitamin B^1 and B^2 (pork, liver, whole-wheat bread, cereals, legumes, cereals); Vitamin C (citrus fruit, tomatoes, strawberries, raw leafy vegetables); Vitamin D (milk, fish liver oils, sunlight); Vitamin E (dark green vegetables, wheat germ whole grains and vegetable oils). One could take one-a-day multipurpose vitamins or specific supplements such as Omega 3, Borage Oil, Alpha Lipoic Acid, Mega E and Ester C (the DeVinik mix) and mineral tablets to insure getting the minimum but the FDA recommended more importantly they have been found to kill radical free elements in the body to protect cells. Vitamin K (leafy green vegetables) but any more may be wasted unless advised by the physician who would have some special reason for prescribing them. Too much intake of Vitamin K can interfere with Coumadin use as it reduces the coagulation of the blood. The doctor might give injections of Vitamin B-2 and other vitamins occasionally for medical reasons, but fad diets, weight losing pills, and supplementary vitamins, etc. for elixir unfortunately do not exist. Everything being equal (that is without restricted diets) a good balanced diet follows for the in-between years.

Suggested Diet for the Middlescent

2 servings of fresh fruit or fruit juice
2 servings of green or yellow vegetables
2 servings of fish, lean meat, eggs or cheese
3 servings of bread, potato, cereal, roll or crackers (6-8)
6 glasses of water, diet or non-sweetened drinks—coffee (caffeine free) or tea.

If a person works very hard physically with much lifting, walking, climbing, etc., additional food is indicated. Calorie requirements can be judged from the following tables; however, individual differences should be noted.

Daily Caloric Requirements Occupation	
Secretary or Office Clerk	1000-2000
Housewife	2500-3000
Factory Worker	3000-4000
Laborer, Farmer	4500-5000

Calories needed for Women Weighing 130-132 Pounds Daily. (If 10-15 lbs. over this add 100 calories to maintain weight.)

Age	To Maintain Weight	Calories Needed to Lose 1 lb. per week
30	2100	1600
40	2000	1500
50	1900	1400
60	1800	1300
70	1700	1200

Calories Needed for Men Weighing 160-162 Pounds Daily

Age	To Maintain Weight	Calories Need to Lose 1 lb. per week
30	3000	2500
40	2900	2400
50	2500	2000
60	1800	1300

1. Vaccination against Influenza, Pneumonia and for Foreign Travel
   This is particularly needed where one has a chronic health problem as diabetes or bronchitis. A variety of shots are needed for those going abroad other than northern Europe where conditions are similar to those in the United States.

2. Immune globulin injections for those contacting persons with hepatitis.

3. Wearing of seat belts when driving particularly when driving on the open road at considerable speed. Automobile accidents are a major cause of death.

4. Periodic Tuberculosis skill testing or chest X-rays to identify contact with this disease in time to reduce its ulterior effects on the body.

5. Periodic Pap Test and Breast Examination is a must, an early warning is the best protection against the possible ravages of cancer. One suggested schedule for mammograms is as follows:

   A. At no extra risk for breast cancer:
      1. Baseline at age 35;
      2. Every 5 years until 40;
      3. Every 2-3 years until 50;
      4. Every year after 50.

B. At risk for breast cancer:
 1. Baseline at 25-30;
 2. Every 2-3 years until 40;
 3. Every year after 40.

6. Heart Disease:
 The Massachusetts program based on recent research there indicates that to help prevent heart disease, cancer, and stroke one should:

 A. be a non-smoker
 B. have a cholesterol level of below 200 mg/dl calories derived from % of fat to be less than 20%.
 C. have blood pressure less than 130 or less mm systolic and 80 or less mm Hg. diastolic Hg.
 D. exercise vigorously for 20-30 minutes 5 to 6 times a week.
 E. minimize exposure to environmental or occupational toxic substance.

7. Avoidance of noxious fumes—acids, gas, etc., and other air impurities such as smog, smoke, dust, asbestos, coal dust, etc.

8. Avoidance of foods which have been labeled carcinogenic—such as cyclamates, betel nuts, smoked fish and meats.

9. Avoid taking laxatives habitually—these lead to rectal problems. A proper diet including plenty of fruits, fibrous foods as cereal, lettuce, celery, etc., liquids (mainly water in quantity) and vigorous exercise will usually suffice to allow avoidance of medicines which in time get the body out of its natural rhythm.

10. Avoid taking pills on your own advice—No drug should be taken even aspirin for a long period of time without consultation with the physician. You are usually just treating the symptoms. The use of analgesics (painkillers—Demoral, Meperidine or Codeine) have the potential to cause dizziness, abdominal distress, nausea and impaired consciousness. Anti-depressants like Siequan, Tofranil and Vivactil can work wonders but should be administered by the physician. The sedatives like Phenobarbital, Amobarbital, Membutal and Butisol are agents which reduce anxiety and promote sleep but over-dosage is a constant threat particularly when allied with alcohol. The diet pills (as Dexedrine, Tenutate) are also contra-indicated without the doctor's advice. (CF the appendix for information on

pill taking conditions, generic drugs, etc.) Beware the use of illegal drugs and alcohol for depression, etc. These can kill.

11. Have a regular routine of exercise—being in good condition, keeping your weight down, burning up calories and possessing good muscle tone, one must work the body, exercise the skeletal systems, stretch the muscles, get the heart beat up (typically 150 beats per minute for the 40 year old, fewer for the over 50-60). The routine you use can be jogging, tennis, brisk walking calisthenics, swimming or whatever puts some strain on the system. Remember, build up the pace of exercise gradually and only after you have conferred with your physician. As an idea of how many calories are burned per minute of activity, consider the following: mopping the floor, 5.3; chopping wood, 4.9; brisk walking, 6.0; shoveling snow, 9.0. Dr. Kenneth Power, Chief Behavioral Epidemiology, Division of Health Education says exercise benefits prevention and control of hypertension, osteoporosis, diabetes and certain psychiatric and psychological conditions. Even low level, he says, physical activity reduces the risk of coronary heart disease. It is believed that no more than 10%—20% participate in physical fitness activity.

12. Keep in touch with your doctor—the doctor is not solely responsible for your health, you are; don't wait until you're sick—those with chronic health problems need to see the doctor regularly—at least every three months if they are under control, like diabetes, high blood pressure, anemia. Even more often if out of control. For the reasonably healthy, one should see the physician once every year in the early middlescent period, after fifty more frequently. When you see your doctor you need to know what to ask him and what to tell him.

Tell Him About

Any fever, level and length
Any pain, or tingling in the arms or legs
Any change in weight or swelling
Bleeding (unexplained)
Cough shortness of breath
Change in urine color or amount
Vision difficulties
Marked weakness or fatigue
Change in bowel habits

Ask Him About

Eating habits, diet, and medication
The state of your health—sugar level, blood pressure, lungs (clear)
Exercise routine
Mountain climbing trip or undertaking of a project involving strain
If you have doubt, worries, or questions about health, ask your doctor
Use of tampons, contraceptives

Sexual Problems (see chapter on love, sex and marriage)

As important as it is to know about the problems and rules of health, one should recognize that a seasoned body that has been carefully tended in young adulthood greatly increases the changes of surviving ailments of the middle age and reducing the effects of the aging process. The natural aging process can be slowed with sensible everyday living patterns. Most of our bodies don't wear out; we wear them down. The person who follows sound health maintenance programs—adequate nutrition, sufficient mental and physical exercise, rest and moderation in living habits would respond better to an unusual physical or emotional stress than those who have not. The latter person, though free from impairment, may not have the built-in reserve, which can handle an emergency situation. Complete well being in the middle years may be defined as a state of maximum resistance to disease, injury, or other abnormal stress.

Capabilities in order to be kept at their peak must be used. The muscle that is not used will weaken. Mental capabilities not employed to their fullest will decline. The circulatory system not subjected to the demands of regular exercises may decrease in pumping capacity. Capabilities must be constantly used to remain at their prime throughout one's life.

Researcher Lester Breslow, Dean of the School of Public Health at the University of California, Los Angeles, questioned 7,000 persons (1975) over a six-year period about their living habits. He found a relationship between good health and common sense and that it may have more to with health than science marvels or a check-up! The forty-five-year old man if he has followed six of the seven rules adds eleven years to his life. The seventy-year-old man who has followed all 7 is probably as healthy as a forty-year-old.

Survival of the Middle Years Depends Upon These:

1. Sleep between seven and eight hours each night
2. Eat breakfast
3. Stay within 10 percent of your proper weight.
4. Don't eat between meals
5. Don't drink excessively
6. Don't smoke cigarettes
7. Exercise regularly

A follow-up study of the Almeda County, California completed in 1985 showed the same results as the earlier 1975 report.

The greater the number of rules a person follows the less likely he is to have an illness. The two most important health rules, this research says, relate to exercise and avoiding cigarettes. The good life during the in-between years can be yours if you take care!

Appendices

APPENDIX 1

HOW TO USE MEDICINE

Follow your doctor's or pharmacist's instructions explicitly and phone him or her if you have questions or notice any side effects. Carefully read the medicine label before you take any of the drug.

Note the following:

1. Note whether your medication should be taken on an empty stomach (1 hour before eating or 2 to 3 hours after eating) or whether you should take it with food.
2. Take pills and capsules with a glass of water. It can decrease irritation of your esophagus an aids absorption by your body.
3. Use all of your medicine, even if you begin to feel better, unless your doctor specifically instructs you otherwise.
4. Do not drink hot beverages with drugs; heat can destroy the effectiveness of some medicines.
5. Take only the recommended dose. Taking more can cause a dangerous reaction; taking less can cause the medication to be ineffective.
6. Never take a prescription drug unless it was prescribed for you.
7. If you take a medication every day, take it at the same time every day.
8. Do not drink alcohol with your medicine (wait an hour between) if you have been instructed not to do so. It has the potential to seriously interact with both prescription and non-prescription drugs and can make you extremely drowsy. Grapefruit should not be eaten when taking Zocor or Lipitor.

Your doctor should know about all the medicines you are taking, including preparations you may not normally think of as medications, such as vitamins, supplements, antacids, eyedrops, or aspirin.

Some people find it easiest to take all their medicines to the doctor's office with them or to make a list of all drugs they are taking. If you have had an allergic reaction to any medicine tell your doctor.

Also, tell your doctor if you:

- Are being treated by another doctor or alternative practitioner.
- Are pregnant or breast-feeding.
- Have diabetes, kidney disease, or liver disease.
- Are on a special diet, or are taking vitamin and mineral supplements.

APPENDIX 2

DRUG INDEX

TO USE THIS INDEX:

1. You can use from the list either the generic or brand name.
2. Look for the name of the medicine from this sample list—the medicine is listed first then the class.
3. The class to which the drug belongs is shown in the right-hand column.
4. Write down each medicine and its class.
5. Use this information to find out more about the drug class or to investigate potential drug interactions.

The Generic name is in **boldface**; Brand name in regular type; Nonprescription in *italics*.

MEDICINE	CLASS*
Alprazolam	Benzodiazepine
Altace	ACE inhibitor
Amoxicillin	Penicillin
Aspirin	Salicylate
Caltrate	Calcium supplement
Cimetidine	Histamine$_2$(H$_2$) blocker
Coumadin	Anticoagulant
Darvon	Propoxyphene
Demerol	Meperidine
Epinephrine	Epinephrine (adrenaline)
Estraderm	Estrogen
Estradiol	Estrogen
Furosemide	Loop diuretic

MEDICINE	CLASS*
Glipizide	Sulfonylurea
Glucophage	Metformin
Humlin	Insulin
Ibuprofen	NSAID
Insulin	Insulin
Lasix	Loop diuretic
Loestrin	Contraceptive (oral)
Maalox	Antacid containing calcium
Mylanta	Antacid containing calcium
Phenobarbital	Barbiturate
Potassium chloride	Potassium supplement
Pravachol	Cholesterol-lowering agent (statin)
Pravastatin	Cholesterol-lowering agent (statin)
Prednisone	Corticosteroid
Prempro	Estrogen
Prozac	SSRI
Synthroid	Thyroid hormone
Tagamet	Histamine$_2$(H_2) blocker
Testosterone	Androgen
Thyroxine	Thyroid hormone
Warfarin	Anticoagulant
Xanax	Benzodiazepine
Zocor	Cholesterol-lowering agent (statin)
Zoloft	SSRI
Zyban	Bupropion

*ACE indiates angiotensin-convering enzyme; NSAID, nonsteroidal anti-inflammatory drug; SSRI, selective serotonin reuptake inhibitor; and MAOI, monoamine oxidase inhibitor.

CHAPTER V

CARING FOR OUR PARENTS

"Tending to Ma and Pa"

For people in the middle years, one of the biggest toll taking aspects of life is that involving caring for parents. It is often energy sapping and emotionally draining. It is said that young people growing up today do not feel they need to care for their parents in a special way. After all their parents have social security, Medicare, Medicaid, pensions, etc. Many youth it is said, are not planning on building houses or having apartments with an extra bedroom for the visiting parent to settle in. They are in many cases moving far away from home. But for most of us middlescent people, we feel an obligation to help our aging parents in many ways—providing money, emotional support, decision-making, and help in planning, etc. For persons 35-40, their parents are somewhere near 60-70; for those of 45 with parents at 65 or 75; for those of 50-55, 75-80, helping our mothers and fathers is an omnipresent problem. With the prospect of later retirement, as written in the national law, some of the matter of time "on their hands" will be at least in part eliminated. For most of us there will be only one parent who will be with us beyond 70-75, usually the mother. But if we are married it would likely leave possibly three parents, certainly two, to concern ourselves with. Some may also have a responsibility for their grandparents who are in their eighties and nineties. I know of one middlescent couple who had the responsibility for four parents and though it was very difficult they managed to survive by utilizing a nursing home for two of them and taking the other two into their home. Deciding who will go where could be a problem!

I am not suggesting that as soon as retirement comes, usually at 65, or maybe a couple years earlier, we will have the immediate burden of our parents. Most of our parents will want to maintain their independence as long as they can; in fact some will not leave their home even under the most extreme circumstances.

We should note that most gerontologists and psychiatrists believe that all people, including the old and the sick, are entitled to control over their own lives. This means choosing the way they live and how they are to die. We as concerned children have no right to impose on frail parents solutions that they will not accept—even where it seems clear-cut that we are right. The pressure on us from many sources to act is constant. Most families do not have a plan that is complete on what to do with our parents in emergency and crisis situations, hence, the reason that so many times social service agencies are called upon to help. Trying to decide what is best when our father is stricken with paralysis and our mother cannot drive to do the shopping and procure provisions necessary to sustain life is a calamity of the first order. Or our mother dies suddenly and our father cannot face the emotional stimulus the reminders of the old home brings and no longer can remain in the house so he must be cared for immediately. In these situations, where there are other persons in the family involved (sisters and brothers), we feel we have to take action and make arrangements as the situation pressure us to do something. These feelings run the gamut from depression (how can I handle it with the other aspects of my life) to guilt (I should have done more or something concrete before now); egos struggle with egos (it may be between you and your parent, or other kin as to who is number one to mother or father, my brother or sister or me? And what reference does caring for the parent have for the division of property and money after their demise? Hostility, duty, the need for family approval, all attend our attempts to help our parents. No amount of advice and outside assistance will ever satisfy what is needed nor make up for the investment of your life in caring. This is unfortunate but usually true. In the long run, it will be satisfaction you get from being a "real person" upon being responsible that makes the difference.

Let us turn our attention to the broader view of changes that take place between ourselves and our parents—attitudes, roles differentiation and what specific help can be given. It is interesting that true friendship between parents and grown children is rare. In many cases, unfortunately there is little or no relationship at all between parents and their children. Partly due to the fact that parents continue the parent-child relationship and the young need to be independent and emancipated. Also they misunderstand the love codes of each other. Parents, however, generally play the dominant, granting and giving role, while children continue in the submissive, receiving and taking role. For the parent who is able, the use of the checkbook is a very powerful weapon and he or she may want to use it as a form of control on a married child. I never will forget my first attempt to get married (I was nineteen and a junior in college); both my grandfather and my mother said that if I got married I would have to support the new wife and pay for my education. This threat along with another thing or two convinced me not to take this step. It was possibly better for the young lady for I was too immature for marriage. But for many the parent-child role continues until in one case I know of the ninety-year-old father, in reasonably good health, and living with his son 65 years of age, forbade him to go with his wife for a day or two visit with friends. The father's complaint was, "I'll be alone and have nothing to do. You can't go." And they didn't.

This type of thing is not an unusual case for persons of this vintage for most rely, due to infirmities, etc., almost totally on their children or nursing home care for emotional support. When our parents become dependent for health and/or economic reasons upon us, the role of parent-child tends to reverse itself. This is not always so and there are a few who think it should not change except under the circumstances where our parents become vegetable-like or senile. This is said in consideration of 'honor our father and mothers' and veneration due them. Typically cultural attitudes and economic circumstances will dictate what is done for our parents when it is essential that we take over their lives—decide the living arrangements, responsibility sharing and planning and establishing a general routine.

There are many groups—Amish, Chinese, Catholics, Greeks, and Jewish people who have a tradition of the three-generation and extended family living together. Some build additions to their homes in anticipation of accommodating the elderly. Even split-level housing in the suburbs is being advertised as mother-daughter homes. I assume these are for any age but certainly for the middlescent woman and her mother and/or father. There are some who are affluent enough to maintain the residence of their parents and provide nursing or a maid to help look after them. If, as in most cases this cannot be done, the parent or parents become a part of the household and they may care for the grandchildren if their parents have to be out working. This is a good arrangement for it gives the older parent something to do. However, many older persons do not want to live with other members of their families. They feel that they will be in the way, or that physically and/or financially they will be a burden on the family. This could be true, however, reassurance on this matter should be given our parents. A recent study indicated a longer life for those maintaining independence that is living alone or with spouse rather than with family or in some other type of care facility.

The Family Round Table

The question often arises who will take care of aging parents who are widowed or ill? In an attempt to solve the issue—enter the family round table. Daughters are the most likely to be assigned to the task due to the former nurturance role, the physical care of the parents, while sons give financial assistance and "moral" support. Whether or not it is the most well off or the poorest child who take the parent depends upon the circumstance. Each son and daughter should take a part that is make a contribution to the welfare of their parents. Approximately what can be expected should be decided early in family discussions about parental care. The personality of the children according to Silverstone and Hymen in the book, *You and Your Aging Parent* is important in how responsibility is assumed. A child who feels very close to a parent and does not resent the extra burden will logically accept the keep of the parent. On the other hand, a daughter or son who feels guilty about their past feelings, the neglect of their parents and lack of concern thinks by taking the care taking role he or she can win approval, heretofore elusive, will do it. Self-centered children may find it easy to break away from caring for their parents. Few, however, are so alienated from their parents that they turn their backs on them completely.

We should remember that many older people do not want to accept their condition—to admit they can no longer care for themselves, be mobile and manage their affairs is too painful to consider. They desire to be independent so they will ignore physical problems, housekeeping ones, etc., in order to continue their lives as usual. They struggle between their need for assistance and their desire to be self-sustaining. You and your parents—and children—must try to sift through conversations, over months and years, the reality of their lives and what should be done. And those things done in haste are often regretted at leisure. Hence take your time to decide what is to be done.

At some point in the lives of our parents they are willing to become the child—when they can't manage getting or carrying the groceries, walk for the newspaper, are afraid to go out of the home in a ghetto neighborhood or can't get service on plumbing or electricity. Sometimes these irritations keep the blood circulating for our parents. However, when these types of things get too much for them, they will usually ask us to intervene. My mother gave up driving at seventy-seven when she recognized it was more than she could safely handle but in no way would she give up her home, even though her only daughter who formerly lived with her had died and she was alone. The principal questions about relocation of our parents is how they regard the quality of life where they are? Frequently when one of the parents dies, the children quickly decide that the bereaved parent should be moved into one of their homes. This movement away from familiar surroundings, friends, activities and sometimes a job, is usually over-reacting, for once things settle down and the shock of loss wears off they become first class burdens, particularly if the parent is in reasonably good health. One such situation existed in our family where my aunt's husband died. Her son insisted she move in with him and his wife and young daughter. Shortly afterwards they built a one floor duplex with an adjoining connection, the living room being the central point between them. The son was transferred to another city where the mother then shared a bedroom in the house. By this time the young granddaughter had grown up and married, leaving—since the son's wife didn't work—the mother-in-law and my cousin's wife together most of the day for weeks on end. This lasted for twenty years and was a constant source of strife judging by the recital of injury transmitted to me both by the wife and my aunt. The aunt incidentally was in rather vigorous health and was mobile until 93. The son was caught in the middle. The lesson I think is to be sure you want to accept the sharing of your home before you make a commitment and consider other options. Remember also that parents often would rather be less well cared for in their homes than be with you feeling they are beholden for everything to you and your spouse. The respect, generally, given old people is not lost on our parents. There are countless situations where parents, old-maid aunt or uncles who have added immensely to the quality of family life, edification of children and joy in general, but these are still in the minority. Frequently when we involve ourselves in a new role with our parents we wonder how our children will behave toward us in similar circumstances.

Getting Help

When we need help in a critical situation in dealing with our parents who may be 1000 miles away and suddenly one is immobile, where should we look? There are a variety of help agencies both public and private who will assist you in making short-term or long-term arrangements. If your mother living alone has broken her hip and you are unable to leave your home for a long period of time to aid her, you can receive assistance from Private Social Agencies or Local Governmental Agencies. Catholic Family Services, Protestant Federation of Welfare Agencies and Jewish Family Services organizations don't require you be of their faith to get help nor do agencies require persons to be poor. (See the end of the Chapter for Sources of Help.) However, one should perhaps start by getting information from friends who have experienced these kinds of problems, from their own physicians, ministers and social workers. You can call one of your local agencies like the United Fund for information. Any city or county with 50,000 population should have social service to help aged persons in their area. Social workers can help arrange, when your parent is a distance away, for meals through "Meals on Wheels," to visit your parent regularly, check on what needs to be done for his or her comfort and keep you informed. They will make necessary arrangements because you cannot be there. And importantly they know what part you are entitled to freely receive from the local, state and federal government. Securing a practical nurse, a temporary shelter and many other services are part of their work. There may be a required payment or donation for this service but you will have peace of mind not otherwise affordable. Private and government agencies are usually found in the white pages, sometimes blue, of the telephone directory under Professional, Business and Organizations, whereas under the yellow pages you will find such agencies as Senior Citizens, Nursing Services, Health and Welfare Agencies, United Way, Social Service Agencies and Homes for the Aged. If you have trouble isolating a person or agency that can give you an answer about your specific problem call a city councilman or mayor, or town alderman. Human Resources Commissions in larger cities can tell you what the Medicaid eligibility requirements in a given state are. For constant (daily) check on your disabled parent, the Red Cross, Volunteer Senior Citizens and many times local police departments will check by phone or ride by the home to check on the security as a reassurance matter. These organizations (Red Cross, etc.) also make provisions for transportation, day-care centers, meals for the homebound, financial assistance and legal aid. Individual churches usually make some provisions for assistance, though they are generally limited; but they frequently do give assistance to people of their own faith who are sick and aged through peer visitation, gifts, reading material, pastoral visits and sometimes meals and counseling.

Nursing Homes and Homes for the Elderly

Most people think of nursing homes as institutions where old people can live and be cared for regularly. To qualify as a nursing home the home must offer facilities that meet the standards and regulations of Medicaid and Medicare as U.S. Agencies. The Skilled-Nursing Facility (SNF) provides 24-hour supervision by a licensed vocational nurse or a registered nurse, the nearest service to hospital care available. Normally a physician has to prescribe admission. At minimum SNF's provide medical, nursing, dietary, pharmacy and activity services. Another nursing home is the Intermediate Care Facility (ICF) which cares for people who aren't well enough for independent living and are not sick enough to require constant medical and nursing attention. They are required to provide 8 hours of nursing. Those licensed nurses are not always available. An ICF should give patients help with bathing, dressing, eating, walking, and other personal needs and provide programs of social and recreational activities. These kinds of institutions usually have agreements with close-by hospitals and health centers to supplement their services or to secure provisions they do not have. This should be checked into when looking into a nursing facility.

Skilled Nursing Facilities for Special Disabilities

This is a facility that provides a protection environment for themselves and others or persons who have mental disabilities. Some have long-term facilities. Besides these types of institutions Old-Age Homes and Retirement Homes abound that are operated by state and private agencies. A number of these are non-profit, frequently caring for the well and not-so-sick old. Many are run by church groups. Before you place your parent or parents in any of these institutions you should investigate the institutions thoroughly. When my brother, a minister, and I considered moving our mother to a nursing home, we looked at a number of places in our local area. He was convinced that some of them offered what we wanted (congenial settings, concerned and adequate personnel and support facilities). However, my visits did not validate this view. The proprietary interest appeared to me to be the dominate concern of the homes we visited rather than patient-centered care. Subsequently instead of moving Mother, we got a home keeper to live with her in her own home. This was the first of many such arrangements, which kept us constantly worried as we lived 400 miles away, for sometimes Mother would keep a helper only a week before something would happen. On one occasion, the lady housekeeper insisted upon having her boy friend into her room; this my Mother strongly objected to and invited her to leave. "No hanky panky here! Not her kind of people," she said.

BEWARE—Be cautious as to hidden costs (nursing, refreshments, games, magazines, shampoo, etc.) and the financial involvement. Sometimes a home will charge two dollars or more for tissue—toilet or facial. The administrator of a home may want a large down payment or commitment of the estate at the person's death—though this is common, however, one should evaluate the agreement before giving a sizable holding, house and/or lot of money. Robert Bua, *Inside Guide to America's Nursing Homes*, Amazon.com, explains nursing home alternatives and ranks and rates all certified nursing homes in the U.S.A. This work will give you help in making a decision in this matter and others which are related to this.

Some general recommendations for the choosing of a nursing home are as follows:

1. Be sure that the home is accredited, licensed by the local and state authorities. If there are any questions, call your local health department. The home you are considering should be certified for Medicare or Medicaid in the case this is to be used.
2. The nursing, medical, therapy, rehabilitation services and the social services should be appropriate for your parent's needs.
3. The home, buildings, and yards should be well-kept and attractive. In addition it should be clean, safe, and meet federal and state fire codes and not located in condemned structures however approved.
4. The room for sleeping should be uncrowded with enough room to allow separate seating, dressing tables, and closet space. The furniture should be appropriate, as should the bathing arrangements.
5. Food should be prepared under the most sanitary conditions and should be attractive, varied and possess adequate varieties in order to cover numerous diet needs.
6. Staff personnel should be well-trained and in sufficient numbers to look after the patients. It should be clear who is the chief and subordinate administrators. In other words, to whom do you look for information and input about the care of your parent or parents. A readily available structure for discussing problems is a necessity.
7. If possible, visit the home with your parents in advance of their entering a home so they can meet personnel and see the sort of living conditions that will prevail. Also this gives an opportunity for them to get accustomed to the surroundings; perhaps several trips would be better, particularly where some reluctance to enter exists on the part of your parents.
8. Make sure that the conditions under which the nursing home operates are plainly spelled out; that is, reduced to understandable English and the responsibility of financial obligation and support is understood by yourself.
9. Is attention paid to the patients' morale?
    1. Are they addressed with dignity?
    2. Do they appear to be on sedatives?
    3. Do they have privacy?
    4. Are they dressed in night clothes or street clothes?
    5. Are beauticians and barber available?

10. Medical services:
    1. Do they have a staff physician or doctor available 24-hours a day? How often does the doctor see the patient?
    2. Are provisions for dentist and foot care available?
11. Do they have group activities, i.e., trips, group discussions, a variety of programs, citizenship participation and social services—are they available?

Make a list of the nursing homes thought suitable, near enough for family and friends to visit.

- Learn as much as possible about each nursing home by talking with:
    - People that have loved ones in nursing homes
    - Ministers
    - Health Professionals such as Doctors, Social Workers, Nurses
    - Long Term Care Ombudsman
    - Nursing home employees
- Review state survey inspection reports for each facility
    - Posted in each facility as required by federal law.
    - Available on the Internet at http://www.Medicare.gov/NHCompare/home.asp

Visit and Evaluate Each Nursing Home

Look for the following:

- Do patients appear happy and well taken care of?
- Is the building clean and well maintained?
- Are wheelchairs and other equipment in clean working order?
- Are activity calendars posted with a variety and sufficient number of activities for patients to choose from each day?
- Are patients involved in activities or just sitting around bored with nothing to do?
- Does the food look appetizing and are patients eating most of their meal?
- Does the dining room and kitchen look clean and are cooks wearing hairnets?
- Do the patients look well fed?

- Are the rooms neatly arranged and individually decorated with personal possessions of patients?
- Do staff members interact cheerfully with patients and each other?
- Are patient call lights responded to quickly?
- Does the facility overuse physical restraints (devices that tie patients to chairs or beds)?
- Are staff members responsive to patient or family needs and requests?
- Are staff members visible?
- Are patients treated with dignity and respect?
- Does the linen look clean and not old and thin?
- Is patient privacy protected during patient care and treatment (are room doors and privacy curtains used)?
- Do staff members stop and knock on room doors prior to entering patient rooms?
- Is the facility well lighted?
- How much time alone with a nurse does the patient receive?

Find out

- Are call lights sounding for a long time before being answered?
- Are patients calling out for help?
- Is patient care and information being discussed within hearing range of others?
- Is there an excess amount of noise in the facility caused by staff, intercom, etc.?
- Notice if nurse relation to patients is friendly, supportive and helpful.

Smell

- Do patients smell clean?
- Are there any strong odors in the facility?
- Are rooms well ventilated and kept at a comfortable temperature?

Taste

- Ask to eat a meal and evaluate the quality and taste of the food.

As increasing numbers of our parents are going to live into their eighties and nineties, we may be called upon to assist them in relocating their homes. In the past several decades there has been a movement to the Sunbelt—Florida, Arizona and California. Florida, Utah, Texas, South Dakota, Alaska, Washington, and Wyoming have no state tax. The decreasing metabolic ability of the body as we age makes it difficult for older people to keep warm; the climate compensates for this. Many older people suffer from heart disease, emphysema, and rheumatism which makes physical exertion difficult, hence these locations serve to reduce needed labor—shoveling of snow, handling coal, putting up storm windows, etc. Clothes are cheaper, fuel use cut down, organizations abound which provide many activities—cultural, recreational, and political. Robert Havighurst states that the principal values older people look for in housing are (1) quiet, (2) privacy, (3) independence of action, (4) nearness to relatives and friends, (5) residence among own cultural group, (6) cheapness, and (7) closeness to transportation lines and communal institutions—libraries, shops, movies, recreational centers, churches, etc.

The best types of housing arrangements for older people other than independence in their own homes according to Havighurst seem to be:

1. Small villages or communities in warm climates specially planned for old people. The communities should have shops, movies, churches, a library, restaurants and allow children and pets.
2. Housing units specially designed for older people in all parts of the city, with laundry facilities, adequate protection, and special ramps for the wheelchair persons, elevators, etc.
3. Dwelling units (small apartments) in single-family residences designed for three-generation families. The grandparents have a small apartment of their own which gives them quiet and privacy, and yet they are in the same house with the rest of the family and can help and be helped as need arises.
4. Cooperative housing projects for older people with communal eating, laundry, and other facilities. The Federal Housing Authority has built and is building such projects. Many of these will be close to their children.

5. Old people's homes that are specially equipped to handle those with limited ability to care for themselves.

Three-fourths of the non-institutionalized disabled persons receive all needed assistance from the primary family and friends. Forty percent of nursing home care payments are private and direct out-of-pocket expenditures. Catastrophic costs of long-term nursing homes require in many cases that the patient spend down their resources to become eligible for Medicaid. When Medicare runs out and when all the resources are used up Medicaid becomes the payer. The elderly frequently believe that Medicare alone or combined with private insurance will cover most or all of their long-term care. Unfortunately, this is not usually the case. Recently some communities have developed what is called Life Care Communities also known as Continuing Care Retirement Communities (CCRS). These provide housing, health care, social activities, supporting service and meals. The typical campus consists of independent living units, a nursing facility, a contract with the residents which guarantees health care for more than a year and where the long-time care is shared by the entire community. No one, therefore, has catastrophic expenditure or goes on Medicaid for the expenses are paid from pooled funds from monthly and entry fees. Entry fees range from $100,000 and monthly fees from $1,800 to $3,000 in 2002. There are hundreds of these facilities in the United States and by 2005 or 2006 these are expected to expand to thousands. Unfortunately, a few elderly can afford this type of care. New York State prohibits these contracts in order to protect consumers from unscrupulous operators.

Another type of care arrangement is the Life Care at Home (LCAH). Entry fees range from $5,000 to $10,000, monthly fees from $150 to $200 per month. The service provided is for the lifetime. Therapies at home are provided, such as physical, speech, occupational, electronic monitoring, respite and day care, personal care, and homemaker services. Physician and hospital care is also given to the elderly.

In a work by Vivian Carin and Ruth Mansberg entitled *Where Can Mom Live?*, the authors discuss several arrangements for living. One is Group-Shared Homes—this arrangement allows for 5 to 15 persons to buy a building, renovate it or build another. Share-a-home began in Florida as a non-profit organization banding compatible persons together to pool their resources to pay their living costs. A smaller version of this is where two or three women rent an apartment and share the expenses. The work required is shared as is cleaning responsibility and meal preparation. The group is supportive of individual members' problems and health needs. A greater degree of independence is available in this setting as opposed to the institutional home or to live with children or other relatives. The secret here is to find persons of common background, flexibility and interests. Saving a large entry fee payment to a Care Community such as the LLC or LCAH's is a distinct possibility.

A second type is the Congregate Community. This arrangement provides a studio apartment with one bedroom. There is a monthly fee covering rent, two meals a day (noon and night), housekeeping services and a variety of social, recreational, and cultural programs. A person must be over 62 and ambulatory to enroll. Individuals have the freedom to come and go as they want and the community has a residence council composed of the renters which meets once a month to discuss programs and problems of the group.

Another type of arrangement allows for the individual to remain in their home (28 million live in their own home or a realty one—8 million alone) and use the mortgage equity of the home to pay their living expenses. This plan is known as the Home Equity Conversion plan. It usually pays rates adjusted to the forecast of the owner's longevity. The money is given on a monthly basis and begins once the contracts are signed following examination of the deed and appraisal of the home. These opportunities have been available in Buffalo, NY, in Wisconsin and California and are available in other places. However, due to the possibility of heir suits contesting the sale of the home and lenders concern for fixed rates many are wary of this type of loan.

The Mobile Home Pool is a situation where many elderly persons are now living. It is not age specific and not organized for the elderly but many retired and older persons (often a majority) are living there despite the high density. There is the advantage of paying low rent, opportunity for developing friendships and finding a support group. Usually located near towns and cities where there is access to supplies, health facilities, churches, and recreational opportunities.

Alternatives to Nursing Homes

Assisted-living facilities: If your loved one doesn't need the level of medical care offered by a nursing home, consider an assisted-living facility, where residents get help with tasks such as cooking and laundry. These facilities are listed in the Yellow Pages of your phone directory. But be aware: They are less tightly regulated than nursing homes.

Home health care: This is an increasingly available option that its advocates say is more cost-efficient than nursing-home care and more supportive of an elderly person's dignity and independence. For more information and an agency locator, contact the National Association for Home Care and Hospice. www.nahc.org/

Sun City (Arizona) and Leisure World (California) are for those who can anticipate retirement early. The age requirement for living in these communities is too young and requires too much outlay for most people to consider. One must be between 48-55 years of age. Children under 18 are not allowed. One must purchase a condominium and pay certain homeowners fees. Climate and recreation are the principal calling cards but the expenses and age requirement prohibits the average families from this arrangement.

Things You Should Know

1. Medicare is divided into two parts:

   Part A—it is a federal insurance for those on Social Security or with permanent kidney failure. Typically it pays most hospital care cost.

   Part B—medical insurance is paid for by monthly premiums for your doctor's services, other medical services and supplement covered by Medical A.

   Under Part A hospital can help pay for in-patient hospital care, in-patient care in a skilled nursing facility, home health care, and hospice care. Part B can help pay for medically necessary doctor's services, outpatient hospital services and other medical services and supplies not covered by the hospital insurance part of Medicare. Medicare supplemental insurance covers most of the medical expenses Medicare does not pay.

2. Each elderly person living alone should have a pill container with compartments for each day, support rails, and a bathing tub with safety features, and a large calendar for medical appointments. Many counties have mobile medical van units such as exists in Broward County (Ft. Lauderdale, Florida). Florida dispenses optometric services, dentistry and medical for the elderly poor and those on Medicare.

3. If your parent(s) becomes or is disabled, you may obtain assistance from a Client Rights Advocate in counties and cities usually operated by the state. These agents can often represent people having difficulty with a grievance over services and their delivery. You can solicit the help of an Ombudsman who is empowered by federal law to inter-

vene on the patient's and/or families behalf in regards to nursing home problems. Confidentiality is maintained if patient or family request. The Ombudsman will investigate your problem and assist in resolving the problem on your behalf with the nursing home.

4. If the cost of medication is prohibitive, low-income eligible persons can get money from state pharmaceutical programs.

Most medical plans—including Medicare—cover very little long-term care, if at all! In general, they cover your stay in a hospital, but provide limited coverage, at best, for nursing home and home care. Medicare (for people 65 and over) only pays for a limited amount of "Skilled nursing care" which is NOT the same thing as custodial care (which is the kind of long-term care most people need). And what Medicare doesn't pay, your Medicare Supplement won't pay either.

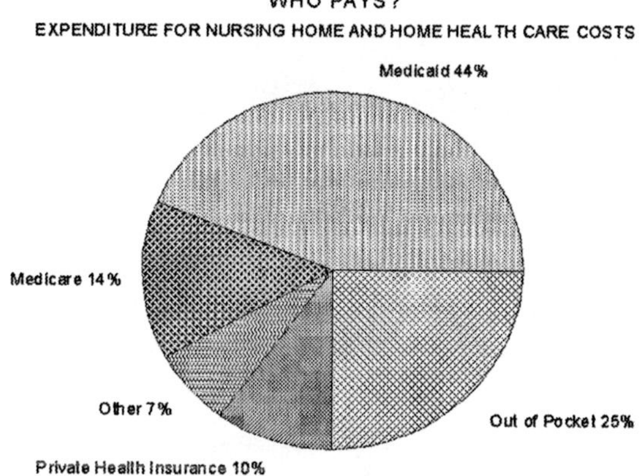

Source: Department of Health and Human Services, HCFA, Office of the Actuary, National Health Statistics Group, Personal Health Care Expenditures, 2001.

Long-term plans cover different types of care. Some only pay for long-term care in a nursing home. Others also cover long-term care you receive in your own home or other settings.

The AARP Long-Term Care Insurance Plan underwritten by MetLife pays benefits for the following kinds of care: in a nursing home, at home, in an assisted living facility, in an adult day care facility and even for something called "informal care" (when friends or relatives provide care), depending on the plan you select. In Massachusetts, assisted living facilities are referred to as "alternate facilities" and adult day care is referred to as "adult day health."

The Income of Average Persons Needs Protection

The average length of stay is 2.4 years.[1] And that's the average. Multiply that by the national average cost of $52,000 a year[2] and you'll see the cost of that stay can exceed $124,800!

1. National Center for Health Statistics, U.S. Department of Health and Human Services—The National Nursing Home Survey—June 2002
2. Mature Market Institute, AMetLife Market Survey on Nursing Home Home Care Costs, © 2002

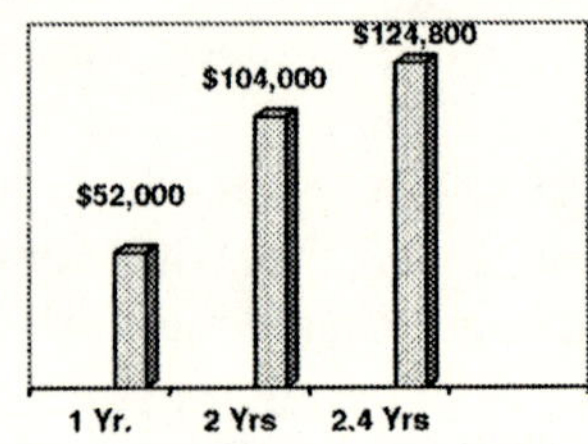

According to an AARP Study (2002) a majority of the 50 or over have at least one chronic illness among Medicare recipients. Eighty-two percent of those 85 or older have at least two ongoing problems.

Women are Vulnerable

Seventy-five percent of nursing home residents are women, two-thirds of home-care participants and more than seven of ten unpaid care givers. Women are the main caretakers. The average woman can expect to spend 17 years caring for a child and 15 years caring for a parent (U.S. Department of Labor, 2000).

Alzheimer's Covered

Virtually all plans, including the AARP Plan, cover care needed by an insured customer who *develops* Alzheimer's. Coverage you can buy will provide Automatic Inflation Protection. 1) Automatic Inflation Protection (your initial premium is higher, but your benefit amount increases every year like clockwork) or 2) Periodic Inflation Protection (each year you get a choice to increase your benefits, at an additional cost—or let them be). Automatic inflation protection could be the best way to help you feel confident that what you buy today will be what you need tomorrow. This is AARP's plan. Others operate similarly.

Who Will Need A Nursing Home?

People of age 65 face at least a 40% lifetime risk of entering a nursing home—10% will stay 5 years or longer.*

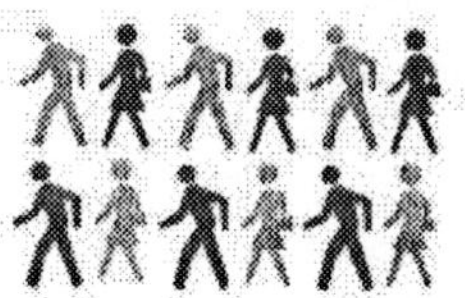

*HIAA, "Guide to Long-Term Care Insurance," 2002

Don't Wait Until You're 70

If you buy it younger (in your 50's or 60's, for example), it's usually much less expensive to buy insurance. With most plans, the longer you wait to buy, the more it will cost you—for the exact same coverage. And you also run the risk that something will change in your health and you won't be able to qualify—at any price.

Remember

Long-term care can help save retirement, assets and aid in your independence at a time when you're most dependent. Most long-term care insurance policies provide coverage to assist in paying for care at home, in adult day care centers, and in assisted living facilities.

THE BIGGEST FEAR/Loss of Independence

In an AARP survey, older Americans with disabilities expressed their biggest worries about the future.

	All Respondents	Ages 50 to 64	Ages 65 and Over
Loss of independence	26%	27%	25%
Loss of mobility	28%	24%	32%
Being unable to pay for the cost of care services	20%	19%	20%
Becoming housebound confined to living quarters	8%	8%	7%
Loss or decrease of financial assets	8%	10%	7%
Not applicable	10%	12%	9%

About Costs and Finances

Long Term Care Insurance

Of those 65 nearly one in three will spend three months or more in a nursing home, and one in four will spend one year or more. Nursing home care can cost 30 to 60 thousand dollars a year—the problem with long term care is the lack of preparation for the costs incurred when someone you love requires assistance. Some people can pay the bill themselves, others will qualify for Medicaid (welfare), but most will fall somewhere in between.

When shopping for long-term care insurance, keep in mind

* Is the daily benefit going to cover the cost of a nursing home stay in your area? Remember, New York City is twice as expensive as Des Moines, Iowa.
* A policy with lifetime coverage is expensive. A policy with a three or four year benefit period is probably a reasonable gamble. Inflation coverage, a 5 percent compounded option on the whole is best.
* During elimination periods, usually 20, 30, 60, 90, or 100 days, you must pay for the nursing home. The larger the elimination period

(deductible, the lower the premium. Keep your elimination period low. And answer all health questions truthfully. If you're not sure of an answer write, "Please see the records of Dr. Jones" or write "I do not recall" (not "I don't know").

* Long-term care policies vary in how they determine that you are sufficiently disabled to required long-term care—make sure you understand this. And know how to file a claim. Many policies require written notice to the company within 30 days of disability, a difficult task for someone who may now be seriously disabled. Make sure your premium payment is automatically deducted from a bank account.

In the future, if you find you or a loved one are in need of skilled services, you may wish to make the Medicare program an important part of your insurance coverage. Since Medicare is a complicated program governed by numerous rules and regulations, many of which change from time to time, I will try to explain some of the more frequent misunderstood aspects of the program, as well as the benefits of Medicare. I want to help you take the guesswork out of Medicare.

Medicare Benefits Can Help You to Live and Recover at a Skilled Facility provided

- You have been a hospital patient for 3 consecutive days, not counting the day of discharge.
- You are admitted to the skilled nursing facility within 30 days of your hospital discharge.
- The services you require are related to the condition for which you were treated in the hospital.
- You require skilled nursing services or rehabilitation services on a daily basis.
- These services, as a practical matter, can only be provided on an inpatient basis.
- Your doctor orders and certifies at time of admission that you need skilled care services on daily basis, and again, certifies your need 14 days after admission and every 30 days thereafter.
- A Utilization Review Committee of professionals regularly reviews and approves your continued need for skilled care services.
- Your stay in the skilled nursing facility is 100 days or less.

You May Receive Help From Medicare On All These Services:

- a semi-private room
- all meals, including special diets
- nursing care
- rehabilitative therapies
- drugs prescribed by a physician
- medical supplies
- use of appliances and equipment

What Kinds of Illnesses or Disabilities Does Medicare Ordinarily Cover in a Skilled Care Facility?

Many different illnesses or disabilities can be covered by Medicare hospital insurance—Part A. Your eligibility for coverage depends on your need for skilled care services on a daily basis. A skilled care service is defined as a service that is provided on a daily basis directly by or requiring the supervision of a licensed nurse or registered therapist. The following services are considered the most common skilled care services: decubitus care; Levine tube; intravenous therapy; sterile dressings; tracheostomy care (if surgery is recent); daily multiple injections; physical, speech and occupational therapy which must be required on a daily basis. The facility's staff should be glad to assist you in determining whether an illness or disability qualifies for Medicare coverage.

How Many Days of Service Will Medicare Hospital Insurance—Part A, Help Pay For In A Skilled Nursing Facility?

Medicare hospital insurance—*Part A* helps pay for up to 100 days in a participating skilled nursing facility in each benefit period. The 100 days of coverage are not automatic since continued eligibility for coverage remains in effect only as long as the preceding conditions are met and skilled care services are required on a daily basis. The foregoing information explains the maximum coverage under Medicare hospital insurance—*Part A*. However, actual experience shows that patients receive an average of about 24 days of covered care. For health plan choices use the Medical Personal Plan Finder, for help call 1-800-Medicare, and the Medicare and You 2005 handbook.

HOSPITAL INSURANCE—PART A (MEDICARE)

Service: Skilled Nursing Facilities Certified By Medicare (Inpatient)

First 20 Days: You Pay Nothing, Medicare Pays 100%

Next 80 Days: You Pay $105.00 a day, Medicare pays balance of covered charges. Typically the number of days likely drops and costs rise somewhat each year.

Requirements

Admission to a skilled nursing facility must occur within 30 days of a hospital confinement of 3 ore more days; must be an extension of the hospital treatment; and must be for daily skilled nursing and/or therapy services which as a practical matter can only be provided on an inpatient basis.

Not Covered

Private duty nurses, first three pints of blood, personal convenience items such as barber, beautician, personal laundry, private telephone and television.

MEDICARE INSURANCE—PART B

Service: Skilled Nursing Facilities, Certified By Medicare (Outpatient)

Doctor's visits; physical, occupational, and speech therapy; lab and X-ray services; prosthetic devices and some supplies and equipment.

Unlimited Time Limit: You pay one annual deductible of $100 plus 20% of the balance of reasonable charges, Medicare Pays balance of reasonable charges.

*Beneficiaries of Medicare Insurance—Part B must satisfy only one $100 deductible. All products or services covered by Part B count toward that deductible.

Requirements

Not eligible for Medicare Part A (Hospital Insurance) benefits.

Not Covered:

Most central supplies, pharmacy, personal items, and room and board.

*If you want more detailed information about your Medicare benefits, contact the administrator of a nursing home you are considering or other homes you know something about.

It should be noted that whether or not your parents live with you or live alone they are entitled to claim on the federal income tax up to $3,750 at 65; a couple can claim $6,200 if they do not itemize their tax and $9,400 filing jointly. If both were under and both retired on permanent and total disability, a claim on federal tax can be made for $7,500. Also if one was 65 and lives apart from the spouse or under 65 on permanent and total disability. Single and 65 can claim $5,000. As one under 65 retired and on permanent and total disability. A thousand dollars for qualified contribution if your AGI (adjusted gross income) is $25,000 or less.

Your parents do not have to file any income tax return if their taxable income is less than $8,850 single and jointly $15,650 if under 65, $7,700 and both over 65, $13,850. You should check retirement income credit (designed to help people who do not have tax-exempt social security income, Medicare or Medicaid). Give attention to medical and drug expenses as deductions if itemizing special tax breaks like some states (Minnesota, Connecticut, North Dakota, etc.) give to elderly renters and assess the cost of your care for your parents. If you contribute over fifty percent of their living expenses the IRS allows you to claim them as exemptions. A word about health plans, frequently insurance companies enroll those 65 or older; the coverage should be broad for if you count solely on Medicare there is usually a gap between the cost of hospitalization and what it pays. One such plan is the AARP's (American Association of Retired Persons) plan underwritten by the MetLife Insurance offering protection to members and their spouses over 65 if covered by Medicare Part A and B. Membership in AARP is available at low rates (recently [2004] $12.50 for a year) for those over 50. In 2003, the Medicare Supplement II cost $11.95 per month. Medicare M6 Supplement (AARP, 1909 K Street, NW, Washington DC 20049) with increased benefits costing $25.95 a month.

Medicare Update—New Preventive Help

Beginning in 2005 New Cardiovascular Screening blood Tests. Ask your doctor what is included and how frequently available. Also, included is colorectal cancer screening.

Certain people with Medicare who are at risk for diabetes starting 2005. Provides self-management training, glaucoma testing, PAP tests and pelvic exams and breast exams.

Prostate Cancer Screening
Screening Mammograms
Physical Examination for those with Part B Medicare within the first six months
Shots (vaccinations, Flu and Pneumococcal Shot)

Prescription drug plans starts January 1, 2006. You must register. Talk to Social Security and Medicare about cost for general information call 1-800-633-4227, they will help you find the answer to most questions you have.

NOTE: Medicare Drug benefit starts in 2006, offers extra help for people on limited incomes. Registration and enrollment open from November 2005 to May 2006. A review follows. Applications will be sent in Spanish and English.

CAN YOU QUALIFY?

Who Can Enroll	Level 1	Level 2	Level 3	Level 4
In addition to being on Medicare, in 2005, you must be receiving the following:	Full Medicaid benefits and income no higher than $9,570 (single) or $12,830 (couple)	Medicaid (but with income higher than level 1); **or** SSI (without Medicaid); **or** Medicare premiums paid by your state	Income no higher than $12,919 (single) or $17,320 (couple)	Income no higher than $14,255 (single) or $19,245 (couple)
Value of assets (holdings but not including your home, vehicles, burial plot or personal possessions)	Not applicable	Not applicable	No more than $7,500 (single) or $12,000 (couple)	No more than $11,500 (single) or $23,000 (couple)
Eligibility	Automatically enrolled	Automatically enrolled	Must apply	Must apply
WHAT YOU GET				
Drug coverage	Full (no gap)	Full (no gap)	Full (no gap)	Full (no gap)
Monthly premium	$0	$0	$0	Reduced on sliding scale based on income
Yearly deductible	$0	$0	$0	$50
Co-payment on prescription	$1 for generics, $3 for brands ($0 if you're in a nursing home)	$2 for generics $5 for brands	$2 for generics $5 for brands	15 percent of cost of each prescription
Co-payment under catastrophic coverage	$0	$0	$0	$2 for generics $5 for brands

SOURCES: Centers for Medicare & Medicaid Services; Social Security Administration; AARP Public Policy Institute

Some people will be fearful of registering due to the complete questions asked and the length of the application (4 pages). They are afraid to reveal information they think may hurt them in getting other help.

The Parent in the Home with Children

For one reason or the other—custom, economics, or compassion, we decide to move our parents into our home. Frequently, we have at the same time preteen or teenage youngsters also to look after. And, top compound the difficulties, it happens when we as middlescents are also trying to forward our own interests. As mentioned earlier, we are destined to serve a middleman function. Sometimes parents refuse even when it is affordable to enter a nursing home saying "you just want to get rid of me" and "I'll never survive the experience." Few middlescent children can withstand this sort of appeal.

Many of our parents can make a good adjustment when moved to our home. Helping services in the home offer an advantage in that they are free due to the use of unpaid labor of household members. The children often love listening to the grandparent or playing cards and games with a companion. Grandparents frequently relate well with the young, even teenagers; for one thing they do not have the ultimate responsibility and sometimes they form an emotional tie with your children against the establishment, meaning you and/or your spouse, unfortunately. This comes out usually as being more permissive with your kids or a desire to rearrange something in their daily schedule or to do something special for them. One lady told me that her mother lived with her for twenty years—we had to take her in because she couldn't afford to live by herself. My mother, she said, followed me around from room to room always wanting to know what I was doing; consequently, I grabbed every opportunity to get out of the house. But my husband was a 'saint' with her. My five children loved her dearly and they all came to her funeral when she died. Some youngsters!

When I was a boy, my family—mother, a brother and sister, moved in with my mother's parents following the death of my father both for economic reasons and to care for them. I delighted in listening to the stories of old times from my grandfather; my brother, a pre-theological student discussed the Bible with him to their mutual joy. My sister had been a favorite of grandma and had visited her on many previous occasions took naturally to looking after her. All was not tranquility, however, for even though we made a separate apartment including a living room, bedroom, porch off the living room and private bath for my grandparents, the noise in the other living room with visiting teenage friends got a sharp proclamation from grandma or grandpa at 9 o'clock—"It's time for decent people to be in bed!" Mother also had to always prepare two breakfast meals—one at 7 a.m. for the grandparents and one at 8 a.m. for the children. Lunch was another matter and served twelve o'clock sharp—(This took some running from school at lunch to make it.) and supper at 6 o'clock. The diet needs of the old folks were sometimes inserted into the common meals for all of us much to our chagrin at times. Later my grandmother suffering the effects of hardening of the arteries had flights from reality; she would get up at 2 a.m., go to the kitchen and initiate a series of cooking—frequently country ham which she loved to have but was restricted from by her physician—this often got everyone up—scurrying downstairs when we heard her rattling the pans or smelling smoke in order to save her from fire or choking to death! For myself, I wouldn't have had anything different for I, like many people, loved my folks!

It does require some planning to make things go reasonably well. In the first place, our parents need privacy. If an apartment or additional room can be built to your home for them, then this can serve as a retreat and a place to visit with their friends who come to call. One thing about our older people is that they require a routine; irregular meals are a no-no; the same is true of noise, a lot of people coming and going, the slamming of doors and revving up a car motor are taboo. This is not because old people are cranky. Their sensory systems do not accommodate to high decibel and cacophony of sound like the young. Even though this is true, it isn't fair to re-organize everything around the life of our parents and require younger members of the family to re-style their lives to accommodate our parents. A good place to start is prior to their becoming a part of the household if this is possible. This conversation should include expectations freely given—you have your life, they have theirs and the children have theirs. Hopefully with a good deal of respect, you can have but a common life and individual ones and things will go smoothly. The following are some general principles which could help in these matters:

1. It should be understood that you have some things to do: social affairs, church obligations, visiting, vacationing time for children, and work tasks which will have to be attended to by you and/or your spouse without them being included many times. The close-knit family of the Waltons rarely exists, in fact, but if it does with you then you have less concern here.

Ann Landers once reported a situation where the wife's husband's mother and grandmother moved in with them. They had an apartment built off the kitchen for Mama and Grandpa with complete cooking facilities. They prepared their own breakfast and lunch. The wife cooked the dinner for all of them. The problem was that the wife worked all day surrounded by people.

When she got home, she wanted peace and quiet—time to be alone. But Mama and Grandpa insisted on having the door open all the time so that they "could feel a part of the household." It drove the woman crazy for they not only watched her, they asked questions by the dozen which interfered with the dinner preparation. She writes to ask is she selfish to want some privacy? The reply was that Mama and Grandma need to know this is one of your ways to get some relaxation and you need peace and quiet when you prepare the meal; therefore, the door will have to be closed.

2. It is not selfish to ask for some respite and to be alone because you need some peace to survive. Many, many different kinds of irritations like this one occur in these situations—husbands and wives both need some time when they are not on call and this should be understood by our parents. (If not, a talk about this will generally insure their cooperation and support.)

Rules When Parents Live With Us

1. If your parents can help financially, accept it, for it will give them a feeling of self-respect by knowing they are helping. If they want to give this on a regular basis, do not spurn it.

2. In the same manner, the help that can be given with the chores around the house should be welcomed; this tends to ward off their over-dependence and has the effect of bolstering their egos.

3. Privacy should be given—children, should along with other adults, respect our parents and allow them to have their own social and individual lives. This means also that our children do not have access to their possessions and belongings.

4. Do not give advice except as a last resort. When your idea is wanted or needed, your parents will come to you. Remember, they respect you for taking your own medicine—so don't give any more advice than you yourself are prepared to take—in short, be gentle with criticism.

5. It should be understood by both parents and children that sharing is expected and that no one is a privileged character in the home. Rules for meals, times to do certain things, use of the bathroom, tidying up, consideration by youngsters at night or loud talk and c.d.'s playing and the reverse for older par-

ents in the morning when they are about earlier than most everyone else in the household.

6. It has been said that "no roof is big enough for two families" and there is some truth to this saying. When irritation builds, as it will from time to time, maybe a visitation to other relatives and friends can be arranged. I remember a situation where a mother once or twice a year would say she and the daughter-in-law were at an impasse (she had it up to her throat), so she'd go visit a sister or friend for a couple of weeks. When she got back, the air would have cleared and life once again was livable.

The understanding of these rules should be accomplished early in anticipation of moving parents in with your family. Our children constantly need to be reminded of these rules. Initially cooperative, they come to view, when frustrated by certain restrictions, their grandparents as interlopers. We know, however, that older folks need more psychological stroking (praise and kind words) than do the young. They have fewer friends, activities and opportunities through which to be complimented. As they get very old or sick, their perceptions turn inward due to increased body monitoring—their sleep, digestion, pain and irritations from being unable to get around as well as they would like. The physical needs come increasingly to dominate their lives like the baby whose needs and developmental level make him completely oblivious to his social surroundings—he cries, vomits, urinates, and defecates at will with little control, no concern. The very old at some point approach this situation—so we need patience to tolerate and function—in short to survive. Understanding their problem should prepare their sons and daughters mentally to undertake the care and assist you to survive yourself in better fashion. Hopefully, good luck!

Abuse of the Elderly

The last thing a child would want to do would be to abuse his mother or father. Nevertheless it happens one way or the other with a spouse or child being equally the perpetrator. The elderly are often like children, they have limited perspectives and cannot decenter but they should be treated with care. We need to remember that abuse is often related to neglect. Neglect—depriving the parent of medicine, food or care ten times a week is considered abuse through neglect. Remember 4 hours a day for each patient is the usual standard for one-on-one care in a nursing facility. Physical abuse can range to being pushed, grabbed, shoved to being assaulted with a gun or knife. In a study reported ten or so years ago (Gerontologist Journal) the elderly (2,020 surveyed) were at greater risk when they lived with others and conversely of lesser risk when they lived in their own place even with their spouse. The abused represented the major religions, 62% had incomes under $15,000, 35% had incomes over $15,000, 40% lived alone and 40% were over 75. Finally, men are more at risk than women though women abuse is more serious. Where you are having a problem due to long-time frustration, sick/lack of resources or burn-out and are peaked to strike out or deny care to your kinsman you should counsel with a minister or call other family members or an agency for instant social agency whose number you can find in the phone directory. The crisis help-lines is another source of help. Some relief is needed in these cases or assistance to get things going normally again. Guidelines on these matters follow:

Suspicion or Knowledge of Abuse or Neglect Should Be Reported Immediately to the:

- nursing supervisor on duty.
- nursing home Administrator and/or Director of Nursing.
- local police.
- State Department of Human Services, Adult Protective Services.
- State Ombudsman.
- State Survey Agency.

Definitions

Abuse: the willful infliction of injury, unreasonable confinement, intimidation, or punishment with resulting physical harm, pain, or mental anguish.

Many states have laws requiring reports of abuse and neglect.

Neglect: the failure to provide goods and services necessary to avoid physical harm, mental anguish, or mental illness. Neglect occurs when nursing home staff fails to monitor and/or supervise the delivery of patient care and services to assure that care is provided as needed by the patient. Some examples of neglect might include: lack of assistance in eating, drinking, walking, bathing, toileting, or ignoring call bells/lights. Neglect can cause depression, dehydration, incontinence, and/or pressure sores.

Verbal Abuse: the use of oral, written, or gestured language that willfully includes disparaging and derogatory terms to patients or their families, or within their hearing distance regardless of their age, ability to comprehend, or disability.

Sexual Abuse: includes but is not limited to, sexual harassment, sexual coercion, or sexual assault.

Physical Abuse: includes hitting, slapping, pinching, and kicking. It also includes controlling behavior through corporal punishment.

Mental Abuse: includes, but is not limited to, humiliation, harassment, threats of punishment or deprivation.

Involuntary Seclusion: the separation of a patient from other patients, or from her/his room or confinement to her/his room against the patient's will.

Misappropriation of Patient Property: the deliberate misplacement, exploitation, or wrongful, temporary or permanent use of a patient's belongings or money without the patient's consent.

When Problems Arise

1. **Speak Directly to the Individuals Involved**

Many times individuals fail to realize there is a problem. Speaking up in a non-threatening way can help focus the staff on the problem and bring about a quick resolution. If the staff indicates the problem is out of their control or too big of a problem for them to handle alone, ask what you can do to help or whom else you should go speak to about the problem. Above all, remain calm and in control of your emotions. Anger will bring nothing more than a negative reaction from others.

2. **Speak to a Supervisor of the Individuals Involved in the Problem**

Ask to speak with the immediate supervisor of the staff members involved. If it is a Certified Nurse Aid, speak to the charge nurse. If it is a charge nurse, speak to the Director of Nursing. Follow the same pattern for other disciplines.

3. **Obtain a Copy of the Nursing Home's Grievance Policy/Procedure**

Medicaid regulations and state law require nursing homes to have a written grievance or complaint handling policy or procedure. Follow the procedures outlined. The procedure will designate a staff person, usually a Social Worker, to review and follow up on grievances brought to their attention. Sometimes the policy will outline other individuals to contact within the nursing home, such as the administrator, if you are still not satisfied after speaking with the Social Worker. The policy may further list individuals outside the nursing home, but still connected to the nursing home, such as an owner or company official.

4. **Contact the State Long-Term Care Ombudsman**

These types of Ombudsmen are interested in protecting the aged and those with health problems. They are versed in state law and licensure of nursing home facilities and will readily intervene for you with those charged with your family member to bring about improvement.

5. **Report Problem to State Survey Agency**

This agency is required to investigate complaints involving the health or safety of patients within two working days. The agency can only take punitive action against a nursing home when during their inspection/visit they prove a problem exists and it violates nursing home regulations. This agency licenses nursing homes and inspects nursing homes on a yearly basis. When surveyors are in a nursing home, take advantage of the opportunity you have to speak with them regarding your concerns. Surveyors are required to interview patients concerning the quality of care they are receiving from the nursing home.

6. **Don't Ever Give Up!**

It can be frustrating at times when you feel no one cares or is listening to you. Don't give up. Find that person in the center or government agency that will listen and help you.

About Our Parent's Money

Perhaps it is more relevant to talk about wills, gifts, and estate taxes in the chapter on death, but it occurs to me that it should be mentioned here. Talks about money with our parents should take place when possible before they are senile, terminally ill, or have mental distortions. In 1976, the Tax Reform Act was passed making gifts given in the last three years of a person's life subject to estate tax laws. Monies and gifts, endowments, etc., given away before this time (three years) will be excluded from tax liability. Inheritance tax can be a very sizable amount. One family looking forward to receiving a fat estate from auntie at her last bequest was shocked at the tax take due to recency of her gift making. If wills are not made, the matter of who gets the property, monies—in short, the estate may very well be up for grabs with you losing out completely. You should gently, tactfully discuss this with your parent and/or parents. Also it is of dire necessity that you insist that they keep or get the records of their stocks, deeds, savings bonds, bankbooks, statement sand insurance policies, etc., and you should know of any contracts they have made. The physician of my mother's father put a tremendous lien on our family estate for bills that we thought had been paid. We had sometimes paid the bills ourselves. But in absence of all but meager evidence we "paid in full." Sometimes our parents decide they would like to give their money (it maybe little) away to a venture, charity or an evangelist. This is a touchy matter, it may be all right in fact commendable, but frankly in many cases it amounts to bilge and smooth glove swindle. The best tactic here is to be persuasive but careful, not losing your cool over it; if it is impossible to convince your parents, then attempt to get them to agree to temporize the matter, to put off the decision, time will usually be a good ally and often circumvent the useless giving away of funds that the parent will need or you in their service.

If you are going to be responsible for your parents there are some facts which can assist you in planning. The requirement of funds is a necessity and whether or not we are in the middle income bracket $30,000 to $60,000 or higher, we need all the help we can get from outside sources—agencies, local, state, and federal.

The typical woman will live nearly 18.7 years after she is 65; for the man at 65, 14.5 years. At age 75, seventy percent of the men still living are married whereas seventy percent of the women are widowed. With two parents (man and wife) it may be more economical to keep them in the home and to supplement their care needs through you. Since forty percent of the homes of the elderly were built before 1939, upkeep could be helped and/or agencies.

HELP AVAILABLE NOW

Program	***Nursing home***	***Home Care***
Medicare	Skilled-nursing care covered only in approved facilities: 100 of eligible expenses for 20 days; all but $105.00 a day for next 80 days; nothing after that; no custodial or intermediate care.	Only part-time, intermittent skilled care and speech or physical therapy covered. Person must be confined to home and care-provider must agree to reimbursement seven days care not to exceed 8 hours per day and 28 hours a week sometimes 30 hours under Medicare rules. Patient must pay 20% co-insurance for durable medical equipment. Annual flu and pneumonia shots, annual mammograms and pap smears for high risk women, once every three years for others (Part B) deductible is waived.
Medicaid	Skilled, intermediate, and custodial care covered once a person's assets and income drop below state Medicaid limits.	Part-time nursing and home-health aids provided if requested by physician for those eligible for Medicaid. States have the option to offer a variety of non-medical home-care services.
Medicare supple-ment policies	Benefits range from nothing to the policy limits for sharing the cost of care for days 21-100; after that, policies pay a set amount each day. Custodial or intermediate care usually not covered.	Nothing covered. Call State Medical Assistance office in your state's capital.
Ordinary health insurance policies	Very limited post-hospital, convalescent, skilled-nursing care covered, but usually no custodial or intermediate care.	Very limited post-hospital convalescent care may be covered.
Veterans Administration	Skilled-nursing care provided only in VA facilities on a space-available basis for eligible veterans. If you are a veteran, call 1-800-827-1000 for available services.	Chronically ill eligible veterans, eligible for medical, nursing, and rehabilitative care.

Additional Sources of Help

The Older American Act provides new services to frail elderly in the home and adult care centers. This law provides for an assessment of the services centers provide and the demand for support services. It also will provide reimbursement or supplements to centers serving 60 persons or more per day and health education programs in centers. My visit to a small community to a senior center (integrated) recently (funded by the State) had a well-organized program of activities running from 8:30 to 1:30 five days a week; included a good lunch, health care information and clinics, recreational trips, tax help, an opportunity to learn new skills. This is an answer for some for a half day relief for caretakers, part-time employed caretakers and those who need a holiday or time to manage their own affairs.

Nursing Homes

The typical home providing long-term care cost at the beginning of 2003 is $4,500 per month or $54,000 per year and up to $75,000 in a metropolitan area (Consumer's Report). This national average figure is higher than in some areas even urban areas it may still be around $1,200 a month (Hampton Roads, Virginia—Norfolk, Portsmouth, Virginia Beach, Hampton and Newport News). In places like New York City, Boston, Chicago, Los Angeles up to $3,500 plus per month. If one gets a private room, this raises the cost. Many homes provide a variety of services—personal care—beauty and barber shops availability, therapies, medical attention with access to physicians, and social and informational program. Medicare pays for 100 days in a skilled nursing facility. You must need skilled nursing or rehabilitation services only provided in an inpatient facility. Must begin within 3 days of discharge from a hospital after a stay of 3 days or more. The average length of stay is 456 days. Hence, the need of a good nursing home policy.

A Desirable Policy

Features of Care	What's Recommended
Daily nursing-home benefit	$150.00
Waiting period	60 days
Maximum benefit period for one stay	4 years
Maximum benefit period for all stays Note: a rider—restoration benefits separate illness, start over with benefits.	5 years
Does it pay full benefits in:	
Skilled-nursing facility?	Yes
Intermediate facility?	Yes
Custodial facility? (Unable to do 2 of the 5 activities of daily living, that is bathe, are incontinent, dressing, eating, toileting, transferring in mobility) (If not, what does it pay?)	Yes
If it has a prior-hospitalization rule, does coverage begin within 30 days after a hospital stay of at least 3 days? Most do not have rule 100% of daily benefits.	Yes
Does it pay home-care benefits?	Yes
Does it pay these without requiring nursing-home care, or a hospital stay?	Yes
Does it have waiver of premium?	Yes
Is it guaranteed renewable for life?	Yes
Is Alzheimer's disease covered by specific policy language?	Yes
Does the premium stay level for life?	Yes
What is the Best's rating of the company?	A or A+
No premium is recommended; premiums vary with the age of the policyholder and coverage.	B

Adult Day Care

In moderate sized cities (100,000-350,000) care can be obtained for $15-$30 a day, however, in larger cities it may range as high as $40 a day. The typical day is from 9:00 a.m. to 5:00 p.m. Services can run from monitoring cardiovascular problems, nutrition, medicine taking, to some therapy, information on tax, exercise programs, to entertainment. Usually one meal is given plus a snack. Some centers are limited to a meal, a place to meet to socialize and play games and perhaps a program or two at holiday time—Christmas, Thanksgiving, and Valentine's Day. Some day care centers are supported by state or federal government and are virtually free to the indigent and low-income person. Sometimes these centers take a daily collection to help defray some of the costs. An example of a center's cost and service can be seen from this report by the director of the Heritage Day Health Center in Columbus, Ohio.

> One of our clients was a 78-year-old man living with his sister, who was herself in fairly poor health. Both wanted to stay together in the community. Because our center is subsidized, we are able to charge fees to clients based on their income. We charged this man only $1 per day because his medical bills were so high and his income low. He had no health benefits and his income was just over Medicaid eligibility. The center also help him control his high medical bills by providing health monitoring through the staff nurse, who reported any change to his physician. Adult day care can therefore enhance the doctor-patient relationship by providing preventive care and education. For example, the nurse educated him about generic medications, which cut his pharmacy bill at least in half. This is one illustration of how cost-effective day care can be.

Many day care centers (20%) are private and non-profit and should be less expensive. Also some centers are not licensed (over 40% said a recent survey by the organization Adult Day Care) and therefore affects the overall quality.

Home Care

The cost of home care may range as high as $40 a day particularly when the elderly need extensive amounts of care. Medicare will pay for speech, physical, therapies, part-time skilled nursing, medical supplies but do not pay for full-time nursing, drugs, meals delivered to the home, homemaker services or blood transfusions. Home care is usually available on once a day basis for helping with a meal, medicine monitoring to check the condition of the patient.

Kelly Girl Assistance

This help is available on a four-hour minimum in a number of cities. This care is found under other names but usually works the same. Assistance is offered 1 to 7 days per week at a cost of $6 to $10 an hour. The aids sometimes are nurses who have had formal training in vocational schools or hospitals.

The Kelly Girl agency requires nursing care experience. Companionship service is offered for as low as $6.40 an hour, however, in some places this can be as high as $70 to $80 a day.

Intermediate Care Facility

Usually requires at least a month's stay with the cost of a semi-private room running from $65 to $85 a day, a private room $75 to $110 a day. A variety of therapies are provided in these facilities—physical, speech, vocational, etc., along with close supervision of medicine and routines and medical care.

Rehabilitation Centers

Most frequently operated on an outpatient basis but are nonetheless usually costly unless underwritten by private and/or public funds. The cost generally is $80 to $120 a day depending on the problem's extensiveness and therapy. If the facility provides resident accommodations, this is added to the cost.

One should shop around particularly if they are a city or build-up suburbs where one can shop and choose. Do not be taken by the outside appearance of the facility. Discover if you can ascertain the quality of care that is available inside.

Nutrition of Elderly Persons

The importance of nutrition cannot be underestimated and caretakers should be aware of the need of a proper diet. The table below prepared by the Journal of Geriatrics indicates the medical conditions and social factors that related to poor diets.

The elderly need a balanced diet and almost all can profit by foods taken from the basic food groups: meat (red and white), fruits and vegetables, milk products, for protein, carbohydrates, fat, calcium, vitamin A & D, breads and cereals, carbohydrates, vitamin A & B complex—4 servings per day—(cereal, potatoes, etc.). Many elderly have lactose intolerance and this may lead to avoidance of dairy products resulting in lower intake of protein, calcium and Vitamin D but this has to be compensated for by other foods. The chronic alcoholic may get by with the calories from alcohol but gets inadequate protein. People who eat plenty of fats and carbohydrates may still have a protein deficiency. Some causes of protein calorie malnutrition are: low socio-economic status, loss of dentition, gastrointestinal malabsorption and other functional impairments. These nutritional problems may be characterized by inadequate intake of both calories and proteins or sufficient calorie intake at the expense of a high carbohydrate, low protein diet.

Common Problems of the Elderly Frequently
Associated with Poor Nutrition

Medical Conditions
Arthritis
Dementia
Drug-nutrient interactions
Depression
Post-gastrectomy or after surgical procedures
Hypothyroiddism
Dysphagia
Neurologic impairment; stroke, Parkinsonism
Malignancy
Vascular insufficiency of the of intestines
Chronic pulmonary

Social Factors
Living alone
Poor dietary habits
Bereavement
Alcoholism
Low socio-economic status
Housebound elderly with poor exposure to sunlight

Some problems of nutritional deficits are reviewed here.

Vitamin and Mineral Deficiency

Toxicity potential—Vitamin supplements have been suggested for the elderly based on survey studies showing subnormal blood levels or low dietary intake, even in the absence of any clinical signs or symptoms of deficiency. Recent surveys suggest that many elderly take vitamin and mineral supplements. Because these supplements are rarely considered by either patients or physicians as drugs, they are frequently overlooked in the patient's evaluation or are taken in excess. Therefore, the elderly patient may be at risk for toxicity, as well as for vitamin deficiencies.

For example, high doses of the fat soluble vitamin D with calcium can promote hypercalcemia. Although the exact does at which this occurs varies among individuals, elderly persons are particularly prone to develop this complication due to increased fat stores. Large doses of vitamin C may interfere with the absorption of vitamin B 12 and has also been associated with a higher incidence of renal calculi. High doses of vitamin A can cause bone and joint pain, skin or hair changes, hepatomegaly, and benign intracranial hypertension.

Vitamin C Deficiency—Blood ascorbic acid levels decline with age in both sexes. This is usually due to decreased intake, although aging may also have an independent effect on blood ascorbic acid levels. Although severe vitamin C deficiency with clinical scurvy can occur, it is uncommon.

Supplemental vitamin C increases plasma and leukocyte ascorbic acid concentrations in those already receiving adequate amounts of vitamin C in the diet. No bad effects have been noted from this but low intake is a problem.

Vitamin D Deficiency—Vitamin D deficiency has been shown to be present in over 45% of non-supplemented elderly individuals living in institutions. Low plasma 225-hydroxy-vitamin D levels have also been reported in elderly persons in the community.

Even though dietary intake of vitamin D has been found to be lower in the elderly, diminished sunlight exposure and declining ability to metabolize vitamin D at both hepatic and renal levels are also important reasons for marginal vitamin D status in many older persons. In addition, a variety of drugs may interfere with vitamin D metabolism or actions, resulting in a deficiency. Examples include prednisone, phenobarbital, and phenytoin sodium.

Clinical Features—Clinical features of vitamin D deficiency are usually secondary to bone demineralization. It is important, therefore, not to consider bone pain, fractures, or loss of height as inevitable manifestations of aging or due necessarily to osteoporosis. Despite a relatively lower incidence in the elderly compared with the young.

Minerals—Apart from calcium, phosphorus, and iron, exact daily requirements for many minerals and trace elements have been difficult to establish. A notable exception, of course, is that decreased intake of calcium has been widely recognized in the elderly and undoubtedly contributes to the high prevalence of osteoporosis. Calcium alone has been shown to reduce the rate of fractures in patients with osteoporosis and to reduce the rate of bone loss. In addition to calcium, a variety of other elements is clearly essential for the maintenance of health.

The situation with other trace elements can become very complicated, however, because a number of them interact between themselves and/or act synergistically with vitamins. Even if coexistent vitamin A deficiency is present, night blindness will not improve until both vitamin A and zinc are in harmony. Zinc deficiency may also play a role in the anorexia often observed in aged patients.

Clinical features of deficiencies of some minerals are listed in the following table. It is clear from that list that many common clinical problems in the elderly including anemia, poor night vision, impotence, glucose intolerance, and cardiomyopathy can result from these nutritional deficiencies.

Fortunately, deficits of trace elements usually do not occur as isolated events, but rather in the setting of generalized malnutrition, malabsorption, or a requirement of long-term nutritional support. Particularly in these settings, assessment of trace element status by appropriate laboratory measurement is essential.

Conclusion—Deficiencies of a variety of nutrients including protein, calories, vitamins and minerals, are not uncommon in the elderly. The clinical signs and symptoms of these deficiencies may be subtle, and often mistaken as either inevitable accompaniments of aging or secondary to disease conditions often present in geriatric patients. Since correction of nutrient deficits can have a major impact on the health of the elderly, all physicians must monitor dietary intake and overall nutritional status of their patients.

Recommended Daily Dietary Intake of Nutrients for Healthy Elderly Persons

Nutrients	Age	Male	Female
Calories (kcal)	51-75	2000-2800	1400-2000
	76+	1650-2450	1200-2000
Protein (g)	51+	56	44
Vitamin A (Fg retinol equivalents)	51+	1000	800
Vitamin D (μg)	51+	5.0	5.0
Vitamin E (mg a-tocopherol)	51+	10	8.0
Ascorbic acid	51+	60	60
Thlamine (mg)	51+	1.2	1.0
Riboflavin (mg)	51+	1.4	1.2
Niacin (mg niacin equivalents)	51+	16	13
Vitamin B_6 (mg)	51+	2.2	2.0
Folacin (μg)	51+	400	400
Vitamin B_{12} (μg)	51+	3.0	3.0
Calcium (mg)	51+	800-1000	800-1200
Phosphorus	51+	800	800
Magnesium (mg)	51+	350	300
Iron (mg)	51+	10	10
Zinc (mg)	51+	15	15
Iodine (μg)	51+	150	150
Vitamin K (μg)	Adult	70-140	70-140
Biotin (μg)	Adult	100-200	100-200
Pantothenic acid (mg)	Adult	4.0-7.0	4.0-7.0
Sodium (mg)	Adult	1100-3300	1100-3300
Potassium (mg)	Adult	1875-5625	1875-5625
Chloride (mg)	Adult	1700-5100	1700-5100
Copper (mg)	Adult	2.0-3.0	2.0-3.0
Manganese (mg)	Adult	2.5-5.0	2.0-5.0
Fluoride (mg)	Adult	1.5-4.0	1.5-4.0
Chromium (mg)	Adult	0.05-0.20	0.05-0.20
Selenium (mg)	Adult	0.05-0.50	0.05-0.20
Molybdenum (mg)	Adult	0.15-0.50	0.15-0.50
Water (ml/kcal)	Adult	1.0	1.0

Source: Adapted from Food and Nutrition Board, National Academy of Sciences

The number of calories per pound for older adults should range between 16-18 per day meaning 2200 calories a day for the average man and 1800 for the typical woman. A 150-pound man would need approximately 2500 calories per day. A woman of 100 would require 1700 calories per day.

Diseases and Symptoms of the Elderly

A number of the common diseases are described in the appendix of this book. Also presented are a number of symptoms frequently observed in the older adult and although sometimes a clear-cut diagnosis of a problem may be identified by the layman the services of a physician or specialist should be utilized to provide answers as to causation and treatment.

Appendix

APPENDIX 1

COMMON DISEASES AND SYMPTOMS OF OLDER PEOPLE

Some of the following diseases may occur earlier in life but are much more likely to appear in the later years. Listed below are a number of common diseases that affect the elderly and some ways in which they may be treated. All patients should, of course, consult their physicians for diagnosis and treatment of their own individual conditions.

ALZHEIMER'S DISEASE

This is a neurological illness affecting the cerebral cortex-the outer layer of the brain. It appears in 2 to 3 percent of the general population and is not recognized in the most common cause of severe intellectual impairment in the elderly. At that event there are only minor symptoms, forgetfulness is one of the most noticeable. As the disease progresses, memory loss increases. Some personality and behavior change appear: confusion, irritability, restlessness. Judgment, concentration and speech may be affected. In severe cases, patients may eventually become incapable of caring for themselves. The causes of Alzheimer's Disease are not known, nor is there yet a cure, but all victims should be under the care of a physician who can carefully monitor their progress and suggest supportive measures as well as procedures that can make life easier for both the patients and their families.

ARTERIOSCLEROSIS (ATHEROSCLEROSIS)

Arteriosclerosis is a general term for hardening of the arteries. Atheroscleria, a type of arteriosclerosis, causes the narrowing and closing of a blood vessel due to accumulation of fats, complex carbohydrates, blood and blood products, fibers, tissues, and calcium deposits in its inner wall.

Arteriosclerosis is also related to hypertension (high blood pressure) and diabetes. The extent of arterial involvement in arteriosclerosis increases with age and can affect all the arteries of the body, especially those of the brain, heart, and lower extremities. When the blood supply to the brain is reduced by narrowing of the arteries supplying the brain, disturbances in behavior and cognition may result.

Arteriosclerosis in the aged is treated by attempting to lower the blood fats by diet when they are significantly elevated. Drugs to lower blood fats at this age are not of proven value. Elevated blood pressure should be treated with a lot-salt diet and, when necessary, the milder antihypertensive drugs. Cigarette smoking should be discontinued. A program of supervised physical activity is helpful, as is the control of obesity and diabetes. Surgical procedures to relieve or bypass obstructed blood vessels in the chest, neck, heart, and extremities may be of value after careful work up and evaluation of the benefits and risks involved.

ARTHRITIS

Arthritis is a general term referring to any degeneration or inflammation of the joints. It is classified according to its acuteness or its chronicity and also according to the joints involved and specific laboratory and X-ray findings. Many older persons suffer from arthritis, some to a mild degree and others severely.

The most common form, called osteoarthritis, involves primarily the weight-bearing joints and is due to the wear-and-tear process that accompanies aging. Osteoporosis, or thinning of the bones with aging, which occurs more often in women, contributes to collapse of the backbone as well as hip and wrist fractures. Inflammatory involvement of the joints, rheumatoid arthritis, is less common in the aged. Gout, a metabolic disease of the joints accompanied by severe pain and signs of inflammation, may also be seen in the aged.

Treatment of arthritis varies with the cause and includes physiotherapy, use of certain anti-inflammatory medications, and orthopedic devices. The use of female sex hormones for treating osteoporosis may be beneficial, but warrant careful discussion with a physician.

BRONCHITIS AND LUNG DISEASES

Bronchitis is an inflammation of the cells that line the bronchial air tubes. It may be caused by infection, or by chronic irritation cigarette smoke or following the inhalation of some harmful substance. Infectious bronchitis may be treated with antibiotics. In the case of chronic bronchitis, cessation of smoking is, of course, imperative. If untreated, chronic bronchitis may progress gradually to pulmonary emphysema.

Pulmonary emphysema, which results when the air sacs in the lungs are distended and damaged, is often found in heavy smokers. The patient suffers form shortness of breath and a cough. Treatment centers around relief of chronic bronchial obstruction by use of devices that help the emphysema patient to breathe. A variety of drugs and exercises are of value.

CANCER

Cancer (malignant neoplasm or tumor) is an uncontrolled growth of a tissue or portion of an organ that can spread (metastasize) to another part of the body. Cancer can occur in the throat, larynx, mouth, gastrointestinal tract, skin, bones, thyroid, bladder, kidney, and so forth. Because cancer symptoms in the aged are atypical, or may be ignored by the aged patient afflicted with other symptoms and often with a poor memory, comprehensive annual examinations are vital for early detection and treatment.

Cancer may be treated with surgery, radiotherapy (X-ray), chemotherapy or by any combination of the three methods. Because life expectancy is limited and the growth of many cancers is slow in the aged, there should be consideration of the value and potential side effects of potent methods before they are undertaken.

CONGESTIVE HEART FAILURE

Congestive heart failure occurs when the heart muscle has been so weakened that all pumping performance is impaired and it cannot provide sufficient circulation to body tissues. This condition may result from many years of untreated high blood pressure, heart attacks, or rheumatic heart disease. It may also be produced by diseases such as chronic lung disease, anemia, infection, and alcoholism.

Treatment for congestive heart failure is directed at improving the heart's pumping efficiency and eliminating excess fluids. Digitalis derivatives are often used to strengthen the heart muscle, and diuretics and salt restriction to remove excess fluid of the thyroid gland, or anemia, may also be necessary.

CORONARY ARTERY HEART DISEASE

This disease, which is present in almost all individuals over the age of seventy in the United States, involves atherosclerosis of the arteries that supply blood to the heart muscle. In older persons coronary heart disease is superimposed on a heart when there may be a general decrease in muscle-cell size and efficiency.

A heart attack (myocardial infarction) happens when a portion of the blood supply to the heart muscle is cut off. In the elderly it is not unusual for there to be hardly any symptoms accompanying an infarction, in contrast to the crushing most experienced by younger persons. Substitution symptoms are also common the elderly. For example, when the elderly heart fails because of a heart attack, blood may back up behind the left side of the heart into the blood vessels of the lungs causing shortness of breath, instead of chest pain. In other cases, the flow of blood from the weakened heart to the brain is diminished, with resultant dizziness or fainting rather than chest pain.

Modern treatment of the complications of acute myocardial infarction (which include irregular heartbeat and heart failure) with drugs, oxygen and clocking equipment is saving many lives and enabling the period of bed rest to be shortened. Patients with uncomplicated cases now get up out of bed and into a chair much earlier than before, and cardiac rehabilitation is begun early with good results. Cardiac shock (intractable heart failure), however, remains a difficult problem with a high mortality rate.

Common in individuals with coronary heart disease is angina pectoris. This condition results from a temporary inadequacy in the blood supply to the heart muscle due to coronary heart disease. Angina is characterized by severe but brief pain near the mid-chest region; the pain may radiate to either or both arms, the back, neck, or jaw. Angina is treated commonly and safely with nitroglycerin.

DIABETES MELLITUS

The common form of diabetes in the aged is Type II diabetes, a chronic inherited disease in which a relative deficiency of insulin or a disturbance in the action of insulin interferes with the body's ability to metabolize carbohydrates. The elderly diabetic may present few or no clinical symptoms of that disease. In fact, complications arising from diabetes may be the first signs of this disease in the elderly.

HYPERTENSION

Hypertension, otherwise known as high blood pressure, when present over long periods of time can lead to arterial disease and eventually to heart failure, stroke and kidney failure. In the elderly, high blood pressure is unlikely to be of recent origin and much of the damage to the arterial system has already been done.

Hypertension in the aged should be treated by moderate dietary salt restriction and, if necessary, by drugs. Only the milder drugs should be use din the aged, since the more powerful ones can cause sudden and severe lowering of blood pressure which may lead to fainting spells or even strokes or heart attacks—the very complications such drugs are used to prevent.

NEURITIS

Neuritis is a disease of the peripheral and cranial nerves characterized by inflammation and degeneration of the nerve fibers. It can lead to loss of conduction of nerve fibers. It can lead to loss of conduction of nerve impulses and consequently to varying degrees of paralysis, loss of feeling, and loss of reflexes. Although the term neuritis implies inflammation, this is not invariably present. Neuritis may affect a single nerve or involve several nerve trunks. Diagnostic work-up by a neurologist is indicated. Treatment of specific causes such as diabetes, pernicious anemia, or alcoholism, may be helpful.

OSTEOPOROSIS

This is a condition of porous bones where bone density and mineral content occurs when new bone is not created as quickly as old bone is lost. Osteoporosis is caused by an acceleration of normal changes that occur with age. Bone tissue and density are lost—brittleness and higher risks of fracture ensue. More women than men are affected. Risk factors include estrogen loss, low calcium and Vitamin D intake as well as body type, heredity, race, smoking and inactivity.

PERIPHERAL NEUROPATHY

This disease involved damage to the peripheral nerves the extensive network of nerves that connect the brain and spinal cord to the rest of the body. The causes of this problem range from alcoholism, diabetes, malignant tumors, Vitamin B_1, B_6, B_{12} deficiency, led poisoning, hypothyroidism, Guillian-Barré syndrome and others. Autoneuropathy affects nerves leading to the central part of the body, i.e., the heart, lungs, etc. and its affects can be cataclymic.

SYMPTOMS AND COMPLAINTS

The following are some of the more common symptoms and complaints of the elderly. Wrongly regarded by many older patients as being the natural consequences of aging and, therefore, not worth mentioning to a busy doctor, these symptoms—and indeed, all others—should be reported to a physician by the older person or his family.

BREATHLESSNESS

Breathlessness, known as dyspnea, is common in the aged and may reflect heart failure, disease of the lungs, or anemia. It is exaggerated by obesity.

CONSTIPATION

Perhaps no part of the body is as misunderstood as the lower digestive tract, which is involved in absorption of nutrients and elimination of solid waste matter. Many people still believe that a daily bowel movement is needed for good health. This belief is false. Not everyone functions on a once-a-day schedule or needs to. It is common to find people in perfect health who defecate regularly twice a day and others who have a bowel movement once every two or three days with the slightest ill effects. There are some people who have regular bowel movements at still longer intervals, without any health problems.

CHAPTER VI

RECREATION AND LEISURE

"What's Most Fun?"

For those among us who are middlescent, it is sometimes hard to take vacations, to use leisure time appropriately, or to enjoy recreation. Our adolescent and young adult populations are not spurred on by the "work ethic" by which we were brought up. Our culture put great emphasis on productivity—consequently, we feel we must always be doing something constructive with our time. We have been known to observe our idle child swinging on a gate and say, "Don't you have anything else to do?" They are doing something! And although we have all heard "all work and no play makes Jack a dull boy" we middleagers really don't believe it. At least many of us do not! Many of us have heard that the amalgam of the good life is a mix of work, play, love and worship.

It is, however, generally accepted that play is associated with leisure, and creation is the antidote to tiresome work allowing us to shed the cares and tensions of the work-a-day world. Piaget, the famous Swiss psychologist, believes the child's cognitive development takes place principally through creative play activity in which the child acts upon his environment, that the child's intelligence is a special form of adaptation, which consists of a continuous creative interaction between the child and his surroundings. It is the same ability in the adult—the ability to recreate through play and leisure—that provides the basis of the good life. If one hasn't developed outlets, activities, the avocational interests, then increasingly life will be deadly stifling and narrow affecting ultimately the growth of the person.

Leisure and recreation are usually thought of as being different but tied together. A French sociologist, Joffre Dumazedier, defines leisure as "activity—apart from the obligation of work, family and society—to which the individual turns at will freely, for either relaxation, diversion, or broadening his knowledge and his spontaneous social participation, the free exercise of his creative capacity."

There are a number of theories about play. One major theory is called the arousal-seeking theory. Play under this idea is caused by the need to generate either interactions with the environment or with the individual that elevate arousal. Play stimulates and exhilarates—makes us feel good and recognize what can come from inside ourselves. The need for continued stimulation causes people to search for ways to extend play and the interactions that they involve. These become more complex in time, requiring often subtle forms of gaming, playing, etc., going much beyond just feeling "full of pep" and energy accompanied by the need for physical release. This theory was called the Surplus-Energy Theory. For the child who has had fewer experiences and knowledge, simple interactions are arousing. Repetitions are not as boring to them. Play is the child's way of learning. This is the instinct practice theory. The child's play is an imitation of adult lives and activities. A recreation theory suggests a tired brain turns to play in some form to restore one's energy. The control of this by adults prepares him for their world, but the child's way of playing, using his imagination, creativity, dreaming, helps develop his intelligence. We should recognize that sometimes things that start as play for the adult become something less than this—routine and work and even emotions that are negative. When the cognitive need for competence becomes too great in an individual, then it may happen that the once entertaining and relaxing act of dance or social doubles in tennis becomes work. In other words, if our recreation becomes making everything a matter of doing it perfectly the leisure for many evaporates. Most people remember a social game of cards that became ego asserting—win or else! I played a little bridge in my college days, sometimes seriously, sometimes comically. A few years ago I was invited, after a period of absence from the usual "game" for social enjoyment to a card party. Before the evening was finished, one of my partners said to me, "You missed my cue!" but, I said, facetiously, I didn't trump your ace, to which she countered seriously, "I should have stayed home!" For some, even this approach is probably enjoyable and considered leisure, but it should be recognized for what it is. How does leisure and recreation relate, we may ask? In the twentieth century two theories suggest self-expression of the individual's personality by appropriate outlets and another—social necessity—the development of parks and playgrounds due to the importance of play in child development.

What one does in his leisure time could be called recreation and, in another sense, recreation can be leisure in that one form of recreation is relaxation. Ordinarily leisure is defined as free, unoccupied time during which a person may indulge in rest, recreation and the like. On the other hand, recreation means refreshment in body or mind as after work by some form of play amusement, or relaxation used for this purpose as games, sports, hobbies, reading, walking, etc. Perhaps in no country in the world is there more money, time and energy spent in search of recreation and leisure with less success than in America. And it is no wonder, for in the United States there is no other people put under the strain from the constant radical change which occurs with increasing rapidity than here. Alvin Toffler called this the "orientation response," the inexorable interaction between organism and environment. So it follows that we make the horrendous rush to socialize, isolate, travel, play, rest, or whatever it takes to settle the nerves, reduce tension and relax the jaded self. Despite the use of the word "rush" more Americans take their leisure time and recreational activity in mostly sedentary ways.

The American worker has more leisure time judging by statistics from the National Bureau of Economic research and the Bureau of Labor Statistics which reveal that in 1870 the average weekly hours per worker has 53 hours plus whereas in 1970 it was down to 39.6 hours per week. This has changed in the last several years with time spent working increasing. Max Kaplan in his book, *Leisure in America*, says that based on a six-day work week the number of free hours after working, eating an attending to other necessities has gone up in 1850 from 2.3 hours to 7.8 hours in 1960, an increase of approximately 350%. Generally it is thought that leisure time is increasing though that has been disputed. In 2000 *U.S. News & World Report* concluded that Americans were working 208 hours more a year than in 1980 and work more than any country in the advanced industrial world. The equivalent of 8 more weeks a year than the average western European country. Robinson of the University of Maryland concludes leisure hours have generally risen by 16 percent during this period. The allocation has changed in fitness where participation activities only increased in walking, bicycling and basketball with drops in gardening, yard work, calisthenics and general exercise, jogging, and swimming, dancing, aerobics. Robinson says some Americans do have less leisure due to greater work pressures. Single parents working jobs and tending to children—sometimes two jobs. The Bureau of Labor survey of production and non-supervisory employee, non-farm business and thousands of randomly selected households of some 400,000 suggests average workweek 34.9 in the mid 1980's and 34.6 in 1998 both down from 36.1 in 1970. Fewer than one third of all employed Americans over 18 have standard work week (35-40 hours) Monday to Friday on a fixed daytime schedule twenty-four hour shifts, workaholics, non-traditional schedules. It should be pointed out that many professionals and heads of businesses unknown to many people work much more than the hours suggested by research as the average. And herein lies the answer to the frantic getaway for many and the submerging of oneself in frenzied activity in distant hideaways.

How to Get Started with Play

Psychiatrist Henry P. Ward said, "Inside each one of us there is a child trying to get out." This child doesn't want to be responsible and he hates the monotony of routine housework or jobs. There are times when the child part of parent-adult-child aspects of ourselves has a part to play even among the middlescent, especially us. Play is important to us but, as Ogden Nash once wrote, most people suffer from "hardening of the oughteries." Of course we must obey the "shoulds" but too often they become ingrained and the usual. It is never easy to break away from the demands of life and guilt involved in leaving a task undone; fortunately there are some ways of handling this. Check this list.

1. Face our boredom—a certain amount of boredom, ennui is inevitable in everyone's life. The routine job we have to do and other tasks must be done. What if we are bored during our free time? If so, we should change some things and do something about the situation.
2. Dream a little!—we lose our ability to fantasize as adult all too quickly—the real world doesn't allow for dreams. Children daydream a lot and so should we. Faraway places with strange sounding names! Piccadilly Circus…..Rue de la Plais or Siam! The dreaming helps to sort out our lives; dreams reveal our inner selves and they give us a break from the ordinary.
3. Let the child loose—the child part of the adult may appear silly to some—like the old man who wishes to have an electric toy train and the middle-aged father who enjoys playing marbles or rolling in the grass. Let's make ourselves more flexible and emotionally responsive learning to play again.
4. Listen to yourself—be assertive. All too frequently we turn aside from what we want to do during our free time. We say yes to people who decide we will volunteer our Saturdays to help carry a group on the church picnic when we had something else in mind. We confuse virtue with good-natured willingness when we haven't been fair with ourselves because we have been afraid to assert our feelings. To say no

on occasions helps our self-respect and allows that life just doesn't "slip by" without our ever doing what we really wish to do.

5. Keep active—the person that engaged in a variety of physical activities is constantly sending the "septal" region of the brain or "pleasure center" messages through sensory impressions. When alerted the septal region shakes us out of the doldrums that boredom brings. Wrestling with our children, playing a little touch football, tennis, badminton, or tag, are the types of things we can do. The time is now and to get started is half the battle. I have noticed in dancing the young are now watching the middlescent person who learned jitterbugging, two step, Charleston and other dances because they are like Disco dancing, so dust off your shoes!

Many experts think that for the middle ager, far too much time is spent in passive low activity pursuits. There are those such as Dr. Steincrohn who say "too many Americans are exercise mad." It is true as Dr. Richard Miller in the work, *Problems of the Middle Age*, points out, that too much of anything turns gold to rust. One can eat too much, sleep too much, work too much, worry too much, and exercise too much. In this sense exercise madness would be harmful. However, the "bay-windows" and poor physical condition of the average middle-age American male shows no indication toward general "exercise madness." The physical strength and endurance of World War II and Korean War draftees showed unexpected weaknesses. In the Scandinavian countries, Norway, Sweden and Finland, middlescent participation in strenuous competitive activities is a common occurrence. As far as can be determined, this program is not the least bit harmful. However, the important consideration is whether the participant has continuously used strenuous physical activity throughout his life or whether he occasionally competes in strenuous activities.

The United States spent personal spending on reaction nearly 300 billion in 1980. It was 431 in 1996 now much more. The largest item in the leisure budget is recreational equipment—boats, camping vehicles, color-television sets, motor bikes and bicycles. Nearly fifteen million people play tennisBup six million from 5 years ago. This is dropping in the 2000's. Many of these are middle-age husband and wife teams who can manage to learn to hit the ball well enough to make it exciting, yet not strenuous enough to be detrimental to their health as might be singles. It was recently said that golf was the sport of America in the 1950's with tennis coming on in the sixties and now some say paddle tennis looms large for the latter seventies and eighties. Participation in selected sports activities is shown below.

PARTICIPATION IN SELECTED SPORTS ACTIVITIES

(Number of persons over age of 7 participating at least once in previous year, in thousands)

Activity	All Persons		Sex	
	Number	Rank	Male	Female
	237,745	(X)	115,443	122,301
Aerobic exercise	24,119	11	5,314	18,805
Backpacking	11,469	22	7,240	4,229
Badminton	6,084	28	2,909	3,175
Baseball	14,823	18	11,610	3,213
Basketball	33,281	9	22,375	10,906
Bicycle riding	53,342	3	28,595	24,747
Billiards	34,477	8	21,841	12,636
Bowling	42,895	6	22,579	20,316
Calisthenics	10,064	25	5,023	5,041
Camping	44,695	5	24,102	20,593
Exercise walking	73,307	1	26,666	46,641
Exercising with equipment	47,823	4	22,200	25,622
Fishing, freshwater	40,208	7	27,160	13,048
Fishing, saltwater	11,045	23	7,926	3,119
Football, tackle	8,219	27	7,436	783
Football, touch	11,645	20	9,603	2,042
Golf	23,082	12	18,219	4,863
Hiking	26,457	10	14,465	11,992
Hunting with firearms	19,251	15	16,317	2,933
Martial arts	4,673	30	3,286	5,251
Racquetball	5,582	29	3,768	1,814
Running/jogging	22,239	13	12,320	9,919
Skiing, downhill	10,466	24	6,277	4,188
Skiing, cross-country	3,385	21	1,820	1,566
Soccer	13,876	19	8,626	5,251
Softball	19,873	14	10,837	9,035
Swimming	60,223	2	29,145	31,078
Table tennis	9,542	26	5,907	3,635
Target shooting	15,695	17	11,097	4,598
Tennis	11,486	21	6,381	5,105
Volleyball	18,535	16	8,970	9,565

Source: *Statistical Abstract of the United* States (1999) and National Sporting Goods Association

There are a number of good reasons for participating in recreation and leisure. Janet MacLean in *Recreation in Modern Society* listed these. Of course, she emphasized the importance of building leisure skills early in life but appetites should be whetted for recreation, not shoved down the throats of youngsters by organizations at breakneck speed.

The key is balance both in kinds of choices as to recreation and depth of pursuit. The benefits of recreation are:

1. Recreation outlets provide a chance to find meaning and self-expression.
2. Recreation is a means to restore balance—social, mental and physical—the thing that keeps you on even keel.
3. Recreation is an opportunity for involvement in life's issues, particularly for those whose age (teens and aged) narrows their choices in identity in meaningful roles.
4. Recreation is a chance for self-realization—a chance to be me!
5. Recreation is a basic human need as real as food or shelter.
6. Recreation is an opportunity for voluntary experiences.
7. Recreation in the real sense is therapeutic.
8. Recreation serves as a watchdog on our natural resources for the demand of outdoor pursuits of recreating serves to protect our land. We are equipped with great neuromuscular memories so the skating done in youth and riding of a bicycle come quickly back to us. Kinesthetic memory enables us to resume a game at almost any age, so 35, 45, 55, golf or tennis is not too late. As middle age parents in teaching sports skills to children, we should follow these criteria:
    1. The basic skills of the sports should be fairly easy to learn.
    2. It should be possible to teach the skills to large classes in schools, parks, camps or other similar teaching situations.
    3. They should be sports requiring no more than two to play—no sports requiring team organization.
    4. Facilities should be available, so that once the skills are learned there is an opportunity to practice them.
    5. They should be sports, which can be played throughout life.

In studies by the National Advisory Commission on Civil Disorders, the cities considered to be Major Riot Cities were often as unconcerned about recreational facilities and the like as they were about housing and the human condition. The public and particularly the private concern to enlarge the opportunity for the deprived for access to swimming pools, tennis courts, camps, supervised playground programs, are wonderful and should receive greater support. All classes will have some kind of leisure time activity be it as lowly as visiting, religion activity, card playing, crabbing and drinking beer for the poor to polo and scotch for the rich. Programs in education and by community agencies at all levels should get our unqualified support.

Recreation Types and Opportunity

It is not true that those who have failed to learn to play in childhood cannot learn to play in adulthood. As a matter of fact, there is little correlation between childhood and adult leisure. Possibly early introduction and pleasure in outdoor activities has more carry-over than the general type of recreational activity. But for most individuals the scope of opportunity is unlimited even at forty and fifty. Winston Churchill said that "to reach the age of forty without ever handling a brush, to have regarded the painting of pictures as a mystery, and then suddenly find oneself plunged in the middle of a new interest with paints and palettes and canvases, and not to be discouraged by results, is an astonishing and enriching experience." I hope it may be shared by others! My middlescent persons find great pleasure in the joy of creation, also to work with their hands, personal satisfaction that comes from arts and crafts hobbies. Some receive appreciation and recognition and a sense of pride and accomplishment from such activities. This kind of leisure provides many positive emotional outlets and opportunities for meeting other people, traveling to see exhibits or exhibiting and even to participate in organizing Board or Side Walk Art Shows, displays of crafts or town decoration projects.

Local Provision for Recreation

Almost every community has organized opportunity for participating in musical activity. The Recreation Department of Cities can give you information on what is available within the area—community choruses, glee clubs, Sweet Adeline organizations, dance groups, ballet—and they usually know of or produce calendars of events which are published in local newspapers. Another area of opportunity that abounds is in music—community concerts, community sings, civic concerts, operas, listening to stereo records and tapes.

A city of 100,000 population with a low per capita income offers a wide variety of programs for all ages, particularly focused on children and youth.

Many more special events are offered from March to August. After school recreation programs are held at all centers Monday through Friday. They include Karate, cheerleading, open recreation period, field hockey, volleyball, flag football, badminton, sports for girls, physical fitness, "just for the fun of it," learn a new game, creative dance, youth basketball, tag and relay races, computer classes, board games, homework assistance, little artists, kids in the kitchen, crafty afternoon, atrium II afternoons, 4-H, kick ball, Girl Scouts and brain teasers. Supervised overnight camping trips, etc. have fun attached to them but most of the activities mentioned above are free. GED classes, investing, the ABC's of Inventing all cost small fees. Adult therapeutic recreation programs are available, also adult basic educational programs, adult arts and crafts, therapeutic leisure field trips, bowling and many other events.

A town of 5,000 serving their county also has youth basketball, an instructional league 8-9 co-ed, midget girls age 10-12, midget boys 10-12 but with teams, junior boys 13-14 with teams and all star teams. They all have adult men's basketball with church teams and open division and district adult teams. In the spring they have men and women's softball, track for youth with track meets. In summer they offer T-ball, youth baseball with mini mite ages 7-8 and mites 9-10, midgets 11-12, juniors 13-14 and All-Star Teams. Also youth softball in various categories, swim teams and classes for 3 years old and up beginning, intermediate, etc. They have tennis teams. Fall they provide football flag, for second levels, soccer and cheerleading. Many special events are arranged—the City Festival Softball Tournament, Volunteers Banquet, Midget Football Bowl, July 4th Celebration—pool activities and fireworks. Punt, pass and kick contest, hopscotch contest, and District II Basketball, Softball, baseball, and men's Softball Tournament. Basketball and softball have girls' and women's teams. Also during the year they offer tap, ballet and baton classes 3-18 years of age and have a recital.

Besides recreational activities organized in most communities, they have YMCA's, over twenty-two hundred across the country offer sports instruction to child care and in fact several years ago they served more than nine million children in non-school hours. You should know many schools have programs, for after school for several hours for working parents providing free time, games and fun things under trained supervision. Some other things that have been done by the YMCA and also the YWCA are:

1. Serves all incomes, all ages and all abilities. Serve 17 million people, raise nearly 600 million for scholarships, subsidies and community services.
2. Reaches 9 million children in non-school hours with gang prevention programs, literacy tutoring, kid clubs and sports leagues, community service projects and including values of honesty, respect, caring and responsibility.
3. Provides childcare nationwide YMCA's are collectively the largest childcare provider in the nation. Approximately half the children in their childcare come from households with less than $25,000 yearly. The cost is very affordable.
4. Partner's with neighborhood organizations—400 YMCA's work with juvenile courts, 300 with public housing, 1550 with elementary schools, 1033 with high schools and 700 with college.
5. YMCA's encourage volunteers. YMCA is volunteer founded and volunteer led. Nearly 600,000 volunteers ask to help or are recruited.
6. YMCA's live their mission every day. Founded 150 years ago. Together is the largest not-for-profit community organization in America. All 2283 independent YMCA's are guided by the common mission, putting Christian principles into practice that build healthy spirit, mind and body for all.

As a one time member for five or six years and having been to their camp for that some time I can testify that their help and effectiveness did something for me that would have never happened otherwise.

It should be mentioned that many public school systems along with some churches offer programs for children after school hours as a help to parents. These programs kept many children from becoming latch key boys and girls and provide a guard against idle hands and minds. Call the Superintendent of Schools' office and they will give you information on their after school programs. In a large city 400,000 plus selected by the National Recreation and Park Association at their first Magnet City. The purpose of the Association is to develop an outreach model to support parks and recreation agencies to set new standards of community service. It spotlights the critical role played by parks and recreation in delivering programs, which insure the quality of life and lead to healthier communities. The Magnet initiative will focus on four areas—health, sports, technology and youth. What follows is only a sample of their programs, which range from water therapy for people with arthritis, M.S. and other such problems to ceramics, crafts, dancing to learning to swim with countless special events. A registration form has to be filled out and a fee given. Special classes such as Karate demand a fee. Scholarships are available for many programs so upon an application some children may participate free of charge.

Example of Two Locations' Schedules with Fees Required and Waivers

Year-Round Program Information				
Programs & Registration Information	Bettie F. Williams Elem. Sch.	Bayside Recreation Center	Seatack Elem. School	Seatack Recreation Center
Before School Fees Hours	$12/$14 per week 6:30 am 8:00 am	No program	$14/$12 per week 6:30 am-8:00 am	No program
After School Fees Hours	$27/$25 per week 2:30 pm-6:00 pm	*$140 per month 3:00 pm-6:00 pm	$27/25 per week 2:30 pm-6:00 pm	$35 per week 2:30 pm-6:00 pm
Intersession Break Fees/Hours	$55/$45 per week 7:00 am-6:00 pm	$90 per week 7:00 am-6:00 pm	No program	$70 per week 7:00 am-6:00 pm
Day Camp Fees Hours	$20 per day 7:00 am-6:00 pm	Various options available	No program	$20 per day 7:00 am-6:00 pm
Licensed programs	Before	After School/ Intersession Break/Day Camp	Before	After/Inter-session Break/Day Camp
Membership Card Fees	No	Required $15 per year	No	Required $15 per year
Fee Waiver Available	Yes 50%	No	Yes 50%	No
Meals or Snacks Provided	No	Intersession: Breakfast & Lunch (USDA Program)	No	Afternoon Snack
Transportation	No	*Limited, Call Bayside for calls	No	To Recreation Center after Intersession
Registration Day Dates Hours	**Registration** Thursday, June 21 6:30 pm-8:30 pm	**Registration** Thursday, June 28 5:30 pm-8:30 pm	Registration Thursday, June 21 6:30 pm-8:30 pm	Information at Seatack Elementary Registration night
For additional information contact	Community Recreation Services 471-5884	Bayside Community Recreation Center 460-7540	Commu-nity Recreation Services 471-5884	Seatack Community Recreation Center 437-4858

*Call Bayside Recreation Center 460-7540 for start date.
Note: TTY number for all locations: 471-5839

Seatack Gym Schedule

Monday	Time	Program	Gym #
	8:30-9:30 am	Summer Camp	1 & 2
	9:30-12:00 pm	Summer Camp	2
	9:30-10:30 am	Aerobics	1
	10:30-1:00 pm	Summer Camp	1 & 2
	1:00-3:00 pm	Teen Basketball	1 & 2
	3:00-4:30 pm	Camp Hope	1
	3:00-4:30 pm	Summer Camp	2
	4:30-6:00 pm	Open Gym	1 & 2
	6:00-7:00 pm	1st Session Adult Basketball	1 & 2
	7:00-8:00 pm	2nd Session Adult Basketball	1 & 2
	8:00-8:45 pm	Open Gym	1 & 2
Tuesday	6:30-8:30 am	Walk Program	1 & 2
	8:30-12:00 pm	Summer Camp	1 & 2
	12:00-1:00 pm	Summer Camp	2
	12:00-1:00 pm	Camp Hope	1
	1:00-3:00 pm	Teen Basketball	1 & 2
	3:00-4:30 pm	Camp Hope	1
	3:00-4:30 pm	Summer Camp	2
	4:30-6:30 pm	Open Gym	1 & 2
	6:30-7:30 pm	Aerobics	2
	6:30-8:30 pm	Karate	1
	7:30-8:45 pm	Open Gym	2
Wednesday	8:30-12:00 pm	Summer Camp	1 & 2
	12:00-3:00 pm	Teen Activity	1 & 2
	3:00-4:30 pm	Camp Hope	1
	3:00-4:30 pm	Summer Camp	2
	4:30-6:00 pm	Open Gym	1 & 2
	6:00-7:00 pm	Adult Volleyball	1
	6:00-7:00 pm	Open Gym	2
	7:00-8:45 pm	Open Gym	1 & 2
Thursday	6:30-8:30 am	Walk Program	1 & 2
	8:30-12:00 pm	Summer Camp	1 & 2
	12:00-1:00 pm	Youth Activity	1
	12:00-1:00 pm	Summer Camp	2
	1:00-3:00 pm	Teen Basketball	1 & 2
	3:00-4:30 pm	Camp Hope	1
	3:00-4:30 pm	Summer Camp	2
	4:30-6:30 pm	Open Gym	1
	4:30-6:30 pm	Summer Camp	2
	6:00-7:00 pm	Aerobics	2
	7:30-8:45 pm	Open Gym	2
Friday	8:30-12:00 pm	Summer Camp	1 & 2
	12:00-2:00 pm	Teen Basketball	1
	12:00-2:00 pm	Open Gym	2
	2:00-4:30 pm	Camp Hope	1
	2:00-4:30 pm	Summer Camp	2
	4:30-6:00 pm	Open Gym	1
	4:30-6:00 pm	Summer Camp	2
	6:00-8:45 pm	Open Gym	1 & 2
Saturday	9:00-12:00 pm	Teen Basketball	1 & 2
	12:00-4:45 pm	Open Gym	1 & 2
Sunday	11:00-1:30 pm	1st Session Adult Basketball	1 & 2
	1:30-3:00 pm	2nd Session Adult Basketball	1 & 2
	3:00-4:45 pm	Open Gym	1 & 2

Most church groups sponsor hymn festivals, choir singing and competitions and music camps. These activities are largely volunteer and sponsored by organizations that solicit individuals to join. Local drama groups allow outlets for many that are interested; most local playhouse groups invite tryouts; frequently a person who has never participated before finds an invigorating interest in acting or in some related activity. Some activities of the Arts, Dance, Music and are seen below.

Arts and Crafts	Dance	Drama	Music
Basket Making	Ballet	Adult Theatre	Singing
Beadwork	Creative rhythms	Ceremonials	Informal groups
Block Printing	Dance mixers	Charades	Quartets
Candle making	Folk dance	Children's theatre	Choirs
Carving	Hawaiian dances	Choral speaking	Choruses
Cards and Christmas	Tap and Clog	Community theatre	Community sings
Decorations	Latin American	Creative dramatics	Playing
Clay modeling	Rock dance	Festivals	Rhythm instruments
Collage	Modern dance	Grand operas	Bands
Etching	Jazz	Light operas	Orchestras
Fiberglass	Social dance	Operettas	Simple melody
Furniture refinishing	Ballroom	Pageants	instruments
Knitting	Square dancing	Plays	Combos
Finger Painting	Foxtrot	Puppetry	Chamber music
Flower Arrangements	Waltz	Scenery making	group
Leatherwork	Disco	Story reading	One-man bands
Needlework	Charleston	Story telling	Listening
Paper craft	Samba	Variety Shows	Home music
Model-making work,	Rumba	Musical comedies	Radio, T.V.
clay, metal	Two step	Monologues	Concerts
Photography	Cha-Cha	One-act plays	Tape recorders
Picture Framing		Skits	Combined Activity
Pottery		Stunts	Folk dancing
Printing and Book		Water pageants	Festivals
making			Caroling
Rugs, Sewing			Seasonal and
Sculpture			Holiday programs
Sketching			Park Concerts
Weaving			

Music is the universal language of mankind—it rocks the baby to sleep, soothes the savage breast, and quiets the jangled nerves of the middlescent. It is estimated that there are 50,000,000 amateur musicians in America. Music, to me, is as much a part of life as eating and sleeping. I don't have it when I am working at my office but at home—television and stereo during the evening and the radio late at night. I like music in almost any form—the symphonic, operatic, the glee club, the quartet, the dance band and even church choirs. I like to sing along, to dance along, or just tap my foot. Many persons living in metropolitan areas should become acquainted with the presentations and opportunities that exist in the local colleges and universities who present many fine concerts, etc., often free of cost. They also offer short courses on instrument playing and appreciation of operas. Also, one should investigate what is offered through organized recreation programs—private, commercial, public and voluntary.

Some middle agers find sports, both team and individual, an important recreational outlet. Though many may have given up the most strenuous sports like basketball or football, still some younger middlescents (35-45) play pick-up or team basketball and touch football. I have played for years on a tennis team, which is an entry in a regional league. Some of us thought up the idea originally and got city sanction for it and support (use of public courts) from local cities in the region. We play once a week beginning in March or April and play until July. You have to make the team under a ladder arrangement, usually all who make the team play which means the 12 to 14 players usually are on the roster; if not singles, then in the doubles matches. In recent times, the opportunity for playing in tournaments of all kinds has multiplied. Many of the new tennis tournaments sponsored by city and town recreation departments and commercial interests have novice divisions which allow beginners to play other beginners. Usually small entrance fees are charged and require the participants to furnish the balls. Softball is played everywhere in small towns and large. Many church groups have teams and organized leagues for both men and women. In fact many churches now have directors of activities including recreation with facilities which include gymnasiums, gaming rooms, bowling, etc. Volleyball and shuffleboard are played by increasing numbers of people of all ages. It is easy to get a volleyball and net and construct a playing area. I see many people bring their games to the beach or lake along with their picnics and vacation times.

Some good individual sports for middlescent persons are: jogging, swimming, bicycling, fishing, tennis (practice on backboard), golf, hiking, boating, horseback riding, roller skating and shooting (rifle and pistol), skiing, miniature golf, handball. Some sports requiring partners, like badminton, horseshoes, table tennis, racquetball, bowling and shuffleboard, have considerable appeal to many people.

Outdoor recreation is an area of American life that has taken on great significance in the past decade. Increased leisure time and mobility have doubled the numbers of persons involved in outdoor recreation. Most people prefer simple pleasures of leisure. According to the U.S. Department of Interior, pleasure driving, walking, hiking accounts for 40% of the total outdoor participation annually. Other activities that require little specialized equipment are playing games, swimming, sightseeing, fishing, bicycling, viewing sporting events, and picnicking. Fewer, thought in increasing numbers, are participating in skin diving, mountain climbing, sailing, requiring outlay of money for equipment, are being explored.

A partial list of outdoor recreational opportunity is given here.

Astronomy	Flower shows	Nature trails
Backpacking	Gardening	Nature study
Bird walks	Glider soaring	Outdoor cooking
Boating	Hiking	Outdoor games
Camping	Horseback riding	Picnicking
Cave exploration	Hunting	Sailing
Coasting	Ice boating	Snowmobiling
Cycling	Ice skating	Snowshoeing
Driving for pleasure	Indian lore	Surfing
Family camping	Kite flying	Swimming
Fishing	Mountaineering	Target shooting
Conservation sessions	Nature Clubs	Travel

Many of these types of recreation are afforded under the sponsorship of the YMCA and YWCA and under various community organizations as follows. Generally there are four types of organization. We will give what you may expect to be offered by these groups, their facilities, and something about the personnel that staff these programs.

SPONSORSHIP OF COMMUNITY RECREATION

Types of Agencies, Kinds of Recreation, Target Persons, Facilities

Public	Voluntary	Private	Commercial
(City, Town or County) To meet public needs. Provide public facilities.	(Quasi-public, non-profit, providing varied services, often for specific neighborhoods)	Organizations with closed membership designed to meet needs of its members.	Profit-related, privately owned. Provides one or more type of recreation to the public.
Recreation programs through Agencies, Parks and Recreation. Maybe School District, etc.	Youth-serving organization (Boys clubs, Girl Scouts, YMCA, YWCA, Catholic Youth, etc. Settlement houses, Jewish Community Centers	Country Clubs, Tennis, Yacht, Golf, athletic groups or fraternal or industrial associations with close membership procedures.	Miniature golf, bowling alleys, movies, bars, night clubs, pool rooms, game machines, skating rinks, amusement centers.
Usually provide wide range of indoor sports and outdoor—have facilities—Bpools, gyms, golf, tennis, beaches, stadiums, parks, trails, museums, nature paths, etc. Have special events, Parades, Celebrations.	Operates chiefly indoors, may have camps, and tennis courts and swimming pools. Organizations like the scouts depend on other agency for facilities—churches, etc.	They operate their own buildings and outdoor recreation areas usually for a specific purpose like hunting, fishing, etc. Some have club buildings with facilities for sauna, dining and dancing.	Chief concern here is usually on single activity, some sports centers like Tennis Centers have amusement area—table tennis, etc. Water slides, swimming pools. Large Recreational Complexes—King's Dominion, Busch Gardens, Disney World, Disneyland, Six Flags over Texas, Georgia, Carawinds.
The staffs of public agencies are usually certified and under Civil Service requirement.	Usually people here have college backgrounds, some have social work college degrees.	Not college degree oriented, people are employed for a specific reason—tennis pro, dance and swimming instruction, etc.	Persons here are hired to do a particular type of job. In the large complexes many high school and college youth are employed.

We should be aware of what is available in our community, the wider area and our state for recreation. Many states regularly provide and maintain parks that offer sites for trailer parking, tenting and some even have lodging facilities. Many people are unaware of the opportunity for recreation that requires little outlay of money and in some instances none. You can purchase a tennis racket and can of balls for a nominal charge. Take lessons even for free often under public recreation programs. Your tax money helps pay for this so you should participate. An investment in a golf club can give a lot of pleasure driving the ball around a park or open land. Our children can have a great amount of fun joining organized playground groups in the summer or other times. Where we can't afford camps, private clubs, commercial entertainment and the like, there are many fine programs for all ages sponsored by the YWCA and the YMCA, usually after school and evenings for both youth and adults. As a boy I attended summer YMCA camp for four or five years. I learned to swim, something about crafts, play tennis, wrestle, baseball and in general to "take it." For one who was a mother's boy, this was great—being taught skills, to play games, learn about nature and have a chance to compete in organized sports and to be dependent on yourself. The lessons of these years have remained—I still play tennis, swim, hike and have the self-respect of one who keeps physically fit. For those who do not have this kind of opportunity for their children, day camps may be available or scouting activities which often include trips which are overnight providing the kinds of experiences that children need to have to come to grips with themselves and learn special self-enhancing skills. A lot of carry-over comes too, from learning games and activities that provide fun, entertainment and leisure they are valuable for the future.

We should not lose sight of the fact that as middlescents, we have the greatest stress upon us at this time than any other. For many who cannot find ways to cope with the constant drain of energy and responsibility, the prospect for survival is dark. Knowing about opportunities for our children to find recreation that is wholesome and directed by responsible agencies or groups will provide us with a period of relief and time for leisure for ourselves. We must remember that our life in a sense is like an oil lamp, if the oil is always burning and the lamp never filled, it eventually will go out. Only the wick burns like nerves too long taut and jaded. Opportunity is needed for us to have time to ourselves to recharge our lamps; if we have three or four children, the husbanding of our energy is crucial. So for some assistance, see what is available in your community, call or write agencies about their programs for our children or ourselves. Even if we have money for entertainment, vacations, etc., the public offerings are frequently fun and enjoyable, not to say anything of the quality. One can only describe as excellent the Boston Pops Orchestra providing the public with its concerts (the one on July 4th every year that the nation shares via television). I remember in Richmond, Virginia, a few years ago the public sponsorship of summer concerts, plays, etc., at the beautiful outdoor setting at Dogwood Dell where one could lie on the grass or sit listening to the lilting music of Cole Porter or watch the unfolding of a Shakespeare story. These are reproduced in countless thousands of places across the land (New York in Central Park has drama, music, lectures) and forcign places. In England a few years ago I listened to the magnificent concerts in St. James Park, London, at noontime. Other places have these public entertainment—Italy, Germany, Japan, France, etc.

It is perhaps interesting to note the differences existing in the kinds of leisure activities in which various socioeconomic classes participate. Results of one study revealed the following:

	Upper Class	Middle Class	Lower Class
Team Sports	2%	2%	3%
Individual Sports (Tennis, golf, bowling)	30%	20%	10%
Hobbies	20%	23%	5%
Sedentary (Cards, Televiewing)	48%	55%	82%

Television viewing has become the most used way of using leisure time today. Many people read and alternately watch the screen.

Everyone needs recreation and leisure and there should be several activities in which we are involved, regardless of our economic circumstance. A good hobby—stamp or coin collecting, sewing, wood working, gardening, or whatever—should be balanced by the addition of some recreational activity or two. Preferably one indoor activity and outdoor activity—square dancing or bowling and swimming, running, walking or tennis.

VACATIONS

Everyone needs a vacation at least once a year away from their regular work and living place. If possible, besides the longer vacation people who constantly deal with people in their work need other shorter times away, that is, weekends and holidays spaced in between the longer late spring, summer or fall vacation. Increasingly many persons have invested in a second home as a retreat from the work-a-day world and people they see frequently that remind them of problems or bring problems to them other than those at work or the office. The type of vacation and places to go depend upon how many persons are involved, their interests and certainly the types of relations that exist between them. If it is a family situation, then probably the decision to be made has to be fundamentally one that allows for recreational opportunity for children. The place, if possible, in a situation where younger children (3-11) can get supervision without the necessity of your being with theme very moment. Of course, the movie has been used as a place to deposit older children for two hours or so if one is within reasonable distance from your lodging. But this is only good for a limited period of time and concern for safety in its location another concern. Family vacations are fun, particularly where the interests can be easily commonized. If the interests are too diverse, then the problem of satisfying every one becomes an insurmountable one.

Vacations are designed to be fun and something different, a change of pace to provide new scenery and to be restful. If you spend all the time driving, this can be very tiring and make post-vacation effects the opposite of what we intended. For many people simply a good rest is the principal goal they have in mind for a vacation, one, which is away from the cares of the everyday routine. For families going to the seashore or mountains, look for smaller places and towns if possible, other than those known as tourist centers, for this will be in many cases the most economical. Good clean beaches in the south like Rehobeth Beach, Delaware; Virginia Beach, Virginia; Wrightsville Beach, North Carolina (Family Beach); Myrtle Beach, South Carolina; and Daytona Beach, Florida, provide varied accommodations ranging from very expensive to relatively inexpensive. You pay more the closer you get to the water. Many from New York, Pennsylvania and New Jersey go to Atlantic City, New Jersey. With gambling, rates of many rooms are sky high. Travel agencies organize weekend tours to there from several states away. There are good sources for organizing trips any where without paying also AAA members get trip suggestions, mileage, etc.

If you have to pay considerable for a room or two rooms, you can offset this by eating outside (Burger King, MacDonald's, etc.) of the hotel or motel where you're lodging. Bringing sandwiches and fruits prepared in advance will do. Many people eat a hamburger or hotdog for lunch and go to Bonanza, Ponderosa, or a chain restaurant with serving lines for the evening meal. Some motels, etc., have pool-side concession stands with drinks and sandwiches. One thing about staying at large hotels or motels is that many of them have organized programs for children and adults. A number have social activities and directors who plan something special every day. I remember one place (a hotel) I stayed in at Virginia Beach, Virginia, where each evening bingo was provided in the lobby or some game suitable for the entire family to enjoy. Another thing to remember is that often a chain motel like Day's Inn, Ramada Inns and Holiday Inns give special rates for children under certain ages or provide the lodging free with reductions in meals or give them free. Many better hotels have cheaper rooms, so ask, and also what is included in the price of a room a continental breakfast may be a plus! It would be wise if going to a recreation area or seashore to choose one even ten or fifteen miles away and save twenty-five dollars a day on the lodging for four nearer the ocean, etc., then paying $80.00 to $150.00 a day to be right on the site. The people who have trailers and campers can save most all this outlay and reserve it for other expenses. In the southeast United States, less well-known places are fine for visitation in Florida—Melbourne, Ormond Beach, Del Ray Beach, Boynton Beach, Pompano Beach, Deerfield Beach, Boca Raton—all in south Florida north of Miami. Incidentally, these places have Dog Racing, Harness Racing and Jai Alai in the area. The 'Moon may be over Miami' but often the traffic, the cost tab and impact of numbers make other places the recommended place to stay. This may not save much with gas prices as high as they are. From a more distant home base, you can drive in to special places for boat cruises, the Orange Bowl, Disney World (Orlando), Key West, Hialeah and the Everglades. Write to the Chamber of Commerce in cities to get an idea of accommodations and cost. Southern California and Mexico for people living in the west provides many fine beaches at reasonable prices such as Cardiff-by-the-Sea, Hermosa Beach, Luguna Beach, etc. Those nearby California and in California and in the west can make a wonderful trip beginning in Sonoma and going south over a four or five day trip stopping along the way giving a day or two to San Francisco (the cable cars) and Los Angeles—Rodeo Drive and Hollywood, also San Diego with its wonderful zoo. Also on the way there, the birds fly at Capistrano.

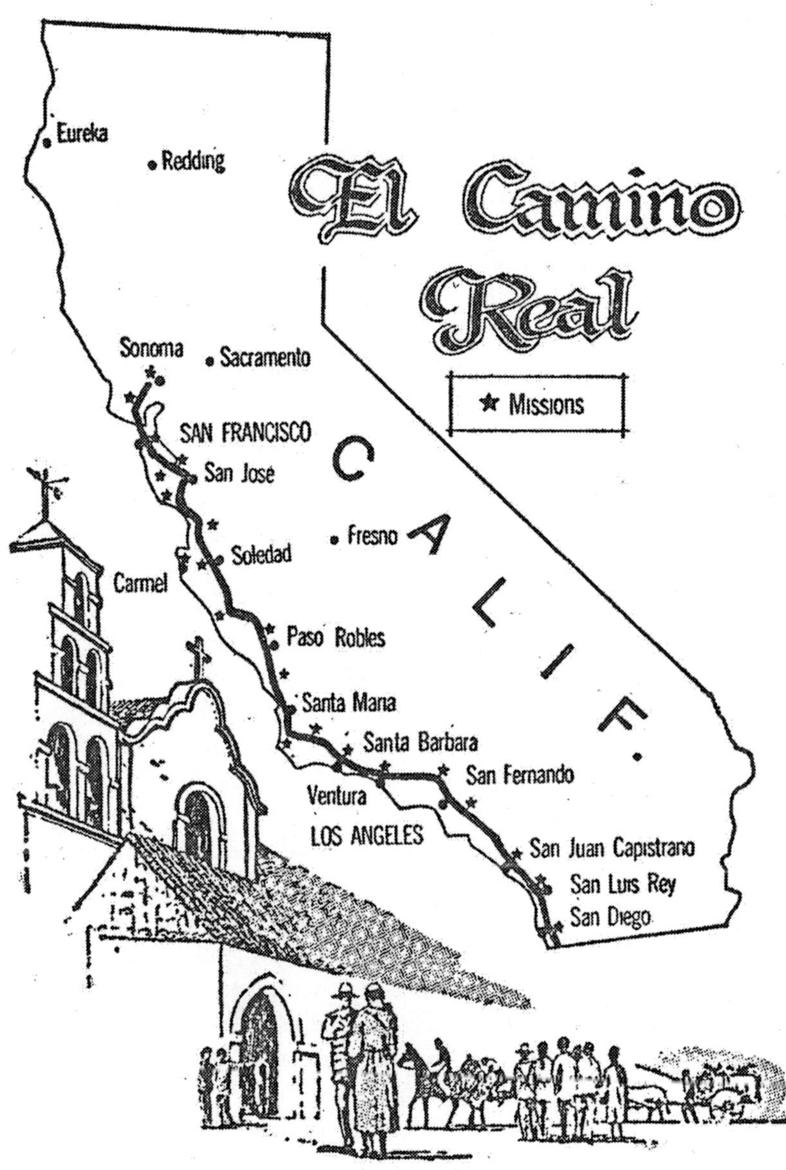
El Camino Real
Missions
CALIF.
Eureka
Redding
Sonoma
Sacramento
SAN FRANCISCO
San José
Fresno
Soledad
Carmel
Paso Robles
Santa Maria
Santa Barbara
San Fernando
Ventura
LOS ANGELES
San Juan Capistrano
San Luis Rey
San Diego

People who are members of the AAA (American Automobile Association) can receive trips planned for them with suggestions on many other things besides road conditions and state police traps. In planning a vacation or when looking for a place to go, write or call a travel agency or two and ask them to send you some literature; they may place you on the mailing lists for periodic trips and excursions they have available. Most of these agencies will handle a number of things for you; and in case you are planning overseas trips, they can be indispensable in arranging for transportation, lodging and tours. Their services are usually without cost to you as they receive their support from the hotels and transportation systems you patronize through them. Whether or not you utilize their services, the free information you may receive is valuable.

There are a number of great parks, government reservations, etc., which are worth seeing. North Carolina Outer Banks has a Federal Park that boasts beautiful beaches and wild undisturbed land. At Ocracoke, on the southern tip of the Outer Banks, the historical lighthouse (1823) is there and occasional skinny-dipping. To the north of Nags Head there is Cape Hatteras Lighthouse (candy cane colored) built in 1870; it has been moved 3 times to protect it from the encroaching sea it is the tallest lighthouse in America. At Kill Devil Hills where the Wright Brothers' first air flight took place and where the recent celebration of the 100th anniversary took place, the first English Colony of Sir Walter Raleigh was located, also where the first white child was born. The Lost Colony, an outdoor drama, is played there during the summer and is a popular visiting place. Innumerable good camping sites are found in the area. To the north a hundred or so miles is Williamsburg, Colonial capital of early America. This is a good family vacation place for Busch Gardens (a major amusement complex—The Old Country) with the Loch Ness Monster and the Budweiser Brewing Company is near by, plus Jamestown, founded in 1607, 13 years before the Pilgrims came to Plymouth. One could take in Washington, DC (150 miles) or Virginia Beach (60 miles) and Norfolk (Douglas MacArthur Memorial, the Monitor-Merrimac Battle, Chesapeake Bay Bridge [longest in the world], also the largest U.S. Naval base, the Wisconsin battle ship, Naval shipyards), a beautiful new city with reasonable costs. The birthplace of Washington at Wakefield is a beautiful place to visit within several hours of driving and near the birthplace of Robert E. Lee. The entire original layout has been reconstructed plus real simulation of the early manufacturing, raising of livestock and gardening. For persons coming from the west a vacation centering around Washington or Williamsburg gives you the benefit of the beautiful Shenandoah Valley, the beaches, a heavy concentration of historical sights, and still only four or five hours drive to New York (approximately 225 miles). A vacation to New York besides the experiences of the "Big Apple" one can take in the magnificent landscape of western Massachusetts in the Berkshire Mountains, Bar Harbor, Martha's Vineyard, Hyannis Port, and Boston are all in the general vicinity. Vermont, New Hampshire and Maine are also in close priximity. In southern New Hampshire, one can visit the famous Lake Winnepesaukee and nearby Wolfeboro. I spent the night, on one occasion, there at the "oldest resort hotel in America"—the General Wolfe Inn. The food and atmosphere were superb at that time.

If one uses Philadelphia as a base of operation, side visits to New York and Washington are convenient, also, the Gettysburg battlefield. On the other hand, you can stay in between these cities and enjoy the mountainous terrain—the Poconos (Pennsylvania). Middlescent couples getting married for the second time can find fabulous quarters in hotels catering principally to honeymoon couples (Mt. Airy Lodge to name one is for couples only). Great sports and entertainment is afforded everywhere with generally reasonable prices. Lake Wallenpaupeck, just a ways beyond are the Catskill Mountains, New York, is noted for its beautiful clear water. The trip from Stroudsburg (Pennsylvania) up Route 209 to I-84 provides all sorts of crafts display, trails, wild animal life, waterfalls and forest; a trip up Route 402 by Magic Valley (an amusement park) to the big Lake.

The Smokies National Forest is another great adventure. Gatlinburg, western entrance, like a lot of towns oriented principally to tourists, is over commercialized and the prices are high. Asheville (60,000 population) on the eastern side offers a greater opportunity base for exploring the area—Blowing Rock nearby, the outdoor drama of Unto These Hills playing at Cherokee near Sylvia (North Carolina). Mt. Mitchell, highest peak east of the Rocky Mountains, is thirty miles away and there are ten or fifteen fabulous golf courses in the area. A visit to the western mountains, the Rockies, with Denver a base from which to operate, with Estes Park, Vale, golf and skiing, etc. is a good bet.

I had a wonderful vacation by automobile from Augusta, GA to Idaho Falls. Great roads, little traffic except Oklahoma (sorry about this but true), St. Louis, Denver, Pocatela, Idaho (a fine small city) and Idaho Falls from there. Two days at Yellowstone then to Cody, Wyoming. There is Buffalo Bill's museum not just about shooting the large beasts but considerable information about Indian tribes, their way of living, etc. Also great rodeo and outdoor drama about "mountain men" who first lived in this area. From Cody the trip to Jackson Hole is wonderful with the Grand Tetons mountain range on your right all the way. The rugged, ragged, snow covered mountains top the Rocky Mountains for grandeur in my opinion and Jackson Hole is a resort for many Hollywood stars in the winter and spring.

Anyway, you get the idea from this incomplete vacation travelogue—take a vacation even if it will be difficult to afford it. Go across town and rent a motel room for two or three days where you can stay in bed as long as you like or eat when you get ready. People with high stress jobs need monthly escapes. It is true we can't escape the reality of a job but the break gives us a chance to regroup and sort things out, untangle the nerves and restore our energy. Wives need a surcease from cooking, house cleaning and respite from total children surveillance.

One parting word, those who have the money but little time can fly for a great change of pace and unique settings to places in the Caribbean. I went with my daughter to Elbow Beach in Bermuda one time to see if the sand there was really pink—you know, it was!! The water and climate make the Bahamas—Freeport, Nassau—ideal also with the islands like St. Thomas. It's cheaper than you might think. The Carnival mainly out of Miami offers reasonable prices, but emphasized rock music and gambling for late nights. Nostalgic music I did not find that is the band people 50-60 would like for dancing. Their ships are large. Holland-America lines though have smaller ships but good food and entertainment.

Another place new for many to go is Costa Rica; many middle class Americans have built homes there and literate people of European origin live there, and the country is beautiful. Lacsa, the national airline, has very reasonable three-night package deals originating out of Miami. Other opportunities like this exist out of Dallas and Houston for trips to Mexico and Central America.

For those who can take a trip to Europe this can be the ultimate. I went by boat (the Queen Elizabeth II) from New York to Cherbourg, France, and then visited fifteen countries via the Eurarail pass (Express train transportation at a reduced rate, purchased from two weeks or for longer periods) and finally after a week in London flew back to New York. Through the Cunard Lines, my daughter and I got a reduced rate for flying British Airways on the return trip. Her rate was reduced initially because of age. Even greater reductions are presently being advertised. But for the five to six days at sea, there is everything to do, movies, games, swimming, dancing, bridge, live entertainment, discos, gambling a library, and time to relax. The Eurarail travel is first class and fast (three hours from Paris to Amsterdam) and dining on the train is unlike that in our country is a treat. Families can get excellent accommodations reasonable or even cheaply when special rates are offered (tourist), the entertainment and access to almost all of the facilities on board. The trains in Europe typically go to the heart of the city like in Paris, Frankfurt, Stockholm, Rome, unlike the airports that are usually 15 to 20 miles out. The Queen Elizabeth II food I found was not as good (variety and amounts) as that on the Greek and Italian lines, which may be expected as these and many other cruise ships project this as their principal forte. Hotels in Europe are there in quantity that cater to every pocketbook—even the less expensive are clean. One striking out to Europe on his own should be well advised to research his trip carefully. I don't mean every detail, time should be left to do nothing or to explore unfettered by a schedule. Tours can be found in the principal cities that run close by your lodging and the local concierge will assist you at a hotel.

Recreation and leisure are too important to be left to chance. They should be planned for mainly in terms of having them. Having them regularly on whatever basis we can. A visit to good friends, even our children, can be fun. Even a work convention can be fun for the family. We shouldn't plan every bit of our time and if it's over-planned, then it may become work with the planner calling for us constantly to get and keep on the schedule. And we shouldn't decide we want to go to the Grand Canyon 2000 miles away when we really want to play a little tennis or golf down at the seashore or up in the mountains. I believe the amount of time spent on vacation is not the most important thing, but how it is spent. Don't go somewhere just to have a topic of conversation or as a status stripe on your sleeve—go because you want to go to see or do something that's not possible at home. Don't make it a rat race and plan more than you can do!

Learning to have leisure has kept many a person from the sanatorium or emergency ward. Middle age people have tough times taking time out, for we're the people who because times were bad in our youth and since only the rich could play, we weren't conditioned to leisure. We need to learn to take our turn at play—all of us—the taxi driver, the store clerk, the bank clerk, the teacher, the physician and whether poor or not so poor, there is something we can do to give ourselves a time of relaxation and quiet. For every hour of work there should be an offsetting hour of rest and play so that our days should be divided by thirds—one-third for work, one third for rest, one-third to play and for time to be alone—to worship and for reverie.

CHAPTER VII

GETTING A JOB AND SECOND CAREERS

"Bringing Home the Bacon!"

In America most men and women are engaged in work or careers outside the home during their middlescent years. In the age bracket 35 to 65 a large majority of women and men hold down regular jobs, some of them working at several jobs. Women nearly equal the number of men in the work force, not only in numbers entering but 82 million are bosses of small and large enterprises. Recently noted is the fact that more women now are applying for medical school in America than men. In Russia seventy-five percent of the physicians are women. Medicine in Russia is considered a technology more than a profession. Interesting is the fact that a college professor's status there ranks him higher than a medical doctor. The figure of women working outside the home is over sixty-seven percent of 125 million in the work force (more than half of the total force) and growing, of this number one-third thirty years of age or over are divorced or will get a divorce. Add to this the fact that one third of all wives with children under three and up to school age shows fifty percent or more work outside the home. The rate of women working outside the home drops from twenty-four to thirty-five (the child bearing years) then rises again.

Frequently at the present time people find it essential to change jobs, careers for the first time secure a job, some because of changing technologies, competition from abroad, the downsizing of manufacturing, shifts in consumer interest and obsolescence. In short, the nature of work is in flux!–smaller families, new fields of work, general change in a major way through the information, service and communication sectors. These economies are salient feature in the new environment of work. One third of all women 30 years of age or will be divorced, add this fact that 70% or less of the children will live with two parents. The divorced woman of 35 to 45 hardly gets enough money to raise two or more children. Even with support they can't cover the needs so work on the outside is imperative! To begin a new career or start a second career makes planning essential. Even this can be traumatic. Retraining is difficult for it entails (1) some loss of security, (2) loss prestige, (3) the competitive market.

The middle-aged person, man or woman, faces a struggle for jobs in many instances as they will be in competition with the young who have been more recently schooled and the computer society is a hand maiden second hand ability. Hence, looking for a job other than employment in basic labor, clerking, sales, care taking, or industry (frequently they have their own training programs) will find a need to go back to school! Certainly they need to have more money than the minimum wage. Women, especially those who have worked in the home for years will have many fears associated with entering work on the outside or enrolling in courses in a community college or business school to prepare themselves for employment. There is some good news some business concerns allow work to be done at home and one can start their own business at home. More about this later giving details.

Those considering or preparing to enter the work force needs to have confidence in their abilities. The middle age employee is really the "cream of the crop" of the job market. As I have pointed out earlier the middle aged person is not hobbled by the immaturity of youth nor the infirmity of many older persons. Their chief assets are: maturity, experience, stability and wisdom, also their outlook is generally more purposeful because they are playing for keeps and have more at stake. In a study a few years ago the National Association of Manufacturing rated 23% of older workers superior, 70% equal to the younger worker and only 7% poor. Somewhat like this study was one done at the University of Illinois utilizing data from 3,000 employees found 69% of the older workers had fewer absences only 9% had more than younger workers. Some 34% turned out better work, 59% turned out the same quality of work with 9% producing poorer work. Even though this is true getting a job won't be easy unless you will be working in a fast food place or a super market.

There are some special problems, particularly for women (men also who are over fifty) who are in their middlescence years and seeking jobs for the first time outside of the home. There is the bias against those fifty or over although Federal Law since 1968 forbids discrimination of those 40-65 years of age.

Some things to consider according to *Christian Life Style* pamphlet for women working outside the home includes:

1. Does the need for money justify the extra effort? Having to work outside may bring unhappiness with working when considering its affects-hurried life style, less time for self and children, strain-relationships with husband particularly where he doesn't take part of the home work load from the wife. Studies show little changes for the women who with a job rather two jobs, one for which she gets money and the other a no pay job-home care.
2. Family support and appreciation may offer the necessary encouragement for a woman to find fulfillment in work outside the home.
3. A woman may go to work outside the home when she receives family support. Studies show that when the wife works she gets some additional help form the husband at home but not much in most cases.
4. Obviously a more demanding routine must be ordered when the wife works outside.
5. Work outside the home should be suited to her aptitude and be meaningful.
6. A major consideration is whether or not satisfactory arrangements for the care of children can be made. Inadequate care for children can be brutalizing.
7. A final concern involves the woman recognizing her limitations as well as strengths. If the work leaves a woman exhausted with no reserve remaining for home and family then the returns will cancel the positive affects.

There are some other hazards that face the wife and mother who works. It could mean postponement of having children, it could mean the neglect of children already in the home; it could result in extraordinary strain and tension within the family, little time could be left for the fine art of living, communication problems with children and husbands could grow. There is also the possibility of tension due to larger income and higher job status for the wife with the resulting challenge to the male ego. If so this will have to be worked out. Most people know about an extra-marital love affair that has developed as a result of the wife's working outside the home. CNN network on a recent program said 50% of women who have an affair met their new love at work. This hazard must be acknowledged. There is also the hazard of the wife's making social ties with fellow workers that may exclude the husband or drive a wedge into the family's social life. In men this situation has existed particularly in white-collar jobs, i.e., in factories, teaching and social service.

If you absolutely have to have a job, take any kind of job that provides remuneration beyond the minimum wage. Over two million jobs have been lost in manufacturing over the past two years. The unemployed figure continues upward with 82 million listed now (recently the percent is down) besides those who have quit looking for the time being and those coming from prisons and many thousands more from rehabilitation, new high school and college graduates, etc., making the true number something like 12 million. The first goal for most of those wanting to be hired immediately is how to get a job. We'll provide that information after we discuss what kind of work and where do you want to do it. Relevant and crucial is what do you want to do? What and where are inextricably bound. In the case of the young student who wanted to be a teacher from early grade school. She graduated with a degree in English but couldn't find a job nearby so she took a job a good distance away in a small mountain village. Unfortunately the mountain children had no use for her teaching and there wasn't any support among their parents. Her intentions to teach good grammar failed and she gave up after a term. Where you want to go can affect what you want to do. Perhaps the teacher of English will have learned that from her experience.

WHAT TO DO

To begin to find out what do I want to do, one must examine those aptitudes you have, talents, gifts and skills. I'm not gifted or talented you claim. I may have skills I'm not sure! What to "do" is tied to skills that you possess skills that relate to people, facts-data and things. Skills are found in people that they do not recognize. People think of skill like the doctor's use of a scalpel used in an operation or the precise cutting of a stone by the diamond cutter. Examine the often used diagram (that follows) to see and ordering of skills of people examining what to do–those categories listed are connected with the job you want. For the essential skills in the three categories are required or prescribed and those at the top a discretionary nature that is to be used at your liking or wanting. For dealing with data the higher level is synthesizing; for people mentoring and for things is setting up. These like lower level skills are called transferable skills. They are functional skills. The ones you use to accomplish a task. The simpler skills are those at the bottom and those more complex skills at the top, it is assumed one has/can use skills that are below.

Schema of Skills
HIGHER ORDER SKILLS

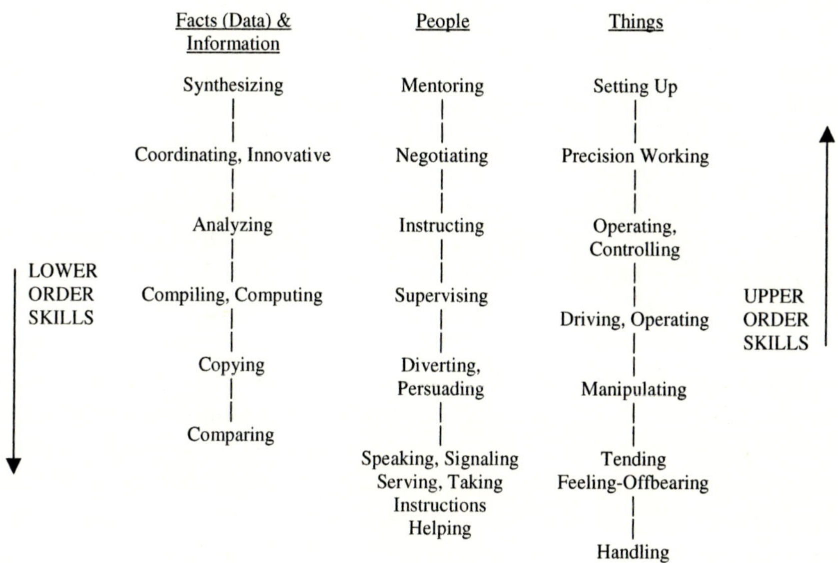

Adapted from *What Color is Your Parachute?* Bolles, 2004.

LOWER ORDER SKILLS

These skills are not traits, that is like energy, ability to get along with people, gives attention to detail, dynamic, good personality, is persistent and dependable. Traits are important in choosing a job for instance if you are shy and the projected job requires meeting and dealing with people you may need to reconsider foregoing those types of jobs. If you have a trait of being persistent then that would subserve the skill of problem solving. With use of the computer there are tests that will give you a clue about your traits or "type" one is the Personality Questionnaire (http://meyers-briggs.com/info.html) costs 3 dollars. Another is the Keirsey Temperament Sorter (http://www.keirsey.com/) and it is free.

On the basis of your experience you can always claim the highest skills you can rightly have. The greater the skills you can transfer the more leverage you will have in seeking and on the job. You will also have less competition than otherwise. Along with searching for a job there are accompanying fears that because of some minuses you possess or biases that exist for you to secure even lower level positions like the racial bias, foreigner bias, physical handicap, prisoner, possess no degree, or I'm too young, too old and I'm shy.

You must, even if doubts about looking for a certain niche trouble you, make wheels of your difficulties and ride on to success. In short, mustering up your courage. Remember—faint heart never won fair lady! I remember the French phrase "Fortune favors the brave"! If you can't think of anything you would like to do if you will invest some time and a little money in looking for the job of your dreams then see Bolles, in his book *What Color is Your Parachute?*, 2004 (Ten Speed Press, $17.95) and do the Job Tree Exercises (adapted from The Flower) you will get an idea. In this diagram there are six branches with a trunk in the center. The branches represent Living Locations, the place you want to work; your Main Interests, Salary Level and Responsibility; My Ideal Job Conditions; My Favorite Type of Personnel Environment; and the things, purposes, etc. that mean the most to me. In the trunk, your main competencies are listed first. This, if utilized, will help in a definitive way get to the result of locating your ideal job and at the very least help identify your skills and put into perspective the entire employment picture for you, that is your abilities, your ideal working place and the way in which you should organize your search for a position. Many times people have the ideal job in mind but unfortunately it is in an ungodly place or too far away from your comfort and family responsibility location. Only you can decide where you will work, at what you'll do and the conditions necessary for your employment.

If the level of the pay and location is not a big deal but you need to make $20,000 or $30,000 the hottest markets across the country are in the following cities:

Ft. Myers, Florida and Bonita Springs close by
Houston, Texas
Phoenix, Arizona
Fargo, North Dakota—fine if you like a long winter and short summer
Fayetteville, Arkansas with Bentonville close by it's the home of Wal-Mart. This area will have nearly 700,000 people by 2025
Atlanta, Georgia—its still the hub of Southeast US of A
Reno, Nevada—It is becoming a large city with new opportunities not just gambling halls and strippers or easy marriage!
Norfolk, Virginia and surrounding close by cities—Virginia Beach, Suffolk, Williamsburg, Portsmouth and Chesapeake—combined with a population of over a million and a half.

Low unemployment, government installations—naval and air bases. The best state for Federal employment—they have more government agencies, more facilities and provide more grants and monies for bases, warehouses, armies, parks, military reservations, etc. Virginia Beach had an average family income of $52,000 in 2004 making it fourth in large cities in the nation. Two other cities are in California-San Francisco and San Jose. Another place is Alaska. These three had higher costs of living than Virginia Beach does.

<u>States With The Most Jobs</u>

District of Columbia
California
Illinois
Maryland
North Carolina
Virginia

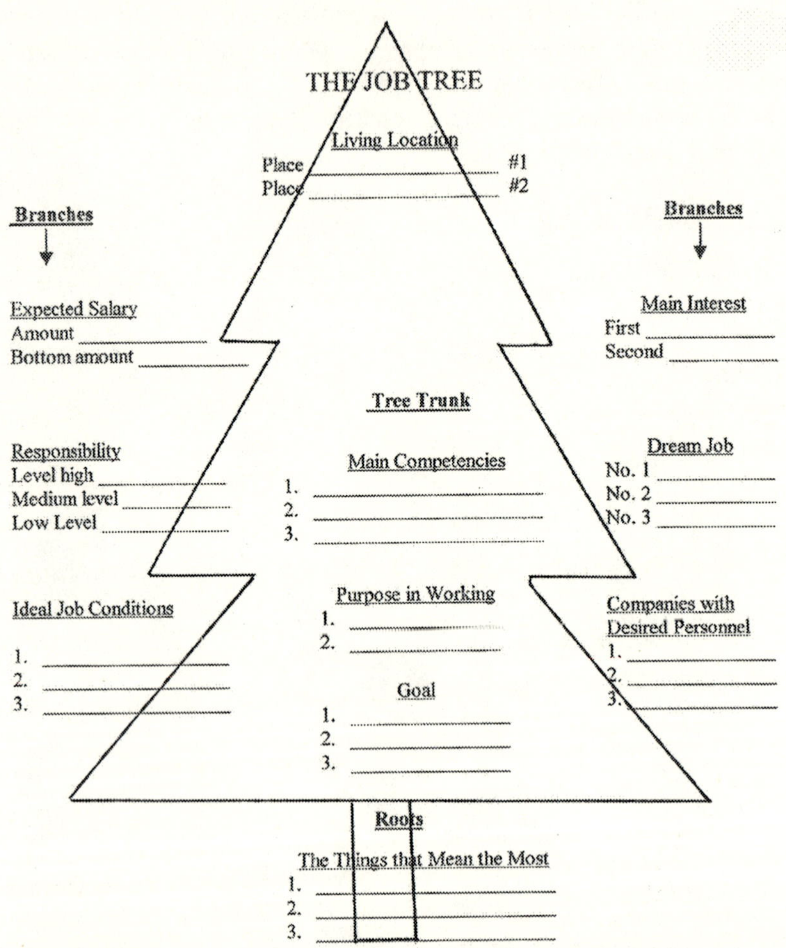

All parts of the tree (roots, trunk and branches) represent aspect of the working situation. Each component is important, but compromise will be made through trade-offs, i.e., the salary is great but the location not so good or the skills you have don't match the requirements too well but the organization is very supportive.

Adapted from *What Color is Your Parachute?* Bolles, 2004.

The Federal Government Employment Agency provides consultation for those without jobs who are citizens about available job openings, vocational training and general guidance. Also there are over 2,000 State Employment agencies affiliated with the U.S. Department of Labor, which provides the following services without charge. One or both agencies (federal and state) provide these seven features:

1. Intensive review of qualifications to discover new skills or refurbish old ones.
2. Careful appraisal of interests and aptitude.
3. Evaluation of physical capacities and activities with the help of the family physician.
4. Informs the applicant about career opportunities and job requirements.
5. Counseling to assist the person in choosing new fields of work or retraining to broaden skills in old fields.
6. Consultation with workers having common problems in job seeking to help them plan and conduct a job search.
7. Selective placement, whenever there is evidence of physical disabilities or slowing down, to protect the worker and the employer for health and safety hazards.

Hunting for a Job

How Employers Like to Fill a Vacant Position

Employers seek to fill vacancy in their business by going with the tried and true. That means hiring someone known to them to be effective workers. That heads the list of methods they use, here is the list in order of importance as adapted from *What Color is Your Parachute*, Bolles, 2004.

1. Hiring from within the firm, a part-timer, or person whose track record is a proven one or if it's a promotion pick from those already employed.
2. Using the evidence of work from an unknown person who brings proof from their record that they have the skills necessary to the job.
3. Using the word of a trusted colleague or best friend who has first hand knowledge of a candidate having employed them or seen their work.

4. Using an agency they trust. This may be a recruiter or search firm or regular job agency. It represents a way to save time and eliminate biases they might have in advance and it keeps them from hiring via a neutral source the best person.
5. Using an ad published in a newspaper or on-line, etc. They then pick from those who respond who are the best suited or whose background fits to come for an interview.
6. Using a resume even if it were unsolicited but only if the employer has to have someone now, in other words the job must be filled pronto!

<u>The way the usual job hunter seeks employment.</u>

1. Send many resumes to employers even if they aren't requested. Unfortunately only 4% gets jobs this way according to Bolles (2004).
2. Put a job wanted ad in the newspaper, on-line, etc. Employers are wary of these kinds, having recognized the overblown, the untruthful and exaggerated hype sometimes used.
3. Use an agency, this will cost you a fee. Some agencies will allow you to pay them over a few months when they get you a job. This is not perfect but if you are a teacher, technologist, researcher, etc. this may be the only way to find a job in an area you want to locate and you know no one there. Many state and federal agencies are required by law to advertise positions. These ads elicit many responses but unless you know that many are foreclosed you will be disappointed for all too often jobs are given to the insider.
4. Use your network of friends or co-workers. These people sometimes know of positions available and have information of their accessibility.
5. Submit to a business concern in writing or in person their ability to do the job they think you need usually illustrating with examples their expertise.
6. Finally many people think last of the company they work for or want to work for. They may try to get a position as a part-time worker, consultant or maybe they have had experience with a similar company, with this parlay it into getting an interview. The known quality of a worker is the chief factor but without a contact unless you're on their payroll or have a like work record you'll be out of luck.

> Employers hiring within their organization look around to see you they don't have to take a chance on failing.

Adapted from *What Color is Your Parachute,* Bolles, 2004.

Most employers begin with a resume in filling some slot to working. Most job seekers recognize this, the question is what kind of a resume? The answers here are difficult because you are trying to guess what type of vita, in this case a succinct note of what you want, your qualifications (education, experience, special expertise, etc.), how you would fit their job description and perhaps what would you bring as intangibles to the firm and facts of your personal life (information about your family–wife and children if any, health, something about your desire to work in a certain field). Then maybe a brief summary relating your persona–work style, effectiveness and willingness to learn. This may not do it, some people put a picture on or with their resume. Of course you run the risk of someone not liking that personal introduction to you. Some will probably like it. Some employers do not like résumés but most employers use it to screen out those they are not interested in hiring. One thing is sure do not submit a long resume, this is a cul de sac! Check the spelling for accuracy and the sheet for mistakes is crucial. However if you are an educator, writers, management at a high level, more detail is desirable so to include what you did when pointing out accomplishments and experience and in general knowledge you have about the position sought is important. The résumé is usually used by those looking for work and the most by all odds as the entree to a job by most employment seekers. Unfortunately only about 4%, as mentioned earlier achieve success this way. One problem is that you do not know whether the bosses or the person they report to wants a man or woman employee, a brown, black or white person, older or younger that you, male or female or even religion and don't overlook nation of origin. In sales work employers usually want a diverse group hence they would look at all the attributes possible such as mentioned above. In other positions where cooperation in paramount, how the prospective employee fits in is moot. This is very important.

If you find an employer's ad on their Web site or one from the better known Internet boards such as Monster, Careerbuilder, Job Options or even a newspaper ad send your resumes to them by E-mail by an address you have. Follow this up with the mail that is formatted in good taste giving the employer a chance to see what your resume looks like. After a week call their number and see if they indeed have both of your resumes. Ask then about setting up an appointment for a face to face interview. They may try to do this over the phone, avoid that if possible for it eliminates the possible opportunity to present yourself. Most first impressions are crucial in getting attention and eventually a job. All of these things are helping you to escape the employers attempt to screen out most of the inquirers.

If you get an interview there are several aspects upon which you will be judged for the job. The aspects are: skills you possess, initiative, your knowledge, your persistence, experience, who you know (or about whom) and the persuasiveness you exhibit. Being too aggressive will turn off many hirers as will too much talk on each of the items discussed. Your résumé should be in their hands if not bring a single page one and hand it to the interviewer. Who you know is not generally important but if your field in editing, writing, book agent or marketing director, consulting (who and what, why and when) and etc. are. Suffice it to say you need to be prepared to discuss, and talk about these topics.

We should talk more about first impressions. Joyce Brothers, famous psychologist, says that the first 30 seconds of the interview is the most important and she says most decisions on hiring is made then. Dr. Brothers calls this the "halo" effect–it is the what we radiate from ourselves–it can be positive or negative. God forbid you stumble on the rug upon entrance to the interviewer's office. The "halo" effect is the first impression we have of a person when we meet them. To demonstrate the psychologists affirmation of this Dr. Brothers asked a friend of hers (owner of an electronic firm) to interview several people on the effect of first impressions or the "halo" effect. What he didn't know was she fooled him by sending the same man to interview with him twice. For each interview he changed himself–once unshaven, hippie look, sloven, wore sneakers, tennis shoes and had shaggy hair. He did however speak intelligently about his interest in the field. Also though rumpled he was clean! On the second interview the plant was clean-shaven, had a standard haircut, had a dark business suit on, looked the electronic chief in the eye, had a firm hand shake and spoke intelligently about the prospective field of work. These visits were on subsequent days. The interviewer didn't recognize the men were the same individual, if he had the plant was prepared to say the other man was my cousin. Later Dr. Brothers' friend reported to her that the gentlemen he interviewed last would be hired by him for his company but the first man never. The electronic chief couldn't believe he had validated her principle of first impressions. Psychologists had isolated two facets of the interview for a job, first, the "halo" effect and secondly the interview itself. This latter aspect is composed of three factors–these are questions from the interviewer; assuming usually he has seen and read your resume. (1) So you're interested in our opening? (2) Why do you want this job? and (3) What can you tell me about yourself?

Regarding the first query the answer is not just "yes" but yes plus like I'm very much interested in this position for it's the kind I've been looking for quite a while. Response of the second question cannot be that I think it would be interesting or because I like working with people–most personnel executives would write you off on that answer for they would assume you didn't really know what you wanted to do. You should be able to tell something involving the nature of the work in which you would reveal your fit with the job offered by the firm. The final questions about yourself–your life history won't cut it! The interviewer would think "oh hum." What he or she is looking for is a clue to your motivation, character and ambition. One night say, if cars were his interest, I've liked to sell or repair cars ever since I tore one apart and put it back together. Or ever since I was a little girl selling lemonade, I've wanted to sell things, to display things, to organize things, etc. Your replies cannot be simply yes or no but something also but not too long, keep you answers to two minutes or less. If they want more information they'll ask. If you've had some activity or lost a job because of being fired don't bring it up–you deserve another try. If you are asked directly about a certain job, which didn't turn out so well, be truthful but put the best light you can on the experience. There was a man I knew who was a principal of a small high school from which he was fired. The Superintendent interviewing him in another school district asked him, why are you leaving the job you have? The principal simply said he was fired and gave briefly the situation he was in at his school. The Superintendent was impressed with his honesty and hired him. He also knew something about the setting unstableness in the other district before he met his new principal. Nevertheless one should accentuate the positive, eliminate the negative and stay away from Mr. In-between!

It is well known by psychologists that there are certain features of the first impression and interview, which is understood, will help you get the job. Dress for success not overly, conspicuously nor too casually, for men wear a white shirt and tie and for women a nice fitting dress with pleasant colors and design but no high heels, glamour is not what they are looking for on most jobs. Now if the job is for acting maybe creativity and some outlandish outfit is suitable to demonstrate a part or dialog you'll present, or other effect. When you arrive for the interview be sure your hands are not sweaty, dry them if they are before you meet the hiring person. Also when you shake hands make sure your shake is firm–many a person lost a possible job because of a weak handshake. Upon entrance to the office make sure your head is raised and look the person in the eye and continue that throughout the meeting. You may not be able to choose the sitting location but if you are to the left of the interviewer you're in luck! People, studies show, pay more attention to you if you are to their left. But even on the right there should be no barrier between you and personnel, interview. In general the closer (not right upon them) you are to the speaker the more equalized is the relationship. When entering the room for your talk about the job hold you head up high, smile and stand straight. Check your clothes before the interview for dandruff, wrinkles, slip showing, hose sagging or hair out of place. Remember you need to have everything going for you that you can and that also means being on time! One final note be sure to rehearse the presentation you will make ahead of time–even go over it several times for practice makes perfect! Soldiers who are preparing get basic training and they soon master it adequately but to get them ingrained so they become automatic takes time and practice. Having attended to these suggestions you should have your halo in place to begin a successful interview with confidence!

Getting Interview and To Enhance Your Prospects

There are several things you need to keep in mind in finding a job. From Bolles, 2004.

1. Seek a position with a small organization (25 or less), two-thirds of the new jobs are there.
2. Seek help for finding interviews from friends and other people you know. You need many people to help for it increases your chances.
3. Do your homework on a company after you have looked the place over, using the library-their encyclopedias on Careers, Dictionary on Careers (5 vols.) and Informational Interviews. The library resource has hundreds of occupation sketches, which are detailed and have crucial information.
4. Find out if possible who will in fact hire you for the company. Lean on your friends and contacts to see that you get to see that person.
5. Ask for only fifteen or twenty minutes of their time when you get an appointment and if arranged keep your word.
6. Make them aware of your potential and knowledge of their organization. After leaving the meeting write them or call them to thank them for their time.

On the other hand, six factors that you should recognize which militate against you getting employed are:

1. Forget large organizations, they typically hire within. Go beyond the NASDAQ group of companies.
2. Find by yourself places to interview using ads, resumes and career notices.
3. Do your homework before going there to apply for the job.
4. Allowing Personnel Department usually in a Human Resources Department to interview you. Their job is to screen you out, theirs is a negative approach so avoid this if possible.
5. Set a time limit on the appointment you make with a company. Do not beg for a job or say any time suits you to visit them.
6. Send a think you note or make a call to the reviewer.

A mature worker should never hesitate to take further training in refresher courses or in a new occupation. Further training is greatly appreciated by personnel managers or employers, because they realize that such a person has the stamina necessary to fight and not let age (middle) become a problem in making a living. For those of you who have never completed their education evening schools can prove a big second chance. Vocational Education through Public School Systems offers wide varieties of opportunity. Evening college and programs like those at community colleges, Teletechnic courses from universities like Old Dominion University which provide a variety of programs the M.S., continuing education programs and workshops. City school systems have special vocational programs available. A chance to complete high school work and begin a college degree is clearly there. Counseling is available and tailored to the needs of older people. There is research which shows intelligence doesn't evaporate at forty or fifty. Even gains are reported. So you want to go to work, make your plans and start. America's labor force will require nearly 200 million people by 2020–you could be one!

Here are some among many jobs you can get with training or college credits.

Assciate Degree (AA Degree)
Community College

Paralegal
Dental hygienists
Registered nurse
Health information technician
Respiratory therapist
Cardiology technologist
Radiologist technology
Middle management jobs in sales and business Office worker

Bachelor's Degree (B.S. or A.B.)
College or University

Data base administrator
Computer resource
Computer engineer
System analyst
Physical therapist
Occupational therapist
Special Education teacher
High School teacher
Elementary School teacher
Records in schools, hospitals and businesses
Communications

Adult Education Training
Often receive a Certificate

Dental Assistant
Hair dresser
Auto mechanic
REALTOR7
Nurses assistant
Opening a small business as
Home cleaning
Child care and baby sitting
Sell goods made in the home—quilts, baskets
afghans, etc.
Carpentry
Sheet metal

Trade School
Award a Diploma with Study Completion

Auto mechanic
Data processor
Dental assistant
Desktop publisher
Food service
Hair dresserBstylist, cosmetologist
L.P. nurse
Air conditioning and heating
Secretary
Telephone repair
Electrician
Plumbing

Adapted from Bolles, 2004.

To review and to supplement the best ways to secure a job again,

1. Through friends, family, community contacts, career centers, community college and college or high school where you graduated. Has a 33% success rate.
2. Going to the employer's place, the factory or office where you want to work even if there is no vacancy. Unbelievable 47% success rate. Again the saying "fortune favors the brave"!

3. Using the yellow pages you locate the position or job you like in a town or city where you are. Call them and ask if there is an opening in the type of job you are interested. Sixty-nine percent success rate!
4. With a group repeat the advice given above using the Yellow Pages to isolate the jobs the group is interested. The success rate is out sight—84%.
5. Do a life-rearranging job change, this is by far the most difficult method to seek a job and get one. It entails additional education frequently moving, cost schooling, franchising, starting a business of your own, etc. Besides being perhaps disruptive to the family.

The success rates seem unrealistic though validated by some experts but you may not have any positive results with any of these ideas. It is believed that if you use three or four of these methods success in finding a job will come. There are ways to avoid using for a job search those listed as the least likely to bring a happy return. These are the most likely to result in failure:

1. Using the Internet. This method has only a 4% success rate. If your field is computer or technical maybe ten or twelve percent success. Look at present ads from an urban newspaper–most ask you to apply on line, fax and some provide a telephone number and address. These are medical personnel represented here but other jobs are presented the same way.
2. Sending resumes out in wholesale and a random manner. It does improve your chances but barely 7% in this manner of hunting for work with the medical ads is like sending a resume to all of those listed for a particular position.
3. Seeking positions advertised in trade and professional magazines that are in your field. This has only a 7% rate of success. These kinds of job particularly those with high salaries have thousands of applicants. Now most people in their thirties have college work and about half of them have an Associate of Arts or Bachelors degree. Most of those jobs advertised in the professional journal require a bachelor's degree or more.
4. Answering a local newspaper ad have a success rate of between 5% and 20% depending on the job level–those with greater pay have the smaller success rate, the other maybe ten percent or more.
5. Signing with an employment agency has a 5% success rate up to thirty percent, perhaps higher for women. The fee goes up for the better paying positions. To get a job in teaching in another state this may be

an only option although many urban schools hold teacher fairs where they offer contracts to those who come given the proper credentials. Recruiters who are seen mostly in technical fields–laboratory work–geologists, chemist or physicist, technologies and managers find employees for employers who need to fill a post often offer in fast time. The recruiter typically gets his fee from the company or industry that is hiring.

Resume Examples

Name

Address Street, City, Zip
Phone
E-mail, Fax Number, etc.

Your Background

Birthday, location, family
Schooling
Activities: Schooling extracurricular, company, jobs, music lessons or golf or tennis, etc.
Health

Kind of Job You Would Like to Have:

What got your interest about this position?
What skills, insights, abilities, experience you bring to suggest you would be a good fit for company and specifically to the position available.

Your expectations

References: Former employer, school and college, counselors, other prominent persons—physician, Priest, Minister, college professor, etc.

Availability for Interview: Personal, by phone

Available Date for Employment

NAME

Address $ City, State Zip Code $

OBJECTIVE

EMPLOYMENT

JOB TITLE — YEARS EMPLOYED (EX: 1992–94)
Organization Name — *City and State of Organization*

Describe responsibilities and accomplishments here.

JOB TITLE — YEARS EMPLOYED (EX: 1992–94)
Organization Name — *City and State of Organization*

Describe responsibilities and accomplishments here.

EDUCATION

DEGREE EARNED OR MAJOR — YEARS ATTENDED (EX: 1992–94)
Institution Name — *City and State of Institution*

Describe honors, related activities and accomplishments here.

DEGREE EARNED OR MAJOR — YEARS ATTENDED (EX: 1992–94)
Institution Name — *City and State of Institution*

Describe honors, related activities and accomplishments here.

SKILLS

- Bullets may be used here to create an attractive list of skills

The following methods though not as unsuccessful than the five methods listed previously but still know that these offer some work.

- Visiting the place where employers hire. Many companies have signs posted at their offices saying we are hiring and suggests some times to come what to bring for an interview and where. Many colleges and high schools have career days in which many different businesses have information to give out through pamphlets, counselors and representatives to answer questions and provide encouragement to prospects. Where jobs are contracted by unions has a higher success rate up to 20%, remember only 8% for just going to the employment place. The drawback for the union is they may get you a job in six months from now when you need one right now.
- Job hunting through taking the Civil Service Examination has a success rate of 12%. A good score on the test gives a boost to a resume also your age and may help get you the job you want but only one of eight or nine of 100 get work this way.
- Asking a former teacher–high or college for suggestions about a job is successful one out of eight times on average. The nearer the time of your last class with the instructor the better the chance of their having something in mind for you to help you be successful.
- Going to a State or Federal Employment Service Office. This will bring good results in one of several times. There are some collateral aspects to this, that is that you get a lot of information and knowledge of what is out there in terms of jobs and requirements.

In the past three years jobs have been fewer with unemployment having risen, manufacturing, which provides usually higher paying work have lost jobs to the tune of over 2 million. Many more are going to China, Japan, Europe and other smaller countries. There is some good news, however, for in 2004 thousands of baby boomers are reaching the peak of their earnings and job growth is coming alive now, earlier boomers retiring, tax cuts may help, due to low inventories that need filling and retail sales are up in 2003. *The New York Times* reports for 2004 the following jobs in selected professions, provide opportunity. John Challenger, the chief executive of the outplacement firm of Challenger, Gray and Christmas says you can't export jobs like financial planners, physical therapists and others like these abroad.

There are those that believe the economy will be slow (it has not done as suggested by Bloomberg) because of the high rate of unemployment, continuing loss of jobs over seas, value of the dollar against foreign markets, government debt health through Medicare and Medicaid and cost of the war. Nevertheless some new jobs are being created, though at a slow rate, people retire, quit working, high level of productivity and slow rise in inflation. Last year's stock market rise will parallel generally the economy demanding higher numbers of workers.

So, There May Be Jobs After All

PROJECTED JOB OPENINGS FOR SELECTED PROFESSIONS, 2000 TO 2010 *in thousands*	
Nurse	1,889
Pharmaceutical sales rep.	606
I.T. consultant	513
Financial planner	423
Information security specialist	338
Accountant	326
Pharmacist	236
Physical therapist	137
Corporate librarian	111
Investigator	20

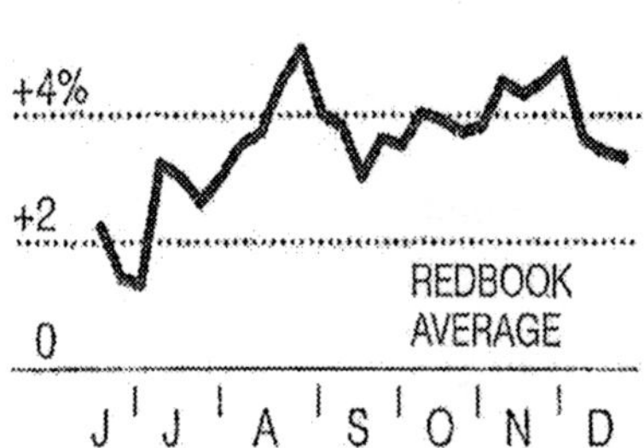

Stocks Through 2004 and Trend Beyond

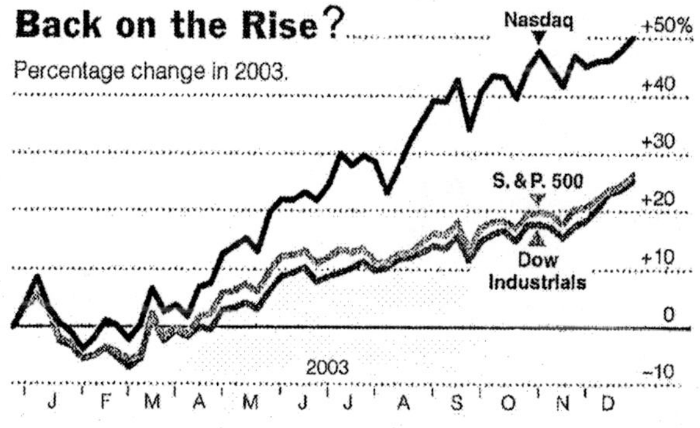

The New York Times 2004

Low paying jobs are easily found–fast food chains, pick-up labor, sales clerking, newspaper routes, yard work, waiters or waitresses, dish washers, child and day care (for elderly persons), supermarket jobs (baggers, stock handling, cashiers, delivery and carry out), janitorial and distributing leaflets, ads for pizza places, home repair, hardware stores, etc., are examples of the easy to find employment. Many of these are posted on the store at their locations.

According to *Time Magazine* (2004) these categories of jobs will grow larger than others. This is projected from 2000 to 2010.

1. Food preparation-Starbuck's, Fast Foods, etc. 673,000
2. Customer Service Representatives 621,000
3. Registered Nurses, biggest gain of all health nos 561,000
4. Retail sales persons, the largest of all occupations..............................510,000
5. Computer Support Specialists 491,000
6. Cashiers, those that have retail and restaurant experience 474,000
7. Office clerks-general 430,000
8. Security guards, low pay around 17,900 per year 391,000
9. Computer soft wear engineers 380,000
10. Waiters and waitresses-has high turnover but with tips okay..........304,000
11. General Operations Manager 364,000
12. Truck drivers-heavy and tractor-trailers...340,000
13. Nurses Aids, Orderlies 323,000
14. Janitors and Cleaners...317,000
15. Post Secondary Teachers and College Instructors 315,000

This is a list of the Ten Largest Losers of the Occupational Groups over the next six years:

1. Farming	318,000
2. Order Clerks	71,000
3. Bank Tellers	57,000
4. Insurance Claim Adjusters	58,000
5. Word Processors	57,000
6. Sewing Machine Operators	51,000
7. Dishwashers	46,000
8. Switch Board Operators	41,000
9. Local Interviewers	38,000
10. Computer Operators	33,000

These figures are probably accurate projections still in these occupations many thousands of jobs are available if one wishes to be hired in these fields. They will not ever entirely vanish. What follows for you is the twenty-five fastest growing occupations and those with the most job openings. This information was provided by American's Career Infonet. On their Web Site you can find this data available for any state you wish to check out jobs of interest to you and other information like wages for specific fields, numbers of jobs and kinds of positions available.

Fastest Growing Occupations

Overall

Listed below are the 25 occupations projected to grow the fastest during the 1998-2008 time period.

Occupation	Employment		Percent Gain
	1998	2008	
All Other Computer Scientists	97,500	212,100	54%
Computer Engineers	299,300	622,100	52%
Computer Support Specialists	429,300	868,700	54%
Systems Analysts, Electronic Data Processing	616,900	1,194,200	52%
Data Base Administrators	87,400	154,900	43%
Electronic Pagination System Operators	225,600	44,200	42%
Paralegal Personnel	136,000	220,400	38%
Medical Assistants	252,200	398,000	37%
Human Services Workers	268,400	409,900	34%
Physician Assistants	66,300	98,100	30%
Data Processing Equipment Repairers	79,300	116,600	32%
Residential Counselors	189,900	277,800	32%
Electronic Semiconductor Processors	63,400	92,000	31%
Engineering, Mathematical, and Natural Sciences Managers	326,200	468,000	30%
Medical Records Technicians	92,400	132,900	31%
Physical and Corrective Therapy Assistants and Aides	82,100	118,000	30.5%
Respiratory Therapists	86,400	123,200	30%
Dental Assistants	228,900	325,400	30%
Surgical Technologists and Technicians	54,000	76,600	30%
Dental Hygienists	143,400	201,400	29%
Sales Agents, Securities, Commodities, and Financial Services	303,100	427,400	29%
Occupational Therapy Assistants and Aides	18,600	26,000	28.5%
Cardiology Technologists	20,800	29,000	28%

Occupations with the Most Openings

Overall

Listed below are the 25 occupations with the largest number of projected openings during the 1998-2008 time period. See Department of Labor data on an occupation to learn more about it, including state data.

Occupation	1998 Employment	Average annual jobs (due to growth replacement)
Cashiers	3,197,800	194,970
Salespersons, Retail	4,056,500	193,800
Waiters and Waitresses	2,018,600	141,520
General Office Clerks	3,021,000	129,960
General Managers and Top Executives	3,362,400	113,970
Food Preparation Workers	1,256,300	113,970
Registered Nurses	2,078,800	79,400
Teachers, Secondary School	1,426,200	77,770
First-Line Supervisors and Managers/Supervisors-Clerical and Administrative Support Workers	1,610,800	67,540
Systems Analysts, Electronic Data Processing	616,900	61,560
Teachers, Elementary School	1,754,500	60,990
First-Line Supervisors and Managers/Supervisors-Sales and Related Workers	2,583,800	60,070
Laborers, Landscaping and Groundskeeping	1,129,900	57,150
Receptionists and Information Clerks	1,293,500	55,300
Guards and Watch Guards	1,026,700	55,020
Nursing Aides, Orderlies, and Attendants	1,366,600	51,510
Computer Support Specialists	429,300	46,600
Hand Packers and Packagers	984,000	45,630
Secretaries, Except Legal and Medical	2,690,400	43,910
Bookkeeping, Accounting, and Auditing Clerks	2,077,600	38,780
Maintenance Repairers, General Utility	1,232,500	37,040
Cooks, Restaurant	783,200	35,090
Computer Engineers	299,300	34,140
Automotive Mechanics	789,600	32,820
Child Care Workers	904,500	32,500

Most Underpaid Jobs

There are jobs you may not want to have but still pay rather well. According to Chris Plummer, a CBS Marketwatch columnist (2004) in San Francisco, the ten most underpaid jobs are: listed below. His view is that it isn't just a matter of how much money she or he makes but it is the function of how valuable or "loathsome" the work is relative to the earnings. Two of these pay salaries greater than the median wage–$37,500. Teachers and Nurses are not on Plummer's list but are thought of as tough jobs. Elementary School teaching–the average salary is 38,000 dollars for nine to ten months. The same rate for a year would be $48,000, a tough job for sure but it has the potential to be fulfilling and enjoyable. It isn't listed among the ten and the following are not listed in rank order. Nurses, in fierce demand, make $49,000 for staff jobs. For Registered Nurses who wish some time off for family, child bearing, etc., they can work two shifts of 12 hours back-to-back and make $40,000.

- Slaughterers and Meat Packers–typical salary is $20,000 a year. If under Union supervision they can usually make more. These heavy lifters are not in our thinking when we eat a marinated steak I'm sure.
- Restaurant Dishwashers–salary is $7.25 per hour–the germs and bacteria these people are exposed to is scary! Garbage to scrap off plates with the grease that gets into your skin pores because the commercial soaps and hot water have opened them up along with the thanklessness makes this a terrible job almost at any price. You can get this kind of a job easily.
- Consumer Loan Collection Agents–salary is $22,826 a year. Most of the people they deal with hate them for calling, talk obsessively to them and many less the half are going to pay nothing. No wonder these agents bash the delinquent customer. Plummer says zero percent financing offer you bought hook, line and sinker!
- Pest Controller salary $24,120 a year. Eliminating rats, cockroaches, spiders, etc., in dark recesses that these creatures inhabit. Imagine the fumes they suck up in terms of chemicals that get into their bodies. Try ridding the noises in the wall in a home. Even snakes have been discovered in the basement and even in living quarters of folks.
- Police Officers–salary $41,950. The strain the job puts on their psyches is immense and we pay them to be society's voice of authority then shy away from them. Their lives are constantly threatened by violence. No wonder some go astray maybe thinking it's a payback for shabby pay.

- Substance Abuse Counselors, yearly salary $31,300. This job is the missionary work of the social-service system rehabilitating the lost souls. Many of these are former abusers who can't find gainful work from suspicious employers and the risk of becoming a doper or addict all over again. They don't save many addicts but the few are appreciated!
- Medical School Residents-$41,000 per year. These doctors have had three or four years in Medical School and mostly have M.D.'s and are doing the required resident work. They give 60 to 100 hours a week, equivalent to the dishwashers pay, to do the dirty work for the medical profession in and around the medical school's community, mainly in urban areas. The Medical Schools call their pay stipend allowing them to give the low remuneration. If they were paid more maybe their desire to pay-back via the greedy grab for money when they do have their own patients.
- Emergency and Medical Technicians along with Paramedics–$25,450. If they help save the patient down the road they will be treated by well-heeled physicians (Top wage earners in a major job category of all). They're under tremendous pressure and now days have to contend with the overweight baby boomers so hope they will get a raise.
- Funeral Home Attendants–$19,200 and Morgue-26,167. A dismal constant reminder of death, the most depressing work environment making the hospice a cheery place in comparison.
- Preschool Teacher–Salary $21,907, Day Care workers-19,900. The Day Care personnel are grossly underpaid but the Preschool Teacher who is responsible for teaching of reading and numbers. These people deal with the very young ages one year to five. These are critical years in the development of the child. They need to have the patience of Job, the knowledge of a trained developmental psychologist, a disciplinarian, social awareness and (loco parentis) a stand in for parents. This amounts to more knowledge than a pediatrician would have in terms of psychology, child development, exempting the actually medical.

Most of you reading this would not take one of these jobs because of the pay or because of what's involved in doing them. But they are very much needed, in fact they are crucial in our society and we owe them a debt of gratitude and they merit a fifty to one hundred percent raise pronto!

On the positive side there are ways to help yourself if you want to go beyond the minimal wage. Many will need to obtain some or more education. Avenues abound for taking courses for new positions at home through the computer or by mail. Even college degrees may be obtained from Universities like Phoenix University (picked at random) who claims to be the largest private college institution in the nation. They state that you can get a degree in two and a half years. Claims of these schools make can be obtained from State Departments of Education in each state's capital. Get their literature and check out what it costs, programs, their veracity, etc. There are many of these types of schools. Business colleges abound offering one or two for diplomas in secretarial work, business bookkeeping, management and a variety of other business related jobs.

Some colleges have programs at their conclusion offer diplomas in a variety of fields. One such school is Stratford in New York State (1-800-363-0058 or www.scitraining.com). They offer forty-five career diplomas (see below) in fields calculated to give you chance of employment and a boost to your ego along with higher pay than the low wage hourly paid groups. Here are the forty-five categories. They also will provide free career information. In yesteryear Universities offered some of this work through their extension departments, some still do, the work is done at home via mail and computer. One note these Colleges and Universities do require work not just going through the motion so be prepared to work if you undertake getting additional education in this manner.

CAREER OPPORTUNITIES AT HOME

Cosmetology/ Esthetics DIPLOMA	Accounting DIPLOMA	Computer Programming DIPLOMA	Nursing Assistant DIPLOMA	High School DIPLOMA
Child Psychology DIPLOMA	Sewing and Dressmaking DIPLOMA	Paralegal/Lega l Assistant DIPLOMA	Psychology/Soci al Work DIPLOMA	English as a Second Language DIPLOMA
Creative Writing DIPLOMA	Child Day Care Management DIPLOMA	Florist/Floral Design DIPLOMA	Business Management DIPLOMA	Auto Mechanics DIPLOMA
Home Inspector DIPLOMA	Administrative Secretary/Secretar y DIPLOMA	Gardening/ Landscaping DIPLOMA	Private Investigator DIPLOMA	Electrician DIPLOMA
Managing Your Own Business DIPLOMA	Veterinary Assistant DIPLOMA	Hotel & Restaurant Management DIPLOMA	Interior Decorating DIPLOMA	Bookkeeping DIPLOMA
Real Estate Appraiser DIPLOMA	Locksmithing DIPLOMA	PC Specialist DIPLOMA	Medical Transcriptionist DIPLOMA	Security/Police Sciences DIPLOMA
Funeral Service Education DIPLOMA	Art DIPLOMA	Travel & Tourism DIPLOMA	PC Repair DIPLOMA	Medical Office Assistant DIPLOMA
Astrology/ Parapsycholog y DIPLOMA	Sex & Drug Counseling DIPLOMA	Internet Specialist DIPLOMA	Natural Health Consultant DIPLOMA	Early Childhood Education DIPLOMA
Physical Therapy Aide DIPLOMA	Medical Billing Specialist DIPLOMA	Photography DIPLOMA	Pharmacy Assistant DIPLOMA	Teacher Aide DIPLOMA

Stratford Advertisement (2004)

Start A Home Business

Many people in hunting for a job they wanted find it is elusive they settled for trying to work at home with a business they organized. Only a few get rich this way in fact what is typically realized is about three-fourths of what regular outside pay provides in the same kind of work. There are other drawbacks mainly in managing time, that is a balance between the needs of your family. Because each success generates more motivation to work harder and longer time for the family might become less and less. Another thing an individual has a job but they keep hunting for customers, better ideas of how to do their work and publicize it, etc. So, in fact they continue hunting for a job to be successful.

If you have thought about doing a business at home but don't know what kind, search the Amazon categories (http://www.amazon.com/) or Monster. Libraries and bookstores will have information you need. Bolles of *What color is Your Parachute* recommends a book *Working from Home: Everything You Need to Know About Living and Working Under the Same Roof* by Paul and Sarah Edwards (1999) in paperback. Considered by many to be the Bible of Information on Home Businesses. Imagine what you'd like to do, even dream of something, but remember you need to study and have considerable information before you get under way. Some people go about this too slowly and inadequately then lose out to someone who beats them to the idea. I knew a friend who talked to me about an invention or an adaptation of an idea he wanted to market. He researched the idea, what would you do to get a patent, how to market and unfortunately numerous other questions consumed his time. The idea was to design a cover for the backs of trucks, which would keep debris from falling out incurring damage to cars or people. Some states had already laid out what kinds of material being transported that had to be covered. After making slow progress he was beaten by someone else who got there first. If you have an idea for an invention, there are funds available for helping inventors, seek the computer site (http://www.oit.doe.gov/inventions/).

Look in your own community for an opportunity. Consider what is needed, what is missing, how to save time and energy for people. Some such ideas are home delivery of groceries, drugs, food from restaurants, cleaning service, home repairs, yard care, baby sitting in your home even for the elderly.

A franchise may be a good investment. One could start at home in a small way and could begin a catalog, which could be sent anywhere advertising a service, product or help. So if your community is small you could reach out by mail or computer. A man I know started a business newsletter providing information about local businesses, how to do things and where to get various sorts of things and assistance in general. It prospered hence expansion occurred and he began to take ads in his letter which now has grown to be a magazine. I visited him in St. Thomas, though he wasn't getting rich he was living well and enjoying it. Nearly everyone on the island knows him also! Working for others in telecommunication is a thought for many had used this to be successful. You can do this along with your regular job. Teach your spouse or children to help and even ask your boss if he could use your services. Ask him if this is possible, also search the following Web Site http://www.workoptions.com/telecom.htm. Chances are high for failure with these businesses when started from scratch: restaurant, dry cleaners, machine shops, baking companies, trucking, car washing, clothing, infant wear and grocery stores.

FRANCHISES

Franchises have a low failure rate (only around 5%) but some do fail. Many franchises are part of a chain of establishments so you get help from a well-known name and likely to be successful if an unknown business may not get the kind of support you thought or advertisement you would need. Naturally the famous names of big businesses like a motel, hotel or even good-sized eating places will cost considerable up in the six (smaller motel) and seven figure bracket and therefore is beyond most everyone's reach. But if you have some money or can borrow some go for it. Caution only after you have investigated it thoroughly, I mean talk to people who know something about it, that is those in the business with a franchise (see people out of your community, they will likely give you straight answers). Research through libraries, consultants and Internet such as the Better Business Bureau (http://www.bbb.or/library/workathome.asp). If you put a lot of money in an enterprise or borrow and you fail to get it back that money may lead to bankruptcy, certainly a quandary and perhaps misery.

These are the things you must consider when buying a franchise also the same for starting your own business. The three major factors are, and you must answer these questions truthfully (for home business franchises, etc.). What knowledge and skills are required to run you business, what do you know about doing this work and what skills will I have to employ to make this work. Answers to the questions are the first step.

When you need to search for an occupation a good start will be to examine the *Encyclopedia of Careers and Vocational Guidance,* 11th Edition in four volumes published by Ferguson, 2000. All the volumes II through IV are devoted to occupations as many as several hundred are given. Each occupation presents some history, information about the job, its earnings, requirements, the work environment are prospects! Also other sources are provided and the Web Site given. Some selected occupations appear here as adapted from the Ferguson publications mentioned above are illustrated here.

FILM EXTRAS

Film Extras called background performers have non-speaking roles in films, stage shows and TV. They work in crowd scenes or in scenes where a few people are needed to fill out the story.

History

Extras have been used for a hundred years or so in the earliest of films like Birth of the Nation, a silent film, produced by D. W. Griffith, which used thousands of extras. Various scenes required people for the battle scenes, dancing, city sidewalks and other where they were needed for background and fill-in reasons. A film like Titanic, used many extras though often through the use of computer generated images to fill out crowd scenes.

The Job

Extras are always needed, some productions have many employed others few depending upon the story. It is easy to become an extra by registering with a non-union extra casting agency, there are several in Los Angeles, New York and frequently ads appear in the newspaper where the locale has been moved to place like Wilmington, NC, Nags Head, NC, Richmond, VA, Atlanta, GA, Macon, GA, St. Paul, MN, Chicago, IL and Seattle WA asking for extras. They provide information on applying, etc. The days you can work you call the recorded line and ask if they need any one of your description. If so call an agent in their office and they will book it for you. You wear your own clothes, paraphernalia (canes, bat, umbrella) and if you have period or special clothes to use see the wardrobe department for costume fittings.

In some instances the film or scenes require action so special extras who have talent are used such as ability to play baseball, dance or act as a stand-in. These extras generally get better pay than one walking, running or standing in a crowd scene. Typically a film must have 30 from the Film Actors Guild–the film industries union before non-union workers are employed. After you have worked for a while (when you receive vouchers for extraing in a major production) you are eligible to apply for membership in this union by paying dues and initiation fees and thereby receive better pay. The job requires a lot of patience for you often stand around for four or five hours waiting the directors decision on re-takes, etc. and you must know what's going on, focus on what the director says and cooperate with the other crew members. You may be used in one scene or many and sometimes asked to speak a line. Which is what you hope!

Requirements

No special training is needed though SAG membership will help. Many children work in form and TV productions. Some classes in speech, acting and dancing might help particularly if you are chosen for a line or two.

Work Environment

Those who do this work are most likely to live around New York or Los Angeles or at locations (found through ads or the Internet) otherwise but special placers are sporadic at best. Some days you may work only two hours on others maybe 8 to 10 hours. Often the scenes are done over and over and waiting for the cast and crew to prepare for a shot.

Earnings

It is rare that a person can make a living on being a film extra. Eighty percent of the SAG membership makes less than $5,000 a year. So it is principally a part-time job, the wage is typically $95 a day in Los Angeles though this may have risen since 2000. In New York City it's $105 a day. If you have a special talent then you get more and also if you supply props such as a pet or luggage. Drawbacks are that you may be required to work in the rain or smoke even perhaps in the water.

Outlook

Something like 400,000 people act as extras in a year and the competition is fierce. If you would like to act this is a good way to learn the business, make contacts and learn about the industry. Many actors have found their way in by being an extra!

For More Information

- **American Cinema Editors**
  1041 North Formosa Avenue
  West Hollywood, CA 90046
  Tel: 213-850-2900
  Web: http://www.ace-filmeditors.org

- **American Film Institute**
  2021 North Western Avenue
  Los Angeles, CA 90027
  Tel: 323-856-7600
  Email: info@afionline.org
  Web: http://www.afiionline.org

BED AND BREAKFAST OWNERS

Twenty to twenty-five thousand such businesses exist in the United States also known as an Inn or small Hotel ranging in size from four rooms to ten. Today they may be found in a large city but more frequently they are found in small towns, in the country along rivers, in the mountains and near the ocean. The owners interact with the guests, provide information about noted places to visit, museums, tours, recreational areas and landmarks of interest. Typically these establishments serve one meal a day–breakfast although some serve two meals.

History

Cottages for rent found in America along its highways in the 1930's were the precursors of the modern tourist motel. In the last thirty or so years the B & B business developed. The idea was an extension of the tourist home or motel business only on a generally smaller scale. Many people who had large homes from the Victorian age 1880 to 1900, some were historic or were located in recreational areas began opening their homes to guests and most added breakfast. Those people traveling found breakfast non-existent in rural settings so homes gave breakfast recognizing the guests via auto could make it to the next destination by the next meal. The hallmark of these places became clean and comfortable rooms, friendly hosts, tasty meal(s) and conversation. Usually these establishments are well furnished and many have special decor and period furniture. I remember going to Montreal on an occasion nearly forty years ago and stopping in St. Albans, Vermont after seeing an advertisement about a

Bed and Breakfast home. They furnished a large room with a double bed and provided two cots for the small children we had. It was a beautiful old Victorian home with a special tone of its own. I found out that St. Albans was involved in the American Civil War. Confederates raiding from a Canada site robbed the bank there and fled back to north of the border. I visited the bank, still standing, and read the memorials, historical signs, etc., that I found.

The Job

Many bed and breakfast homes have well-documented backgrounds as the former home or a famous general or politician. In Cape May, NJ you see them in Victorian homes, brownstones in Brooklyn or a home designed by Frank Lloyd Wright. Many of these are furnished with antiques or special decorations with a theme such as an oriental setting, western motif, southern, puritan or the theme of a well-known book or story or historical incident, like the Civil War or space exploration in Cape Canaveral. They often reek with individuality.

Taking care of business means getting up early in the morning to prepare breakfast, assuming you have gotten the groceries you need the day before, noting special requests of the visitors. Some places cater to wide differential dietary needs. This, however, is not standard. By early afternoon, 2 p.m., the rooms and bath facilities must be ready as many visitors will start their trips very early in the morning and, therefore, wish to light for the night early avoiding also a last minute look for a place to stay. Keeping a register–their names, addresses, any phone numbers–thought a small part of the work demand keeping records such as bills to be paid, cost of operation, social security accounting for those you hire or maybe even yourself. Tax records for paying the local township, etc., state and federal and for adding to the bill of the overnighters. Purchase of new for replacement, etc., or different furniture, linens, toilet paper, soap, etc. Make available business cards with salient features of your home-business. Unobtrusive signs about smoking or no signs. You get the idea. Your schedule would involve the following: wake up at five or six at the latest for breakfast and clean up following it; then begin cleaning the rooms and making the beds, etc., at ten or eleven. Save time for bookkeeping in the early afternoon one hour say 1:00 p.m. then at two or three o'clock shop for groceries and other needs–light bulbs, soap, new towel rack and whatever. Have house ready for occupancy at 4:30 p.m. Be sure vehicles are cleared from the driveway or parking place and have yard tidied and manicured. Managing a place is more than meets the eye. One has to decide what to charge, that is no small task. One needs in summary to be a manager, an organizer, likes people and has some time to interact with the guests. Advertise in a local travel booklet put out by the Chamber of Commerce office or magazine like *Southern Living* or *The New Englander.*

Requirements

One should be able to handle this work with a high school diploma but if they lack skills then they would need to get some training. Training is available through a mail order course or Internet and Teletechnic course from a university and there are many like Old Dominion University in Norfolk, VA (www.odu.edu) which has the largest Teletechnic program in the USA. Willing to work long, hard hours is essential-nothing can be left to chance.

Work Environment

Increasing a home is located in a city or small town although as previously mentioned many are located in recreational areas and historical settings. The work setting is both inside and outside–the home and the yard–drive way.

Earnings

The money to be made is dependent on several things (1) the size of your inn, (2) the amount of funds you charge, (3) your location and (4) the reputation you achieve. Small homes that can accommodate only three or four people–two bedrooms with a charge of $30.00 per night for a couple–children extra and filled three nights a week will probably accrue 8 to 10 thousand a year. A large bed and breakfast home (eight to ten rooms) could make a substantial amount near $100,000 upward if they charged $75 or $85 a night and were filled five nights a week at $75 per night, you could take in $144,000 per year. Many families do this using older children to assist in serving meals, cleaning or caring for the lawn. They usually are paid by allowances. A frequent pattern of ownership is a man and his wife, two old or young maid sisters, or a mother and daughter/son. The reward that comes to this business is meeting people, knowing about them and being stimulated by their conversation.

Outlook

The growth of these businesses will be as fast as many other kinds of businesses–a projection is fifteen to twenty (perhaps somewhat less during this slowdown) percent growth a year. There are too many in some locations but not enough in other places where they could flourish. One needs to check out a location by talking to a bed and breakfast owner in a different location for they are likely to give you realistic information, also the Chamber of

Commerce, if there is one, Better Business Bureaus to find out the businesses who have difficulties (some won't give you this) and seek what occupational guides suggested.

FOOD SERVICE WORKERS

This work includes the following jobs: waiters (men and women), counter attendants, dining room helpers, fast food workers, dining room helpers, and to other work around food, you may, for instance prepare salads or drinks. Today's food service industry is one of the largest and most active in the nation's economy. In the nineteenth century particularly in European cities many large eating places existed mainly in hotels where food was served in elegant style utilizing many employees to handle the lavish setting and food. In earlier times, the American inns dotted the major roadways and usually had lodging and food available for travelers, some states had laws requiring towns and cities to have such establishments. Mobile societies today like in the USA have many varieties in food offerings from Chinese to Sinn Wang, Western cuisine to Italian lasagna and pizza and available almost any place you travel. Increasingly people eat out, even entertain friends by going to a private club or fine restaurant. Many thousands of jobs are available providing an opportunity to interact with people and sometimes be offered a job at higher pay than they have through the contacts they make.

The Job

There are many variety of jobs in food service, the environment may be a small restaurant, a fast food place, a cafeteria, coffee shop, grills, diners, sandwich shops and even stands seen on street corners or in ballparks. In indoor facilities working means more than just waiting on the customers, in slack time they may be required to clean food equipment, mop floors, take out the trash and polish the serving silver, etc. If they add up the cost of meals they may also be asked if the worker doubled as a cashier to sell a variety of goods at the counter such as mints, chewing gum, candies, pencils, chap sticks, crackers, etc. You may be able to eat a meal or two at no expense to you at the establishment. In formal and expensive restaurants the main jobs in serving food goes to the experienced personnel. These establishments follow formal and correct procedures in serving dinners, etc. The Captain or Headwaiter in large eating places usually greet the customers and seat them although they may turn them over to an assistant to seat them.

The Captain takes reservations, phone calls, assign seats and supervise the work of the waiters. These are the men you see in some movies getting tips for finding people a special seat or when crowded find a place for them. The Wine Stewards help the customer select wine from the restaurant's stock. Dining room assistants or bussers assist waiters do their duties, they take away the dirty dishes, carry in trays of food, and clean up spilled food and broken plates or glasses. Sometimes they bring in the bread, butter and water to the diners. In slow periods they fill salt and pepper shakers, dust tables, etc. Another category of worker is the cafeteria attendant who sets the tables, arrange flowers on the table, also sometimes clears the table, even carries dirty dishes to the kitchen, also sweeps, scrubs floors, attends to hygienic care of the food and move food from storage to work areas. Not much chance for advancement here, however, in the larger eating places one may be chosen as a headwaiter, or get a short order cook position or cook's helper. On the other hand if one is interested in a future in the business of owning or managing a food establishment this type of experience of learning from the inside provides an opportunity found no where else.

Earnings

Getting a job as a food service worker can be negotiated by seeing a posted sign in the window of a food place and walking in particularly those businesses that are smaller. Others from newspaper ads or one could have an employment agency search for a job for you. This type of job search is a good one if where you would like to work in is an exclusive place. Waiters in popular with higher than usual prices are also the place to receive more tips. In resort areas many college students like to work these jobs for the tips are very good. Tips usually are ten to twenty percent of your wage. The Department of Labor several years ago stated that waiters made $14,000 per year including tips. The top ten percent in money making earned near $25,000 a year. Headwaiters earn more than this in large restaurants. Dining room attendants earned $13,520 with the top 10 percent earning $21,300 per year. Kitchen helpers made more than these workers. Food counter workers received $11,440 per year. They also were the recipients of tips. Tips in food-drink places operating mainly at night some as clubs with bars provide tips that are much higher than the basic wage. Often tips are pooled with other employees and divided in many eating places. Wages today are probably higher than given above.

Work Environment

The work in food services is physically strenuous requiring one to carry heavy trays, pots and pans and stand on your feet for long periods of time. Rush hours are also hectic with a good sense of humor an asset! The majority of waiters work 40 to 48 hours per week, food counter workers, waiters' assistants and kitchen helpers generally work less than 30 hours a week. Split shifts are common with several hours between them, for some particularly students this can be a boon allowing them to take a course at college during this time or a mother to take their child(ren) from school to a sitter or home. Some hazards exist in this work place as steam tables, hot stoves are about and knives are handled, floors slippery and sometimes broken glass is around. Most restaurants give their workers their meals free or if not at a reduced price.

Outlook

There are perhaps over 800,000 food service businesses in America and this figure will certainly go up in the years to come. The food industry work force should reach 7,000,000 by 2006. Management jobs will grow the fastest to something like 55,000 by 2006. The drawback is that many companies tie pay to the minimum wage scale. On the other hand if you wish employment for a couple months to help with the living expenses or for a season, say summer time jobs can easily be found. The prospect of the cost of living or some raise in the minimum wage is likely over the next several years.

For More Information

- **Council on Hotel, Restaurant, and Institutional Education**
  1200 17th Street, NW
  Washington, DC 20036-3097
  Tel: 202-331-5990
  Web: http://chrie.org/
- **Canadian Society of Nutrition Management**
  P.O. Box 948
  #2G 57 Simcoe Street
  Oshawa, ON L1H 7N1
  Canada
  Tel: 905-436-0145

For information on careers and scholarships, contact:

- **National Restaurant Association Educational Foundation**
  250 South Wacker Drive, Suite 1400
  Chicago, IL 60606-5834
  Tel: 800-765-2122
  Email: info@foodtrain.org
  Web: http://www.edfound.org
- **Canadian Restaurant and Foodservices Association**
  316 Bloor Street West
  Toronto, ON M5S 1W5
  Canada
  Tel: 800-387-5649

CHEMICAL ENGINEERS

Chemical Engineers takes chemistry out of the classroom (laboratory) for use in the real world! Their job is to develop methods and equipment for the mass production of chemicals and other materials requiring processing. They develop products from these materials such as gasoline, plastics, detergents, metals, pharmaceuticals, foodstuffs and caulks and sealants. Chemical engineers or applied chemistry workers have been around since the ancient Greek period of 800 BC when they first distilled alcohol and at 300-400 BC Aristotle wrote of a process of obtaining fresh water by evaporating and condensing water from the sea! The Chinese fermented rice to make alcohol maybe as early as 1000 BC.

The basis of modern chemistry found its roots in the Renaissance when questioning old notions about interaction of materials–air, water, wood and in general many substances. New discovery was afoot like sulfuric acid used for fertilizers, alkaline for soap, and information on gases. John Dalton and Amedeo Avogadro with their atomic theory laid the foundation for modern chemical research and practice. In the mid-nineteenth century large scale manufacturing needed the knowledge of these chemical technicians as they were called then. In 1888 the first courses in Chemical Engineering were offered at MIT. In the twentieth century chemists organized large-scale production of plastics, antibiotics, high-octane gasoline, synthetic rubber and many other valuable products.

The Job

Chemical engineering is the most versatile of the engineering groups–civil, mechanical and electrical. Chemical engineers have substantial work in college in Chemistry, Mathematics and Physics. Besides this they also have usually taken courses in Geology and Biology. Their work is in laboratories where experimental work is done. Many of these experiments die in the lab. If they prove worthy then these engineers run tests on the processes and make necessary modifications. They work to improve the product with an eye toward reducing the cost of production. The project is reviewed by Process Chemical Engineers to see how the product can most efficiently be produced and to insure quality. They also work on the design of the equipment to be used. Project engineers oversee the construction of new plants and equipment. Field engineers test a new operation–its process and equipment. In most cases they periodically check on the manufacturing of chemicals and operation of the plant to insure safety and product facilitation. Production engineers supervise the day to day operation of the manufacturing of a product. Many chemical engineers work with environmental issues such as pollution, water and recycling. Technical sales engineers work with customers about their products to determine what best fits their needs. They also answer questions about products such as: what does this caulk or sealant work when connected to rock or tile? They enroll in workshops and additional courses from institutions to keep up with the rapid changes and discoveries of new knowledge that occur. Graduate work allows for specialization to a greater degree in fields of kinetics, biotechnology and medical technology.

Requirements

If a man or woman wants to prepare for the position of chemical engineer their education starts early, in fact, in high school with if possible, the inclusion of four years of math (Trigonometry, Calculus, Algebra, Geometry), the same for sciences, Biology, Chemistry, Physics and Computer Science. The college work should replicate this only more so with close to forty hours in this field also some cognate courses. There are about 150 undergraduate programs leading to the B.S. degree in Chemical Engineering many require a fifth year of work and some seven six years. These almost always require an internship in an industrial setting. For management an engineer usually needs an M.S. degree in the field requiring two years or if specializing in research, teaching or administration. For managers an M.B.A. would be helpful. License is required top be a registered engineer. Leading to this title means after four years of experience in the field you take a written exam and make the passing grade.

About one third of chemical engineers are registered. All fifty states and DC have specific licensing regulations. In this field problem-solving ability is essential as is flexibility, inquisitiveness, creativity and open-mindedness.

Employers

About 42% of the Chemical Engineers work in the chemical industry, the remainder work in federal and state government and college and universities. The categories where most engineers (Chemical) are employed are: fuel, electronics, food and consumer products, design and construction, aerospace, materials, environmental control, paper, pulp, biotechnology, pharmaceuticals, public utilities and consulting firms. They are trained to be versatile therefore can easily work in several fields increasing their viability!

Earnings

Chemical Engineers are among the highest paid scientists. Salaries vary with education and experience. The American Institute of Chemical Engineers in 1997 gave the following salaries for these engineers–entry level with a B.S. $42,000 in the field; with a M.S. degree $46,500 and with a Ph.D. $63,000 both of these represent starting salaries. In industry the B.S. brings $63,000, the M.S. $75,000 and the Ph.D. $80,000. These salaries are higher today particularly if the work is in the petroleum section. Many chemical engineers in universities earn $100,000 a year and in industry where they have management responsibilities up to $150,000. Experience and being a licensed engineer enables one to argue for and to get more money. Work is typically done in one place under a roof, though some work outside and most work at one location. There are jobs where the engineers of this type move about often, seen in atomic plant inspectors or where the need develops and they may spend two or three months at one place or even a year. Status is high for these engineers. Their work is extremely important, it requires superior ability and dedication and society recognized their work as crucial in the modern world! Many also know of the great work of these engineers in developing and producing penicillin and sulfur drugs making U.S. casualties lower than any in modern warfare.

Outlook

The chance of employment in this field through 2006 should develop at a twenty percent growth rate. This growth should be in line with other occupations requiring college degrees. Due to the compensation given these engineers, newer engineers will perhaps face stiffer competition in the years ahead, however, I believe environmental needs, new products, development of ones that do not exist now should argue for increased demand for those trained as Chemical Engineers.

More Information

In addition to general career information and a job bank, the American Chemical Society offers a directory of experience opportunities that lists undergraduate internships, summer jobs, and co-op programs.

- **American Chemical Society (ACS)**
  Career Education
  1155 16th Street, NW
  Washington, DC 20036
  Tel: 202-452-2113
  Web: http://www.acs.org

A Final Word

There's a job out there for you, it may be less than you desired or more than you expected. In any case you need to invest time and energy into researching the job you want and the kind you can reasonably fill adequately. To repeat what we have said in this chapter related to job finding I will recite some of the salient features you should use to locate a position.

1. Use a placement office–one that's organized both for profit and those for non-profit. Use the college placement office and their career centers. Use also state and federal guidance and career agencies. One of these may not land you employment but it will give you tips and an understanding of the job market and how to find out about kinds of occupations, etc.
2. Use job fairs and workshops that are offered by your local Chamber of Commerce. Attend college and school career days and employment opportunity sessions frequently advertised in your local newspaper. Some are sponsored by businesses who are searching for employees.
3. Network and Explore References. Many jobs are not publicized and must be found, in some instances businesses have not sought help. Use a business card that indicates your expertise and qualifications (briefly told) name, address and email and telephone numbers. Use cards and letters to discover jobs or to learn more about a particular opportunity. Search the availability of jobs that require the use of

your expertise from prospective employers through email or to get information on the parameters of work which interests you!

4. Search the Web, which is the user-friendly part of the Internet for jobs. Use Monster.com or some other clearinghouse for careers and job searches. Be selective, considering the source of information, know the field and protect your privacy.

5. See classified ads and use them. Think about what they are saying about the work, that is, the requirements and the pay. Find out who the employer is–reputation, etc.

6. Read the fine print. If you consider taking a position remember to have someone go over the contract if there is one for and with you. Check the benefits, part-time jobs rarely pay or provide any! Note vacations, sick leave, hours of work (does overtime get extra pay?), total emoluments, etc. and work conditions. Find out who is to be your supervisor, the chain of command and ask about anything else that you are concerned with related to your work.

GOOD HUNTING

CHAPTER VIII

LOVE, SEX AND MARRIAGE

"Do You Like To Kiss?"

If you read books on or about love, you rarely ever see an attempt to fashion a discrete definition of love. This is due in part to the fact that it interfaces with so many other aspects of our lives–marriage, sex, family, loss of spouse, view of self, attachments, and death. Even divorce is not exempt, for in the process of separation one is frequently called upon, at least to himself, to redefine the meaning of love or evaluate what it is not. There are other components–intimacy, passion, and commitment as suggested by Robert Sternberg. Liking to kiss may have reference to love in that we usually like to kiss the love object or express our satisfaction in this way. For many this is motivated by the physical but probably more because in the long run a lot of other harmonies exist between two persons–view of live in general, goals, compatibility and complementary needs projected for each into the other, etc. The kiss, liking or not liking it, comes to be a gauge or mark of how a marriage is making out. When I visit the honeymoon cottage (where my newlywed daughter and husband live), I check to see if the "kissing machine" is still working. Little kissing usually indicates that perhaps little pleasure exists in marriage, a lot of kissing then a great amount of pleasure in marriage! We recognize it can be perfunctory, also. When the kissing stops, whether at twenty-five or fifty-five, for most the party is over–enter a crisis point of whether or not to try anew with someone else who likes to kiss or tough it out because there are offsetting advantages to staying with a union, kissing or not. Intimacy and passion may be gone but commitment remains.

Love is one thing in childhood and adolescence; it is something else in middlescence and this will be the principal reference to love here. In the meantime, there are some things concerning the topic of love that are general and need to be discussed briefly.

THEORIES ABOUT LOVE

According to Rollo May, there are four kinds of love in Western tradition, via Greek literature. One is sex or lust–libido. The second is Eros, the drive of love to procreate or to create–the urge toward higher forms of being and relationship. A third type is philia–brotherly love like the name and meaning of the city Philadelphia or love in friendship. The fourth is agape, the love devoted to others, the prototype of this love is God's love for man. Certainly there is another kind of love–stergo which means patriotic love, the love of one's country which I presume in our time may not mean the same thing as it did for instance when Richard Lovelace wrote the lines in *To Alcastra on Going to War*–AI could not love thee half so much, loved I not honor more."

On the other hand, Dr. William Kroger suggests there are, from the standpoint of the developmental, four types of love–the first one "I love I" is seen in the child who loves only those who contribute to his well being and comfort and egocentricity. The second type of love is projected self-love (I love me as seen in you). This type is frequently found in immature people who see qualities of others that rightly or wrongly they attribute to themselves. Romantic love is a third type and it is the basis of marriage for most persons for they have been conditioned to believe it is the highest form of love. The principal element of this love is passion and idealism. Unfortunately, when sexual drives fade the partners often become strangers to each other with little commitment or intimacy. The final type of love is mature love identified as the condition where each partner thinks only in terms of the other person's happiness–their chief enjoyment is in giving, not getting or possessing. The sexual impetus does not drive them into marriage and those couples with this base to their marriage usually remain married for a long time. Unfortunately, this is a rare type of love, although it is usually taken to distinguish love apart from mere attachments, likings, desiring, wanting, etc., as Freud used the term, although he said, that love is the attachment and not the feeling. There may be feelings associated with attachment but they are not always pleasant. Love can be romantic and lofty, on the other hand, it can be selfish and highly ego-centered. Some of our loves make us happy and provide a great sense of fulfillment; others keep us constantly striving, feeling inadequate and full of anguish. Therefore, feelings associated with love are not dependable as the sole basis of love for they vary too much, as Fromm says, as much as the ways we express love.

Robert Sternberg, IBM Professor of Psychology and Education at Yale University, has formulated a theory (1986) of love in which he suggests there are three faces of love. I believe these ideas are as compelling even today! The three faces–commitment, intimacy and passion. Sternberg visualizes love as a triangle, the more commitment and intimacy and passion you have, the larger the triangle and the greater the love! Intimacy is emotional closeness, sharing, communication and support. Passion is motivational, physiological arousal, intense desire, it develops quickly and involves kissing, touching, hugging, making love. Commitment is cognitive, it starts at zero and grows, it is first short-term commitment to love another then it becomes long-term commitment to maintain that love as expressed by fidelity.

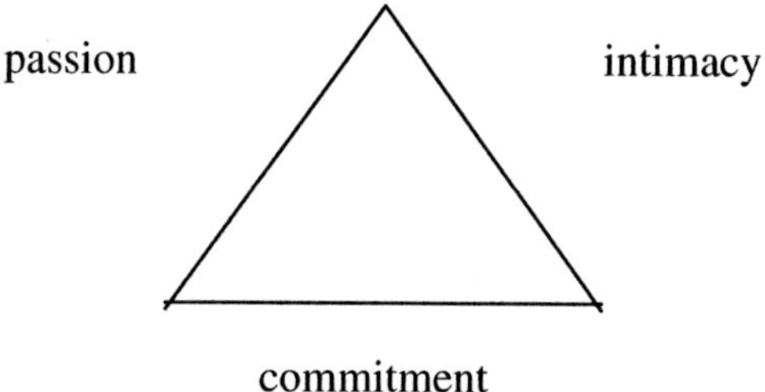

The shape of love based upon this theory says commitment is the cognitive component of love and is all that some couples seem to have left after the intimacy and closeness have been lost and the passion has died down. Intimacy is the emotional component of love. Some people can bare their souls to each other but have little in the way of commitment or passion. This is the characteristic of high-grade friendship. Passion, on the other hand, is the motivational component of love, it calls the tune in some love triangles. This might be an affair or a fling in which there is little intimacy and even less commitment.

Triangles may be used to define various loves beginning with non-love. In this triangle there is no intimacy, commitment or passion. In liking another person, you have intimacy—we can talk to a person, tell them about our life and dreams, there is closeness and warmth but not passion or commitment. With infatuation there is only passion—it is adolescent-instant love upon seeing his dream girl or her dream boy.

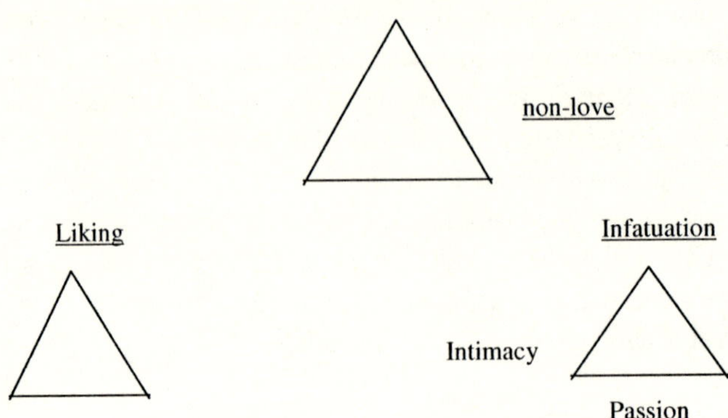

Empty love is frequently called cold love; there's no passion or intimacy, whereas, romantic love has passion and intimacy but not commitment (Romeo and Juliet type). These are like summer affairs which die when autumn comes and vacations are over—she goes one way, he another. Passion plus commitment is what Sternberg calls "fatuous love" (lacking reality). It's the Hollywood type of love—boy meets girl and marries next week—the commitment is to the passion that's aroused them but the emotional core necessary to sustain a commitment is not there.

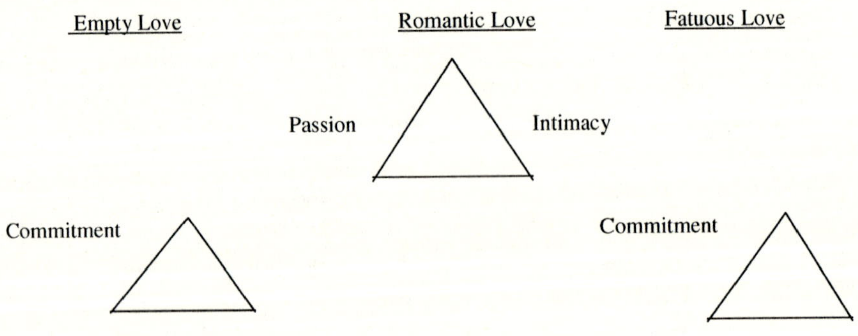

Finally, there is companionate love, which is constructed of commitment and intimacy but not passion. This is long-term friendship—the kind of committed love and intimacy seen in marriages in which the physical attraction has died. Consummate love is where the three forces are all there—passion, intimacy and commitment. Sternberg says this achievement is nearly impossible—like keeping off weight after you have lost it. This love is possible only in very special relationships.

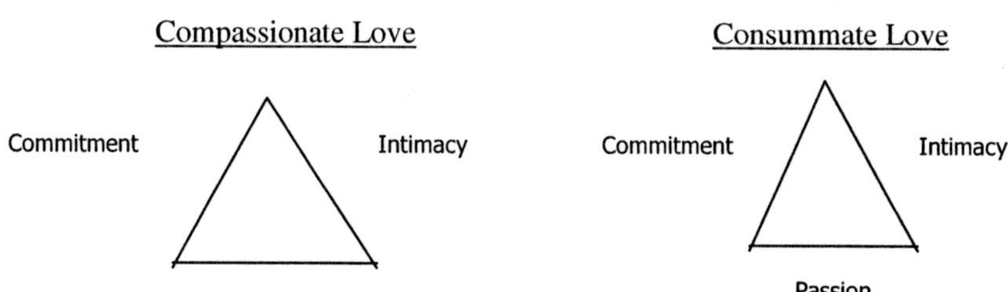

Many theorists believe women are better achieving intimacy than men and they value it more than men. If they fail to get intimacy they desire from a man, they try to find it with women or another man. They establish close friendships and are able to say things to women they can't say to a man. This may account for the fact that women have a much more extensive network of support than does the average man—principally from women.

Passion though initially may be the positive force, which drives people together and though quick to develop is also quick to level off. This negative motivational force, the one that works against the attraction, is slow to develop and slow to fade. The result is first an explosion of passion that is followed by habituation when the more slowly developing negative force kicks in. Like coffee, cigarettes or alcohol addiction that can be rapid once however habituation sets in, increasing the amount needed it no longer stimulates the arousal that occurred earlier. When a person is dooped, they end up more worse off than before—depressed, withdrawal symptoms, irritable, loss of appetite—the negative force is still there after the person or substance is gone. One thing is true, according to Sternberg, the consummate love involves couples who love each other more than anyone else. Among many loves there remain a "lost love" or "parent love" which may never be eradicated.

Love and Sex

One thing should be said, love and sex are not the same. Sex is a way of expressing love to be sure. We should say that love and sex are not necessarily mutually exclusive of each other. In the first place, sex is a basic drive—an appetite like hunger or thirst. Nature made this appetite pleasurable in order to insure the continuation of the race. Sex is physical—it can be identified and measured. Love, unlike sex, is a state of mind and it is much more elusive. Love and sex often occur together, so are mistaken for one another. Love, according to Allan Kaufman in his *Interview with Sex*, is choosy—"It insists on one particular person…sex on the other hand is a passionate interest in another's body." Love may be just as passionate, but its interest is in the whole personality. Love is a deep and constant feeling for another person. The other person's happiness is as important as yours. A person who loves another wants that person to be happy forever—it involves faith in that you allow yourself to be vulnerable to hurt—it involves giving love with conditions—only those imposed by yourself. Like Corinthians I. 13, says Love suffereth long and is kind, is not puffed up, does not act unseemly…

Love gives sex its other satisfactory meaning. There are sinister uses to which sex is put—to achieve power, to trap someone into marriage, to punish oneself or someone else, or to make one feel important. The word itself has become a catchword for advertising. It has come to mean fulfillment, freedom, doing your own thing—the ultimate. Sex is as natural to living as love is to self-actualization, this is the making of one's potential into his best possible self.

When love and sex are intertwined, life is greatly enhanced. The stages through which we develop love start with the child when he discovers his body and becomes attached to it, stroking his genitals and learning to masturbate. It also happens in girls. These attachments are extended to people who care for him and make him happy. The next significant period comes sometime between 5 and 11 or 12 when manipulating his own body is taboo. Attachments are generally reserved for like-sex playmates although this period does not mean everything in the social-sexual area is latent. Many girls and boys in the early part of this period experiment with sex by playing house and doctor-nurse. It is also true that the like-sex attachments are often the source of homosexual contacts. Toward the end of this period, many girls form crushes on uncles, older persons not only their own cross-sexed parent. The adolescent has already experienced many lovers. But when maturity of the sex glands is accomplished, boys and girls begin to notice each other and finally most of them prefer the company of the other sex than their own. This attachment is strong, often called "puppy love." It may not relate directly to strong sex feelings although certainly the physical stirrings are there. Like many attachments of adolescents to objects, ideas, etc., this one too may be idealized. Much like the Victorian Age attempt to express love without sex, some adolescents are not overwhelmed with the idea to initiate sex. A girl may have many puppy loves without participating in direct sex activity or giving up her virginity, and the boy likewise. Most youth will have experienced heterosexual activity by the time they are eighteen. The sense of curiosity and wonderment is woven around the love object and becomes a drive to incorporate the other person as oneself. Aiding in this maturity is the desire, strong in the adolescent, to divest part of his family heritage and try a new attachment—this time in values with another person. The love object partly makes the girl or boy a new personality. When attachments become very special and childhood attachments are gone, then a longer lasting stable love eventually leads to marriage or cohabitation.

DOES MIDDLESCENT LOVE GROW OLDER AND COLDER?

The typical marriage does change over the years. It need not necessarily grow colder as it grows older for among the healthy the ardor of sexuality may diminish very little. Most husbands by the middle of life have mellowed, become thoughtful and tender human beings. Wives have become more understanding though less passive helping to increasingly bear the burden of life. The earlier years have served to iron out many difficulties between husband and wife. Of course, there are many marriages that did not survive to this point. Complete love, according to Dr. Rose Franzblau, a middle years expert, is made up of two components, romantic love and tender love. Both must always be present. There is no doubt that with aging, certain physiological changes takes place that affect sexual activity. At that point, tender love is more predominant, but romantic love is still there. This is now expressed in the mindfulness and consideration that each shows for the other.

No matter what can happen, the statistics tell us the sad tale of nearly 1,126,000 divorces per year in America with a rate of 4 per 1,000 in 2002 (National Center for Health Statistics). It was earlier predicted by 1985 there would be 50% of the married divorcing then an updated projection was 54-55% by 1990. Today of five marriages 18 years old and up 2 will succeed. Three will fail. The heaviest incidence divorce occurs from 20-35 for both men and women. Most divorces occur in the first seven years of marriage. World Almanac 2005 shows marriage and divorce about the same as in 2002, however, many divorces or separations never appear in statistics for one or the other partner just walks or runs and never formalized it legally but in the practical sense are divorced.

According to Joseph Brayshaw, a number of years ago, the serious problems according to the length of marriage were as follows. My research suggests these are still the major issues.

Married Three Years or More
1. Sex
2. Living conditions
3. Parental influence
4. Ill health
5. Incompatibility
6. Infidelity
7. Income

Married Eighteen Years or More
1. Ill health
2. Infidelity
3. Incompatibility
4. Sex
5. Parental influence
6. Living conditions
7. Income

As you can see, the basic problems are the same fifteen years apart only the order in importance has changed. It is not very surprising that problems with sexual adjustment lessen as women are beginning to feel the strength of sexual drives more like men of twenty do and the incidence of extramarital affairs grows. Ill health, of course, can be mental or physical, certainly numerous men and women are alcoholic or drug addicts by forty years of age, have the beginning of a chronic health problem, and many are twenty to thirty pounds overweight and have been under-exercised by some years, therefore, many are suffering from a variety of maladies caused in part by this regimen.

Judging by a number of factors, the American family is eroding according to the second edition of a work *What is Happening to the American Family* (Johns Hopkins University Press, 1988). The so-called traditional American family is hardly dominant as only 56% of Americans are married compared with 75% 30 years ago. If you include families with a breadwinner-husband, homemaker-wife and children much less than 50% reported in the New York Times 2004. Married mothers in the work force represent 70-80% currently against 54% in 1980. It takes two incomes to support the traditional household. Co-habitation and many heterosexuals regardless of income don't want to marry. Demographics say Americans are voting no on marriage. The new economy has eliminated all sorts of traditional values including family wage, job security and money safety nets. It has propelled many women into the work force not necessarily for personal fulfillment. Out-of-wedlock births were 33.5% of all marriages in 2002 in the USA (National Center for Health Statistics 2002). In 1970 only 10%, higher now but were only 18% in 1980—5% in 1960. Co-habitating couples are estimated to have been 2.3 million in 1990 while in 1980 only 1.6 million. In 2004 there are 86 million unmarried adults many co-habitating. Partly reflecting the baby boomers (those born 1947-1965) who were raised in relative affluence only to grow up to find the initial promise not fulfilled. No wonder by mid-life, many of this group at or approaching forty settle for more passion and less commitment.

That infidelity increasingly becomes a problem as ennui in marriage sets in, driving many to have a yen for variety or to enter into a new relationship to bolster their sagging egos, counter burnout or even sexual desire—remember the "Thornbirds" movie and the dowager Barbara Stanwick's desire for the Priest Richard Chamberlain. That family or parental influence is important this late middle age is surprising to sociologist Duane Windemiller who suggests that apparently if parents are interfering in a marriage at the start of it the tendency is to continue. I believe there is something else involved here and it may be more significant. That is that the spouses have not satisfactorily taken care of the unresolved conflicts of childhood. The meaning of my family—its customs, values, aspirations, etc.—have to be consolidated into another set of family values, etc., before reasonable long-lasting harmony can be obtained. Also, too, as psychiatrist Roger Gould states, the illusions of childhood have to be overcome. Growth into persons who are adequate as adults demands that we understand the bargaining we do with our spouses and the negotiations (agreement to allow the wife to go back to school now that the husband makes more money in consideration of her work at home) that we make in continuing marriage. Parents may not interfere so much as that the parent-child is still in the adult and one or both of the other party hasn't acted like their parents.

Besides some of these difficulties, there are those that appear in the developmental life of nearly everyone. These are seen in the middlescent years as problems of confirming or readjusting our identity, the emancipation of our children, evaluation of our careers, status and the growth process which is constantly going ahead, all combine to unsettle our lives and perhaps reduce the joy of life, conjugal love and sexual ardor.

SEX IN THE IN-BETWEEN YEARS

Increasingly, we have come to know more about the sexual lives of the middlescent beginning with the Kinsey Studies of Sexual Behavior of Men and Women in 1949 and 1953. In more recent times, data of importance is available through the *Psychology Today* Survey, *Playboy*, The Hite Report, *Redbook* Report, panels and seminars of *Ladies Home Journal*, Masters and Johnson Reports. The importance and value of sex in American life is too great to be kept a secret. If the Kinsey research seemed flawed due to the sample which included many more college educated than those who had less. It was also suspected that those who were interviewed were the kinds of people who like to talk and therefore somehow these were guilty of overloading the results. We now know beyond doubt that the essential findings were correct and that the results of the sexual revolution have affected every area of our life. It is true that there is some research to show the major change of the revolution is in the way we communicate about sex. Nothing is taboo about sex, even in ordinary conversation among men and women. Although all of this is true, the advent of AIDS has pulled up a caution flag. Easy indiscriminate sex has been stopped in its footstep for most middle-age persons, those from younger adult years, 20-39 for all races contribute the largest total on news cases and old ones excepting among the most foolhardy. There are considerably fewer incidences of AIDS among the middle-aged and those heterosexuals but this group is not exempt. Those involved with casual sex should certainly use a condom–safe behavior–suggests the officials such as Dr. Koop, Surgeon General– abstinence and fidelity.

In 1993 there were about 450,000 cases in this country around 2.5 million people are currently infected with HIV virus, the source of AIDS. Death by HIV is listed in the top ten causes of death. Minority populations are where the disease is chiefly lodged particularly among blacks and Hispanics.

Most AIDS cases reported in this country to date have occurred in the following groups of people in 2001. (Health United States, 2002 CDC National for HIV, STD TV prevention)

- Males sexually active homosexual and bisexual (or men who have had sex with another man since 2001 (57 percent) Women 40%
- Injecting drug use 21%
- Homosexual men, injecting drug users (7.6 percent)
- Persons who have transfusions with blood or blood products (0.8 percent)
- Persons with hemophilia or other blood clotting disorders who have received clotting factor products (1 percent)
- Heterosexual men and women (these include sex partners of persons with AIDS or at risk for AIDS, and people born in countries where spread of the virus by heterosexual sex is thought to be more common than in the United States) (4 percent)
- Infants born to mothers infected with the AIDS virus (1 percent)

About 3 percent of AIDS patients do not fall into any of these groups, but scientists believe that the virus was spread to them in similar ways. Some patients could not be followed up, or dies before complete medical histories could be taken.

A panel on Women and Sex organized by *Ladies Home Journal*, said AIDS has generated an extraordinary amount of fear. But actual use of safety measures—condoms and spermicides is sporadic at best. The press is heralding the new chastity and claiming condoms are in—they may be non-events. Single women walk around with condoms in their pocketbooks but does the condom come out of the pocketbook in a moment of passion and do men accept it, if it does. Said one of the panelists, people feel protected by their community and high-risk areas, but 70% of gay men say they've had a sexual encounter with a married man at least once.

The young middle-aged woman (35-45) reads the book *Open Marriage* may not accept it for herself, but she is apt to look at her marriage with a new and a critical eye. For a segment of society that reads Henry Miller's works, *Tropic of Capricorn* and *Tropic of Cancer*, The Paris Review, or those of this ilk, the new morality has been with us for some time.

Research indicates that among men, they no longer receive their initiation to sex from prostitutes that promiscuity has lessened, and pairing has increased without a necessary commitment to marriage. The young see marriage and parenthood as less attractive than we did twenty-five years ago. In earlier days sex for most women, even though engaged in before marriage, was intimately linked with marriage. Today, this is no longer true for many women. Many of today's teenage girls have been initiated into sex through preventive measures—that is, contraceptive information and its artifacts that are provided by the mother and in some cases school or social agencies. Although the mothers are not saying, now go involve yourself, they recognize the certainty of it. "Turning on" and "making out" is the central theme of much of the media advertisement message, hence adolescents desire to try it out and having done so, they seldom give it up.

One thing that is universally acknowledged in middlescence—that a need exists for sex. The old stereotype of aggressive male and passive female is gone. The sexual revolution, women's liberation movement, and population zero have simultaneously come together to create a changed but more suitable climate for society—more forthright and honest. Masters and Johnson with their stress on mutuality and communication have made a contribution for better inter-sex understanding. Rightfully or wrongfully, sex has become the common denominator of fulfillment for most middle-aged persons, particularly those entering early middlescence 35 to 45. It is true that many who devalue their marriages because of lack of satisfaction have not tried to understand the cause and the effect involved. The range of contrast goes something like this: sex is good when life is good; sex is bad when life is bad, or stated another way, when love exists between people it overrides frustrations with child raising, lack of money, technique in sex delivery is not perfect and other problems. Certainly with the impact of the feminist movement, the rising prowess of women in the work world and politics, women are examining their lives and concomitants (satisfactions, careers, family) with increasing seriousness. Research reveals that the incidence of marital infidelity begins for the men involved in their 20's and continues on a plateau until the early 60's. For men with incomes over $60,000 a year, 70% have affairs. It is believed 20% of married men under age 40 believe they will have an affair. For married women, there is a build-up with the higher percentage of those involved in unfaithfulness coming around forty. There is recent evidence of women in their fifties leaving their husbands to make their own lives, some say this is their last chance to be themselves and in some to find sexual satisfaction. The value of sex tends to go up dramatically after menopause for them and in men it generally lags although their climacteric may occur later than women by some ten years. Here we are equating the male change of life to the time in which the hormonal flow in the female and male is more alike than at any previous time in ratios nearly equal. This is around 60 in men and in the late 40's and early 50's for most women, according to Drs. Masters and Ballew. Steroid replacement therapy is sometimes recommended for both men and women. If physicians give treatment at the appropriate time over a long term, great physical and psychological benefits are received. The dramatic cessation of the ovarian function often within a few months or year for many women does not happen to the male testes, the complementary organ to the ovary. The other endocrine glands (pituitary, adrenal, thyroid, etc.) seem not to suffer essentially and the pituitary stimulation for both sexes is sufficient for most people until advanced age. Apparently, the organ reserve of the testes accounts for the woman-man differential. This does not mean the loss of interest in sex or the ability to have sex. Around forty years of age both in men and women the accessory organs are in weight their heaviest, atrophy is a considerable time in the future particularly for those who have kept their health. The incidence of sexual relationships among married and unmarried couples is basically the function of the man. For women who are chaste in marriage to the middle years will tend to remain so for it is not easy at fifty or sixty to make a liaison with a man as they could have earlier in their life. But there are numerous women who are trying and undoubtedly many are successful. Growing numbers of women and some men who have suffered sexual abuse by their mates due to lack of interest or physical and psychological distractions and due to the sheer boredom associates with their lives will seek extramarital sex. Among women the greatest frequency of extra-marital affairs come among the younger marrieds (20 to 25 years old). Hunt in the *Redbook* Survey a decade or so ago found that by their fortieth year, 40% of the married women responding (over 100,000) had been involved in an extra-marital situation. This figure has risen to 50%. The crucial years are between 30 and 40. The length of marriage obviously increases one's chances of having an outside affair. Working wives also have greater opportunity (greater mobility, working in teams of partnerships with men), for in the above study of those women in their late thirties 53% had participated in an affair as opposed to only 24% of women were housewives. This is beginning to approach what Kinsey found in his male study (1949) about men's extra-marital affairs but we should recognize that Hunt found the frequency of affairs for women to be considerably less than men. In his study (*Redbook*), it was found that of all the women who had had affairs outside of marriage, 50% were involved with only one man. Eighteen percent with one man, one time. Another 33% had two to five partners averaging between two to five times with each. Only 5% had more than 10 partners with another 5% having between 6 and 10 partners. It should be noted that among those having extra-marital sex 65% rated their marriages very poor.

We must not conclude that all women having affairs are guilt-ridden or as the song "Torn Between Two Lovers" suggests. A letter from a woman reported in the published book the *Redbook* Survey on Female Sexuality by Tavris and Sadd suggests even euphoria—

> I'm more fortunate than most in that I do get to meet my lover on a continuing basis...even if irregular. We are both married, have the same number of children, and our families are friends. I feel that I have the best of several worlds really. How long do affairs last? I don't know what lies ahead, but this loving, supporting relationship has passed the nine-year mark.

Another woman wrote, "My extramarital relationship is sexually exciting and an emotional supplement to my marriage. My lover and I have been together 4½ years so far."

Still another woman, who described herself as very religious and anti-feminist, stated:

> I am happily married to a man I love, respect, and am proud of. We have gotten along well for 18 years. I am 38 years old. However two years ago I began having a relationship with another man. It led to love and intercourse. I don't know why because my husband has always been very affectionate and attentive to me in all respects. Even when he is out of town he always calls. I just found myself strongly attracted to this male friend. We get along well in every respect, not just sexually; I feel married to two men.

Another interesting phenomenon I have observed is in separations, the announcement most frequently is made by women which ushers in a variety of liaisons for her particularly for the younger middlescent (35-45). In many of these cases, the women have, after some weeks or months, gone back to their husbands. Most husbands seem slow in announcing their separations, and on the other hand are often caught by surprise when their wives seek a divorce, even those that are actively seeking liaison with other women, for to lose even an unsatisfactory wife has far-reaching effects–on the work life, the wider family and their own ego loss, besides not the least having been looked after for a period of time.

Most persons in the middle years prize sex very highly, viewing it as an expression of love, as real pleasure and/or fun, as providing cement which buttresses them against the outside world and do something that assuages the loss of parents through death and children through emancipation. "That love is here to stay" is more than a cliche. By acknowledging that fact, we are stating something about the strong power it has over us, not only because of the strong desires it generates but also because of the profound satisfactions it can deliver. Rollo May (psychiatrist) says that "an attachment to a human being of the opposite sex potentially offers the maximum physical pleasure; no comparably satisfying way of using the body has yet been discovered. The sexual expression of love brings satisfaction to the loved one, to the self, and to the strongest feelings of attachment that we know." Unfortunately, Dr. Helen Kaplan of Cornell University Sexual Adjustment Clinic suggests that 8 to 10% of all the women have never experienced orgasm and of the 90% who have, only about half do so regularly. A somewhat equivalent circumstance exists, though much less for men for those who have had no climax the incidence is about 5%. Most men experience regularly orgasms but on occasions some psychological conditions create an impasse. Most frigidity and impotence can be helped by what Dr. Kaplan has called no-nonsense therapy.

As Dr. Kaplan tells it, there are two aspects of sex. Sex is composed of friction and fantasy and with deficiencies in either producing unhappy results. If there are sexual malfunctions, it seems logical to check with the physician to ascertain the health of our bodies. There may be a need to check with a psychologist or psychiatrist to see that there are no deep-seated mental problems. There are many clinics available, which specifically deal with these problems.

MAJOR SPECIFIC SEX PROBLEMS

Male: Ejaculation Prematurely—Inability to Control Ejaculation

Men who are plagues with this problem are unable to control their ejaculations. Once they become aroused, they reach an orgasm quickly. They feel guilty because they have been unable to satisfy their partner. The causative factors are debated: some say it is anxiety, others that it comes from hostility between the partners. Masters and Johnson believe that stressful conditions happen during a young man's initial sex experience brings on premature ejaculation. Also many men without a partner complain had continued this action.

Therapy

The best approach is usually found in the clinical situation where psychotherapy is also being administered. This is important and for this reason home-made therapy may not be successful. Usually some kind of stimulation is required whereby the woman eventually brings the man to orgasm with the penis near the vagina. Finally, the woman is told to stimulate the man almost to orgasm at which point he is to enter the vagina with pelvic thrusting. This type of problem is difficult to solve, but patience and outside assistance is usually required to relive this circumstance. Your physician can direct you to a urologist or sex therapist to help you.

Male: Retarded Ejaculation—Difficulty in Controlling Orgasm

The man suffering from this malady cannot control orgasm, the retarded ejaculator cannot trigger it. Some with this difficulty have never had an orgasm. For most men, ejaculatory inhibition is confined to specific anxiety-provoking situations such as guilt feelings about the sexual situation. It may be tied to religious upbringing and some clinicians relate it to an unresolved oedipal complex (in the case failure to attach significance to any woman besides mother) and/or an ambivalence toward one's partner.

Therapy

The best approach is usually found in the clinical situation where psychotherapy is also being administered. This is important and for this reason home-made therapy may not be successful. Usually some kind of stimulation is required whereby the woman eventually brings the man to orgasm with the penis near the vagina. Finally, the woman is told to stimulate the man almost to orgasm at which point he is to enter the vagina with pelvic thrusting. This type of problem is difficult to solve, but patience and outside assistance is usually required to relive this circumstance. Your physician can direct you to a urologist or sex therapist to help you.

Male: Impotence—Inability to Have Erection

Men who are in this category are usually constantly anxious and frustrated. It has been estimated that at one time or another half of all men have been impotent. Even though they are able to be aroused, they cannot have an erection (also called erectile dysfunction). Most men seek help from their physician when the problem becomes a chronic one. For men, it is of signal importance that they be able to perform. In the climate existing today, especially for young men, where women are now often being very assertive and initiating sexual relations, have already, by some accounts, been a factor in the rise of impotence. To perform on demand is sometimes threatening and inhibiting to masculinity.

Therapy—Aid for Impotence

Those with an impotency condition should have a physical examination. Stress, fatigue, undiagnosed hepatitis, high sugar levels, alcoholism, smoking, drugs, low levels of testosterone and other problems (heart disease, diabetes, surgery) may lie at the root of the difficulty. Many therapists think that impotence has at its roots some pathology, that is, Parkinson, neurological problems, etc. Obviously, psychological problems bear on this—fear of failure, conflict, excessive demands by a wife or lover all may be involved. Frequently depression or marital troubles relate to impotence so need treatment. The practice for remedy usually suggests that a couple caress each other in sexual play at home, under quiet conditions, but not to engage in coitus. The middlescent woman is encouraged to accept clitoris stimulation to orgasm if the sexual tension becomes too great. This routine usually builds up excitement in both partners. Eventually, erection and intercourse can be accomplished. Sometimes a period away from attempts at intercourse is desirable. One thing is sure, tension, stress, conflict and hatred are cul de sac where male erection is concerned. The climate for lovemaking must also be unhurried and protected from interruptions and noises—relaxation is an important ingredient.

It's only an estimate, but it is believed that 10-20 million American men are some times affected by impotence. Normally when a man is sexually aroused, nerves affecting the penis triggers a chemical reaction that causes two slender areas of spongy muscle tissue in the penis to relax, then to fill with blood. The engorged tissues press against veins that drain blood from the penis trapping the blood and producing an erection. Failure of the system is often the fault of nerves or blood vessels that have been damaged by disease or injury. Urologists have found that cells lining blood vessels release nitric oxide, which causes surrounding muscle to relax. Since cigarette smoking, high blood pressure and diabetes damage these nitric-oxide-producing cells. They are suspects in any investigation of the causes of impotence. Many doctors are recommending the use of Viagra and/or Lipitra finding help for thousands of their patients.

Medication itself may be a cause of impotence. Drugs for high blood pressure may affect a drop low enough in blood flow to the penis to preclude an erection. These sympathetic blockers as Aldomet, Ismelin, Catapres, Tegament (anti-ulcer agent) and Zantac used widely to neutralize acid may lower testosterone levels. This hormone is responsible for sexual desire in men. Sometimes a change in the drug to alternative ones by the physician can solve the problem.

Drug therapy can be used for men with nerve or blood vessel damage caused by diabetes, multiple sclerosis or a spinal cord or pelvic injury. A major advance in treatment is the use of Sildenafil, which increases blood flow to the penis. It does not help those with diabetes or alcoholics and for side effects—headaches, gastrointestinal upsets. Fatal interactions have occurred in men taking Sildenafil with nitrate medicine. Another drug is Alprostadil that increases blood flow to the penis. It is not absorbed in the blood flow hence has fewer side effects as Sildenafil. It can produce erection in men not excited. The Alprostadil is injected into the base of the penis or placed inside in the form of a pellet. If used 20 minutes before sexual intercourse 90% of men get an erection. In some men it can cause priapism (cause an uncomfortable prolonged erection). This problem can be neutralized with a shot of ephinephrine thus preventing damage to the spongy tissue of the penis.

Some 20 to 30 percent of older males with impotence have hormone deficiencies. For this group, testosterone injections, give by a doctor, may make achieving an erection easier. Spanish Fly, Zinc, Yohimbine, and vitamins (high potency) have not been proved by clinical investigation to be effective.

Surgery

About 10 percent of impotent men can have damaged blood vessels repaired, if the damage is caused by injury to the pelvis. Localized blockages are much easier to fix than those caused by fat buildup, which affects vessels throughout the penis. In bypass surgery, the surgeon grafts sections of an abdominal artery around narrowed branches of the main artery leading to the penis. Where the major veins draining the penis leak blood too quickly, the veins are sewn shut so that smaller veins take over the draining. These vascular procedures are still considered experimental and are performed at only a few medical centers nationwide.

Psychological reasons are often the cause of the inability to have an erection. A single failure to get an erection according to Dr. Helen Kaplan of the New York Hospital (Cornell Medical Center) or alcohol or stress over the ability to perform sexually may cause impotence. Fear and stress all to create more adrenaline, which constricts the blood vessels leading to the penis and results in relaxing it. If a man can have erections while sleeping his problem is likely to be psychological.

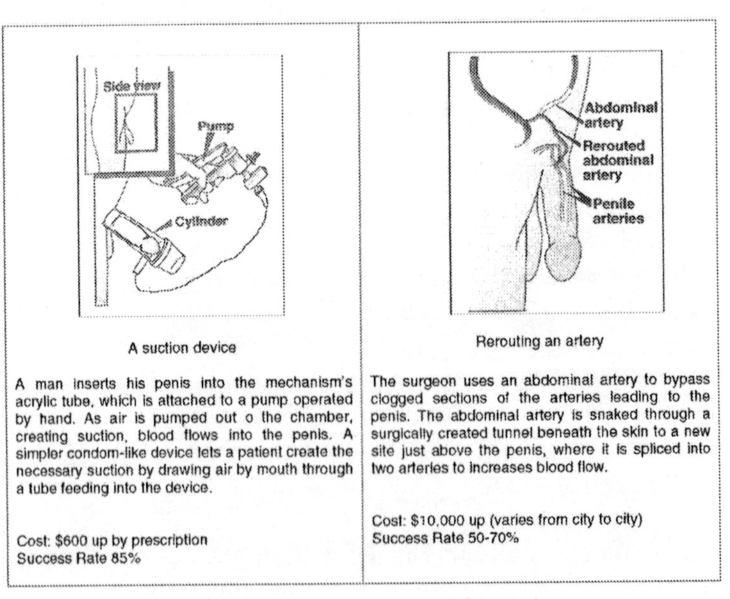

A suction device

A man inserts his penis into the mechanism's acrylic tube, which is attached to a pump operated by hand. As air is pumped out o the chamber, creating suction, blood flows into the penis. A simpler condom-like device lets a patient create the necessary suction by drawing air by mouth through a tube feeding into the device.

Cost: $600 up by prescription
Success Rate 85%

Rerouting an artery

The surgeon uses an abdominal artery to bypass clogged sections of the arteries leading to the penis. The abdominal artery is snaked through a surgically created tunnel beneath the skin to a new site just above the penis, where it is spliced into two arteries to increases blood flow.

Cost: $10,000 up (varies from city to city)
Success Rate 50-70%

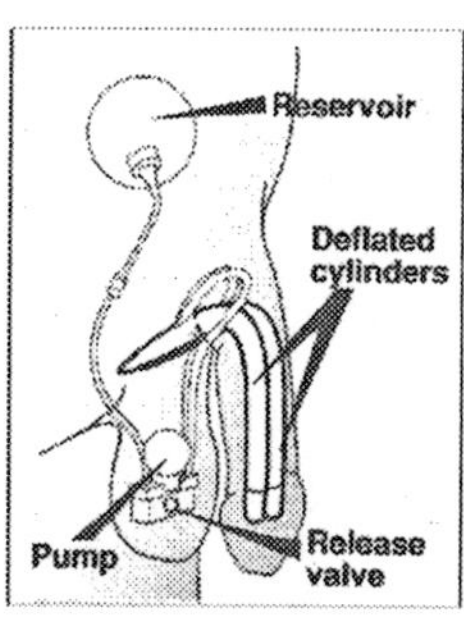

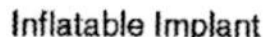
Inflatable Implant

A surgeon implants this three-part prosthesis through an incision in the abdomen or below the base of the penis. When the man squeezes the pump in the scrotum, fluid is forced from the reservoir into thin tubes, causing an erection. To deflate the tubes, he presses a release valve on the side of the pump.

Cost: $15,000 up
Success Rate 90%

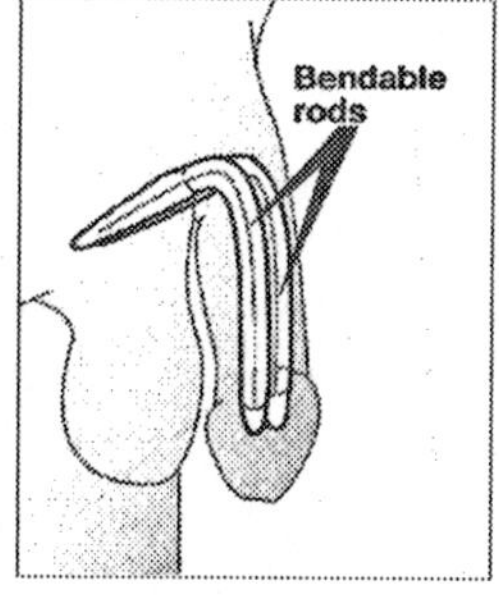

Semi-rigid Implant

The simplest penile prosthesis consists of two firm but bendable silicone-rubber rods inserted into spongy muscle tissue on each side of the penis. Normally, the rods are in a bent position so that the penis lies close to the body. To stimulate an erection, the man can simply extend the rods straight out.

Cost: $8,000 up (varies from city to city)
Success Rate High

Female: Frigidity—Inability to be Sexually Stimulated

Women who have this problem receive little or no pleasure of a sexual nature from attempts at erotic stimulation. Like impotent men who are chronic cases, these women so handicapped view sex with disdain and alarm usually because of lack of sex education and inhibition. In the worst cases, some have never experienced sexual pleasure or have an orgasm.

Of course, as mentioned earlier, some 8 to 10 percent of all women never experience orgasm. One approach to the solution of this situation is a sex therapist technique called sensate focus which consists of having a couple forego sexual intercourse and orgasm while the woman caresses her husband's body, after which he stimulates her by stroking. By having the wife act first, we help counteract the guilt she may have from previous failures and the fear that her husband will reject her. The attempt here is to eliminate the pressure to have an orgasm. When this is done, the woman often can feel sensuous and sexual excitement. The sensate exercise is expanded to light, genital play. The husband strokes the woman's body, touching her breasts, nipples, the clitoral area and the vaginal entrance. The woman guides his fingers and hands by telling him and moving herself to receive the maximum feeling. If the man becomes excited, then the woman is usually told to bring him to orgasm manually or orally after she had had a chance to experience non-pressured and comforting genital play.

Manipulating the penis usually creates a sexual response in the woman. When the woman reaches a high peak of excitement, the couple moves to have intercourse. The woman usually takes the top position initiating coitus slowly and tentatively thrusting at first but focusing on the sensation in her vagina. In this way she controls the intensity and exact location of her clitoral and vaginal stimulation. The man does not allow himself to have an orgasm until the woman is ready. Considerable emotion is frequently generated by these encounters due to their long problematic duration. But, this type of treatment allows a therapist to observe the point of blockage of sensuous feeling. Usually good prognosis is indicated where the husband has patience and genuine care, and pathological conditions are not present.

Female: Difficulty in Reaching Orgasm

Dr. Helen Kaplan suggests that there are two facets to this problem: On one hand the problem is primary orgasmic dysfunction if she has never experienced an orgasm and from secondary orgasmic dysfunction if the disorder developed after a period of being able to reach a climax. The problem of inorgasmic disability is said to be absolute if a woman can't achieve an orgasm under any circumstance (10% never achieve orgasm under any circumstances) and a situational one if under any circumstances can she have an orgasm. Women who suffer only from orgasmic problems often have strong sex drives. They fall in love, enjoy sex play, lubricate sufficiently and love the feeling of intromission by the penis. Nevertheless, they can't have an orgasm, stopping short, only reaching the plateau stage and no further. In the situational case, women can achieve orgasm by self-stimulation, vibrators or by their husbands' manual dexterity or orally. In therapy, the search for conflicts, inhibitions, use of drugs or medicines, also fears are sought as a clue to the problem's cure.

Therapy

In solving the problem indicated here, an attempt is made to eliminate the inhibiting factors of the sexual environment in order to achieve the first climax. Since women are least threatened when at home, they are counseled (the inorgasmic woman) to masturbate at home in a situation where they will not be intruded upon. If their own attempts fail, then generally a vibrator is recommended which can be applied on her genitals, the labia and the sides of the clitoris. Some become hooked on this method so usually after the experience of several orgasms by the manual method—hands/fingers, and she is able to stimulate herself, the husband is brought into the picture to make love with the wife and told not to make any effort to have an orgasm. After he has climaxed and there is no pressure for her to perform, quickly he uses the vibrator or manually stimulates her to orgasm. Usually after a few of these sessions, women climax during intercourse after stimulation.

Female: Vaginismus—Inability to Control Vagina Muscles

This circumstance is seen in the woman whose body is normal but whenever the male attempts penetration, the vaginal muscles involuntarily close off the entrance making intercourse impossible. This is relatively rare. The problem arises as fear of intercourse and its association with pregnancy, disease, lack of experience and pain or abuse. Most women who seek help in this regard are usually sexually responsive and orgasmic. The basis of this problem may be a rigid hymen, pelvic diseases (arthritis) and tumors, childbirth diseases, and hemorrhoids; also guilt, rape and a husband's impotency.

Therapy

After assurance that there are no pain-producing circumstances surrounding the vaginismus, an attempt is made to understand the nature of the fear of vagina entry. A re-conditioning of the involuntary spasm of the muscles is undertaken through having the husband and wife examine in a well-lighted bedroom the opening of the vagina. The woman is then told to put her finger in the vagina. When this is done without pain or discomfort, she is told to move the finger around inside until she can tolerate the touching without pain. The woman is always allowed to control the situation. Following this, the husband inserts his finger or two fingers into the vagina, rotating them carefully and stretching the sides of the vagina. When the woman can tolerate this, a move is made for intercourse. Entry is made tentatively and gentle thrusting proceeds until desire for full vigorous copulation is desired by the woman. If pain is involved, the procedure is slowed or repeated until the woman wishes for penetration. Very good results have been achieved through this procedure which is used by many sex therapists. The process above may require more practice with the woman alone using her finger(s) to rotate in the vagina or a tampon when she feels comfortable with this invites her partner to try it.

It is true that many knowledgeable couples work through their own problems by being patient. Many will have to have help from their physician or therapist specializing in remedial methodology. We should mention that most couples who have sexual problems practice poor, abrasive and non-effective methods. Some poor lovemaking results merely from a couple's ignorance about sex. For instance, it has been observed that many couples do not know where the clitoris is or seem to know that it is the seat of ecstatic pleasure. I have observed that some graduate students in Human Development courses cannot place in the proper position the endocrine glands (including testes and ovaries) when asked to on an outline of the body. Many couples have intercourse as soon as the man has an erection and he climaxes without considering his partner. Then they wonder why the woman is unable to have a climax. Women typically are slower than men in achieving an orgasm but once stimulated are usually capable of multiple orgasms. The circulation of blood to the woman's vagina and the pelvic regions takes more time than it does to engorge a man's penis and women are slower after tumescence has been accomplished in return to normal. The rule for both partners in the sex act is to attend to the enjoyment of the other but at the same time make sure that you receive what you would like out of the lovemaking. Sure it will vary: sometimes an orgasm isn't necessary, but the communion, nearness, stroking or satisfaction of one or the other is usually sufficient.

Women need to understand their needs sexually and many need the help of their husbands and/or partners. Talking and patience is needed. A too-aggressive woman often repels many men as many women are turned off by caveman treatment. Many people need (both men and women) to rid themselves of some prudish beliefs about sexual morality. Some would like to try activities that to them are arousing and erotic but are stymied by puritan partners or their own inhibitions. Couples should invest in a good sex manual like Alex Comfort's *Joy of Sex* that's been on the market for a long time, if for no other reason than to see what is considered normal and the range of possibilities. Psychiatrist David Reuben said he and his wife tried a lot of positions and situations found in a sex manual but that he was not overwhelmed by their effect. This is what most people find, but many may find one or two variations, which they come to enjoy. Good sexual morality between man and woman demands they be supportive of each other; when reinforcement takes place, this motivates the other partner to strive to please and improve his or her performance.

DISABILITY OF SEX AND FREQUENCY

The *Redbook* report on "Female Sexuality" a decade or so ago mentioned earlier involved one of the largest (100,000) number of women ever included in a survey on sex. In this study, some 23,000 or more women who responded were over 35 or in their middlescent years. The desire for sex in women reaches its peak in the late thirties and forties (recognized by some is the fact that many women do not have a man or men to engage in sex and because of religion, moral or fear of disease do not attempt to find a partner, under chemical therapy for breast cancer become highly interested in having frequent intercourse); for healthy men, the desire for sex maintains a plateau from the early twenties onward to the fifties, even then some will not slow down much until their sixties. The frequency of intercourse per month for women is indicated below. The total woman sexual outlet is seen in the figures below.

Times per month

0	1-5	6-10	11-15	16-20	21
2%	26%	32%	21%	11%	8%

It was found that ten percent of the women in the survey reported earlier agreed with the statement that no sex was about right in terms of satisfaction per month. Of those having sex 16-20 times per month, 90% said this was about right. Those having intercourse over 21 times, 11% felt this to be too much. But 6% of the women felt that 16-20 times was too little and 5% thought that over 21 times too little. Most significant was that of those in the 1-5 frequency category, 74% thought this was too little; of the 6-10 frequency group, 41% thought this too little.

A number of studies of frequency of intercourse among men and women indicate usually men are desirous of more intercourse than their mates from 20 to 40 but from 40-60 women who are active desire intercourse more. Many middlescent husbands complain that their spouses lose interest in sex after menopause. In the *Redbook* survey, a number of women cite evidence of their husbands' impotence or lack of interest. In fact, one lady in her sixties mentioned in this survey said she went out with a fifty-three year old man. "We made love nearly every day," she said, and "it is fabulous!"

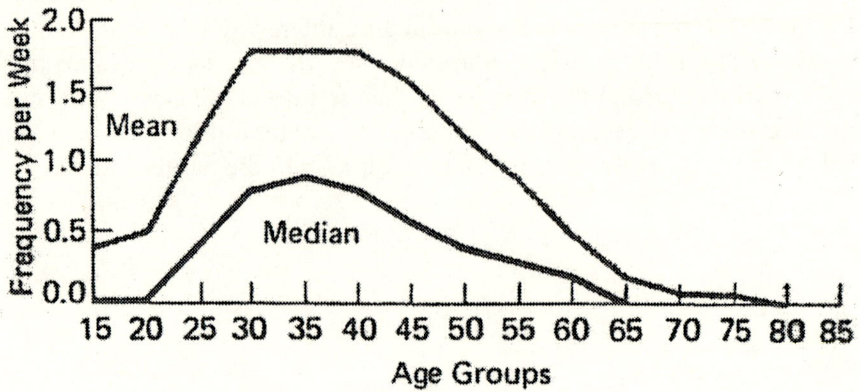

Frequency of total sexual outlet for females, by age groups. (Adapted from Kinsey et al, *Sexual Behavior in the Human Female*, 1953, p. 548. Courtesy of the Institute for Sex Research.)

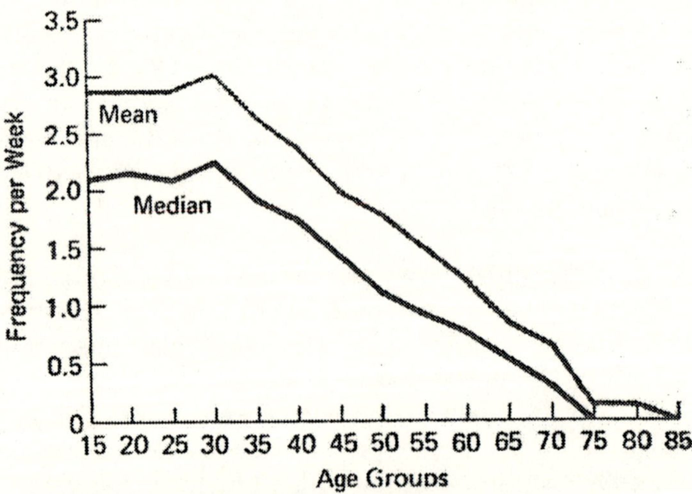

Frequency of total sexual outlet for males, by age groups. (Adapted from Kinsey et al, *Sexual Behavior in the Human Female*, 1948, p. 220. Courtesy of the Institute for Sex Research.)

My mother had an elderly friend of long duration. She was married twice, both husbands had died. I came into possession of a letter from this lady at the time of my mother's death. The friend of my mother lived some distance away and because I wanted to see what conversations were being carried on about my mother's illness, I opened and read the letter. I was surprised to read that most of her letter had to do with her boyfriend. She was explaining some difficulty between them, which if it could be resolved meant all they would have to do would be get the marriage license and jump in bed! The last three words were the actual phrase—and this from an 80-year-old plus lady. Her boyfriend was in his sixties, I might add.

Studies on sexual frequency over the decade show similar results, i.e., Hunt (1974) revealed among 18-24 reported intercourse occurrences as three times a week. In the 1990's sex researchers Michael, Gagnon, Laumann and Kolat (1994) in a national sample based upon the answer to the query how often have you engaged in sex in the last 12 months, the responses possibilities were not at all, once or twice, about once a month, two or three times a month, about once a week, two or three times a week and four or more times a week. The highest percentages came from married men 43% and married women 47% who stated a few time a month. The next most common option was two or three times a week 36% of men responded this while 32% of women did. One percent of married men said no intercourse in the past year while 3% the women, 7% of women and men answered 4 or more times a week. This means these figures are not much different than the Kinsey studies of fifty years ago. However there were flaws in the sample of his studies for instance too many middle class women, lack of minorities and elevated levels of education. For those in middle age or approaching it (mid 30s) the average was found to be 9 times a month those 50-54 5.5 times per month over those in their late sixties reported a little more than 2 times. Increasingly as people age and responsibility grows and inclination lessens sexual activity goes down. This research was done using a sample of 6,785 adults by sociologists Call, Sprecher and Swarts (1995) in examining sexual incidence across the life span.

The Duke University Study (Pfeiffer, Verwoerdt and Davis) completed in the 1970's and a report by Jones (1992) parallels their data shows the middle year's incidence of sexual intercourse. By the time women are 60 many are widowed hence lack of a partner reduces the number responding. Women over sixty married frequently blame lack of sexual interaction on men.

FREQUENCY (IN PERCENT) OF SEXUAL INTERCOURSE IN MIDDLE LIFE

Group	Number	None	Once a month	Once a week	2-3 times a week	More than 3 times a week
Men						
46-50	43	0	5	62	26	7
51-55	41	5	29	49	17	0
56-60	61	4	38	44	11	0
61-65	54	20	43	30	7	0
66-71	62	24	48	26	2	0
Total	261	12	34	41	12	1
Women						
46-50	43	14	26	39	21	0
51-55	41	20	41	32	5	2
56-60	48	42	27	25	4	2
61-65	44	61	29	5	5	0
66-71	5	73	16	11	0	0
Total	231	44	27	22	6	1

SEXUAL ACTIVITY

An interest of sex researchers concerns sexual practices or what people do when they are sexually intimate with each other was reported by Pamela Regan (2003). Michael and colleagues' (1994) national survey revealed that although there are a number of sexual activities from which to choose, the most commonly practiced is vaginal intercourse, with more than 95% of the heterosexual respondents stating that they had vaginal intercourse the last time they had sex. Oral sex, although less common than vaginal intercourse, was also reported by a sizable percentage of respondents. Specifically, about one third of cohabiting men, and one fifth of cohabiting women, reported either giving or receiving oral sex during their last sexual interaction. The numbers were slightly lower for married individuals, with approximately 24% of married men and 17% of married women reporting having participated in this activity during their last sexual event. Other forms of sexual expression occurred far less frequently. For example, only 2% of cohabiting men and women (and even fewer married respondents) reported have engaged in anal intercourse during their last encounter.

Homosexual couples practice many of the same sexual activities as do heterosexual couples but report higher frequencies of particular behaviors. For example, lesbian couples engage in more kissing, caressing, holding, and breast stimulation during sex than do cohabiting or married heterosexual couples (e.g., Blumstein & Schwartz, 1983). In addition, oral sex and anal sex are more commonly used by homosexual couples than by heterosexual ones.

Approximately 40% to 50% of gay male and lesbian couples report usually or always engaging in oral sex during lovemaking, compared with 20% to 30% of heterosexual couples, and gay men are more likely to have anal sex than are heterosexual couples (Lever, 1995; Michael et al., 1994).

The results of two national surveys conducted by sociologist Janet Lever (1994, 1995) suggest that homosexual couples may also be more experimental than their heterosexual counterparts. For example, many of the lesbian respondents—particularly those in their teens, 20s, and early 30s—had incorporated dildos (43%) or food (35%) into their sexual activities, had engaged in bondage or discipline (25%), or had participated in three-way sex (14%). Similarly, 55% of the gay male respondents had used dildos (in anal sex) during sex, 48% had engaged in three-way sex, 24% had participated in group sex, and 10% had experienced sadomasochistic sexual encounters. It is important to note that Lever's question concerned activities during the past 5 years; hence, we do not know how often participants engaged in these activities.

SATISFACTION IN SEX

Most paired couples (Laurence & Byers and others, 1995) report satisfaction with their sex lives. Two-thirds of the husbands and wives in a national survey that they experienced a great deal or a very great deal of satisfaction in their sex lives. Half of married and cohabiting men and 45% of married women reported the relationships were extremely physically pleasurable (Michael et al., 1994). Homosexual men (40%) and women (30%) appear to be equally satisfied sexually rating them good or great these were partnered couples. There is a high correlation between the number of sexual encounters and satisfaction. Among partnered homosexual women 92% of those with sexual frequency of 21-40 in the past month rated their sex lives as great compared with those who had sex 11-20 times only 67% whereas those with 5-10 times 44% and 18% with sex 2 to 4 times. Other factors of sexual satisfaction were:

(1) reaching an orgasm,
(2) engaging in frequent sex,
(3) reaching an orgasm at the same time,
(4) receiving more sexual rewards than costs.

SEXUAL PREFERENCES

When possible sexual activities were elicited by Michael (1994) study these were the suggestions:

- Having sex with more than one person at the same time
- Having sex with someone of the same sex
- Forcing someone to do something sexual that he or she does not want to do
- Being forced to do something sexual that you do not want to do
- Seeing other people do sexual things
- Having sex with someone you do not personally know
- Watching a partner undress or strip
- Engaging in vaginal intercourse
- Using a dildo or vibrator
- Having a partner perform oral sex on you
- Performing oral sex on a partner
- Having a partner stimulate you anus with his or her fingers
- Stimulating a partner's anus with your fingers
- Engaging in passive anal intercourse
- Engaging in active anal intercourse (only men received this item)

Participants were asked to indicate how appealing they found each of these sexual activities using a 4-point scale, where 1 represented *very appealing*, 2 represented *somewhat appealing*, 3 represented *not appealing*, and 4 represented *not at all appealing*.

The results despite the wide variety of acts from which to choose, both sexes found only a small number appealing. Some 96% of younger women and 95% of younger men (18-44 years of age) rated vaginal intercourse as very appealing or somewhat appealing; similarly, 93% of older women and 95% of older men (45-59 years of age) found this particular act to be somewhat appealing. In fact, vaginal intercourse was the clear favorite. Watching a partner undress was the second most preferred activity, although this was rated very appealing by more men than women in both the younger (50% vs. 30%) and older (40% vs. 18%) age groups. This was followed by receiving and giving oral sex, with both men and women indicating that it was more appealing to receive than to give. Other behaviors or events seemed to appeal to only a very small percentage of people, for less than 5% of women and men said that they found using a dildo or vibrator, watching other people have sex, having sex with a stranger, or engaging in passive anal intercourse to be very appealing. No respondents thought being forced to do something sexual was very appealing, and none of the women and younger men (and only 1% of the older men) rated this as highly appealing.

Much less is known about the sexual preferences of homosexual men and women, Lever's (1994, 1995) national surveys yield some insight. For example, her male respondents said that their favorite bedroom acts included hugging, caressing, and snuggling (endorsed by 85%); deep kissing (74%); receiving oral sex (72%); giving oral sex (71%); masturbating a partner (52%); and being masturbated by a partner (51%). Their biggest sexual turn-offs were engaging in insertive anilingus (disliked by 26%) and engaging in receptive anal intercourse (disliked by 14%). Many men selected these two particular sex acts as turn-ons; fully 29% said that they preferred insertive anilingus, and 43% endorsed receptive anal intercourse. Lever (1994) concluded, when it comes to anal play, it appears [that gay] men either love it or hate it.

Homosexual women expressed similar sexual preferences. For example, most participants said that they "loved" hugging, caressing, and cuddling (91%); French kissing (82%); caressing a partner's breasts (82%); and sucking a partner's nipples (80%). About 75% identified holding hands, touching a partner's genitals, and having their own genitals touched as appealing practices. Like homosexual men (and like the heterosexual men and women in Michael et al.'s [1994] study), more lesbians prefer receiving oral sex (75%) than giving it (70%). Women reported that their least favorite activity is anal stimulation, with more than half expressing a dislike for anilingus (both giving and receiving) and anal penetration.

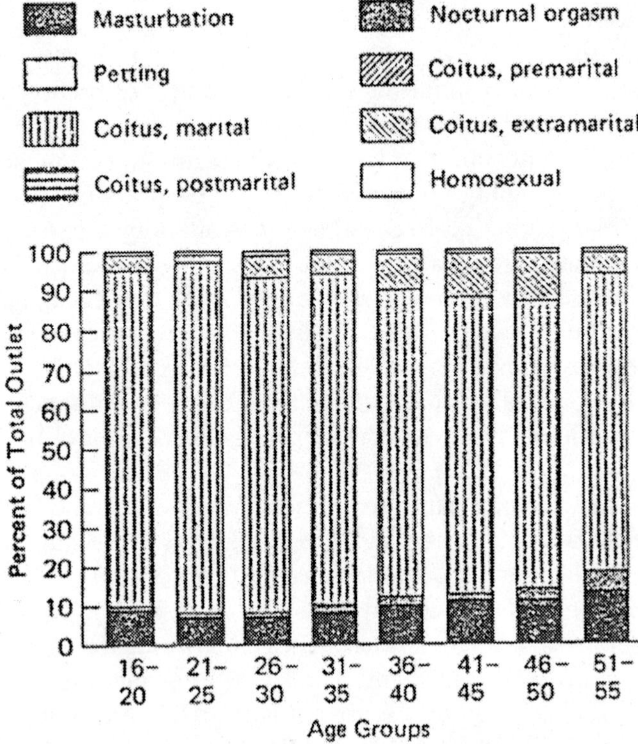

Percentage of total outlet: sources of orgasm among married females (Adapted from Kinsey et al., *Sexual Behavior in the Human Female*, 1953, p. 562. Courtesy of the Institute for Sex Research.)

Evidence from the Kinsey reports (1949, 1953) indicated that in the years 31-35, pre-middlescent married males had 2.1 orgasms from all sources per week; with females, it was 1.5. Of those from 46-50 for women, the frequency of orgasms was only .8 per week and for men 1.2. Greater incidence by men was increased by more use of masturbation and sex outside of marriage. The Kinsey study revealed that men and women reached about the same point fifty years of age with 1.8 per week; at sixty, 1.3 times per week, and .9 at seventy.

The old wag that suggests the history of man's sex life follows these stages—tri-weekly—try weekly—try weakly, misses its mark as does the notion that sex is great at twenty but lecherous at sixty (dirty old man). There may be problems (but more men than women stay sexually active if at a diminished rate) as we progress beyond forty-five and fifty for often there exist prostate problems, cardiovascular difficulties, diabetes and variety of maladies—declining levels of 17-ketosteroids associated with testicular fibrosis and tubular atrophy. For those over 50, about 60% of all men suffer from an enlarged prostate gland; this is no problem unless it blocks urination or has a malignant growth associated with it. Even if it has to be removed, approximately 30% find they have increased potency as a result after an operation removing the prostate. It has been found that at least half of these impotencies are psychological. Many men claim to be impotent when it has been found that they are regularly masturbating or have a mistress. Prostate problems are a serious prospect and can lead to death. Screening by the PSA exam and manual check by a physician is urged for all adult males. Some help from a therapist would probably aid the situation although some men are looking for an excuse not to perform with their wives. Menopause has the same effect on some women what with the hot flashes, weight increases, dry skin, etc., many women think the sex life is over. They do have their difficulties and it should be mentioned that prostate problems for the man may be no laughing matter; before removal if he has sex, it may mean not being able to urinate for the next six to eight hours. He may, therefore, after a couple of bouts with this, decline to engage in sexual activity.

Except in the most severe cases, heart problems should not mean the end of sex. Exercise nowadays is advised for heart patients and sexual encounter is frequently a good muscle-toner; in addition, it is worth about 150 calories loss for each engagement. As for vaginal shrinkage, lack of lubricants, and penis flaccidity due to lack of estrogen or testosterone, Viagra and Levitra, steroid substitutes can be administered to reduce losses and dramatic sexual changes. There is no reason for the majority of people not to have sex regularly though, unfortunately, many are affected by cultural taboos as: after menopause you don't have sex any more, or our children or kin to say you're too old to be doing that stuff and when a spouse dies in the middle years, many think their sex life is over, so dismiss it. Young adults who suggest this kind of advice should try giving up their own sex lives. Undoubtedly, the best evidence we have at the present time tells us that to sustain more fully and increase the length of life, the best guarantee is a regular effective sex life. The lack of partners, though little research has been done on this, doesn't keep most people from sex, be it by masturbation, a close friend, or by some other manner (vibrator, dildo). Various avenues open to women are discussed in the work, *Our Bodies, Ourselves* by the Boston Women Collective (2000) which has been through many editions. Many sensitive matters related to sex are discussed here that will be of interest to most women.

SUMMARY ON SEX

Men and women cannot share equally in the privilege of a mature sexual relationship until each understands that sexual function is truly the birthright of both—something that a man and woman are privileged to do with each other and for themselves, not something a man does to or for a woman. It should be remembered that sexual response is solely the function of the individual—it evolves from within from the mind. It starts with a proper mental outlook. The physical processes begin in the mind which then relates the message to the pituitary, hence to ovary and testes. What the partners do share is responsibility for their emotional environment, which in turn is an expression of the emotional bond of the marriage itself.

Without mutual consideration based firmly on each individual's assumption of sole responsibility for his or her sexual function, there rarely is sexual security in a marriage. When male or female fears for sexual performance intrude upon or even dominate a marital relationship, the partners are denied the incredible value of confident sexual expression, which is the essence of interpersonal communication. Without a secure opportunity for sexual expression in marriage, tensions that the partners can accumulate from every complexity of contemporary living rarely have sufficient outlet. Without full sexual accord, couples contending with marked personality differences or handicapped by dissimilar social backgrounds generally can find no common denominator through which to mediate their social tensions, their personal differences, or their natural sexual demands.

The transition years are usually designated as the decade between 35-55 years of age. This is a period when women and men become their own person. Obviously, some men and women transit from 35-45, others from 45-55, and some refuse to be pigeon-holed. What changes are to be expected in the quality of life when and if we do transit? How does aging affect sexual interaction and, therefore, affect communication between men and women committed to each other.

As we age, there are only two factors necessary for continuation of effective sexual functioning; first, a reasonably good state of general health and, second, an interested and interesting partner. It must be remembered, experts tell us, that as every man ages he may notice some combination of (1) delayed erection time, (2) reduced ejaculatory volume, (3) reduced ejaculatory pressure, (4) reduced ejaculatory demand, and (5) some degree of penis flaccidity.

As woman ages, she may be aware of (1) slowed production of vaginal lubrication, (2) reduction in volume of lubrication, (3) thinning and loss of elasticity of vaginal walls, (4) shortened orgasmic experience, and (5) some shrinkage of the vagina. Knowledge that these changes in sexual functioning are to be anticipated during the transitional years is only important in that such knowledge is real protection against the fears for performance that develop when uninformed men and women are naturally concerned or disturbed by the onset of any alteration in established sexual response patterns.

MARRIAGE

The elements of remarriage in the in-between years are not the same as they were the first time, for usually the first marriage involved a high degree of intense physical attraction and the projecting of one's self image upon the desired person. Both of these may be involved in the second marriage but also of prime importance is communication, companionship, good mother or father-ship to children, economic status, and the provision of an added dimension to life. There will not be many persons who, having been single all their lives, marry after forty. It is a fact that women who are thirty and divorced have a better chance to remarry than those who have never married. There are also those who never try to marry and they succeed!

Marriage in the U.S. has a joined partner—cohabitation as an almost equal experience. Cohabitation is an alternative to marriage, it is almost a universal experience, it resembles marriage in that it is essentially a pair bond or monogamous union between two individuals who live together. This couple coordinates their economic, social and sexual, also sometimes reproducing children. Cohabitation has increased considerably from those born in 1933-42 (10% men, 6% women) had cohabitated before marriage. Among men and women born from 1943-1952, 33% men and 24% women had cohabitated. Of the 1955-1962 53% and 43% men and women whereas two-thirds of both men and women had cohabitated prior to marriage if born in the years 1963-1974. Now we find many middle years men and women divorced, single, never married, losing a partner, etc., find cohabiting a way to "try it out" those many for economic, social and sexual reasons expect it to be lasting. Cohabiting is characterized by a more equal division of labor than in marriage both homosexual and heterosexual couples have a more egalitarian attitude toward division of household labor than married couples as mentioned earlier this is a more peer relationship than in marriage. In Norway and Denmark gays and lesbians according to Lever (1995) find a majority of these would marry if they could (gays 59% and 70% lesbians). In these countries gay and lesbian couples are permitted by law to register their relationship, these socially sanctioned partnerships provide access to many of the legal rights held by heterosexual married couples. Dual and triple women in a marriage to one man (polygamy) is allowed in some countries outside the U.S. even in Utah Mormons have practiced many wives for one man. There are problems by increasing restrictions for law and societal concern. Increasingly across the world regardless of traditions and ethnicity women and men seek romantic love the basis of marriage.

Most middlescents will marry for the second time, either for reasons of divorce or death of a spouse. As mentioned earlier, Health, Education and Welfare predicted that by 1985 one of every two marriages would end in divorce. This projection has come true and is now (2004) edging upward favoring divorce. By the time middleagers reach fifty, there are many more widows than widowers. To point out the problems of women beyond forty getting a second husband, one need only think of the population differential of men to women; in the United States there are some 6 million more women. True, many are in the upper age brackets but the influence of these numbers filters down to the middle age groups. Men divorcing or becoming widowers at 45 rarely marry a woman their age; the typical liaison is with a woman three to ten years younger. In some instances, the woman is 15 to 20 years younger. Even for the 50 to 55-year-old men this holds true. One bright spot for the ladies, is in England where there is a surplus among younger males in the age bracket 20-40—something like a million. A visit to central London for a few weeks might result in an opportunity to meet eligible males. Also, Australia and Alaska. Of course, if the prospective male has a reasonably good job, you may have to live there. But it's worth a try!

According to the Census Bureau, in 1972, the percentage of those with five or more years of college, 35-44, who have never married was rather astounding. See for yourself—overall those that never marry, up to 44 years of age, represent about 13% in 1972 and 16% in 1985. Since then decline in married numbers have nearly doubled (U.S. Bureau of the Census, 1998). Nevertheless marriage is a common event as 9 of 10 marry at least once in their lives—most are adults who expect to marry at some time though many do not.

Never Married 35-44

Race	1972 Female	1972 Male	1985 Female	1985 Male	2000 Male & Female Combined
White	20%	8%	13.4%	18.7%	
					25%
Black	11%	11%	--	--	

Advanced education is a drawback to marriage. One thing may be the self-imposed limitations that one makes or that a choice has to be made either/or have a career or marriage. The highly trained woman professional is not likely to choose a husband several educational and class levels below her—maybe one level lower. No where is this more evident among black women in high salaried jobs or ones requiring masters and doctorate degrees unless they reverse the old time order of men marrying up and women down. They will experience a problem some one marrying other minorities or whites. Men see no handicap in marrying generally and may easily accept a woman from a lower socio-economic class. Men see marriage as an asset in business, social community affairs and most communities for the ministry, school administrators and teachers. Although in 1969, 93% of all men and 95% of all women by the time they were 55 had married, this heavy trend toward marriage has reversed itself as evidenced by the above figures for the 35-44 age group.

No longer do social and economic factors push people into marriage. The scorned single woman of yesterday who was relegated to an inferior position, stayed at home to do menial tasks and came in time to fulfill the prophecy of the neurotic spinster, busy-body prim and proper "old maid" exists no longer. Women at one time had only several alternatives for careers—school teaching, to be a nurse or secretary. But today successful single women are in business, education, medicine, engineering, government, the professions, and the arts which serve to counteract the idea that a woman is a failure if single and proscribes the housewife role for work outside the home. Many persons have raised their voices in the women's liberation movement and out of it to assure women that singleness is a worthy alternative to marriage, point out that the single-life style can in many cases expand a woman's opportunities for self-fulfillment and development in a way that would be impossible were she to assume the traditional role of the wife. The single woman can have children, many men friends and even live with a man or woman according to her desires. That many women are following this trend is seen in the fact that by

1976 nearly 25% under 25 were still single and by 1986 26.4% under 30 had never married. Now some 28% never marry.

The Other Woman

In competition to the never-married middlescent widowed and the divorced looking to remarry there is a phenomenon of the new other woman. These people are likely to be our neighbors, friends, even sisters or our daughters. She is usually not a "kept woman" but typically works and often is a career or professional person. A "new" other woman, and the advent of single woman—married man liaisons is more and more widespread. As with any new social pattern, it reflects the demographic, social and cultural changes of the previous decade and forecasts the future as well. There are not enough single men for all single women. One out of five females do not have a potential mate. Currently 40% of American women are single. There are 33 million never married, divorced and widowed in America. Many of these will spend long periods of their life single. In fact as mentioned earlier only 56% of all adults are married in the U.S., in Sweden and Norway less than that.

For the single woman over 25 and 30 there is a serious under-supply of men, and as she ages that supply rapidly diminishes; for the older the woman many fewer men. This is the result of the very large differential in mortality, the preference of men for younger women and the fact that divorced men marry more quickly than divorced women. In 1980, widows outnumbered widowers six to one. In 1983, there were 91 single divorced men for every 137 single divorced women. Divorced men ages 25-44 are twice as likely to remarry as divorced women, while in the 45-64 bracket men are four times as likely to remarry than women. For every 223 unmarried women in their forties there are 100 unmarried men in their forties. The men who are available draw from a wide range of women, including the pool of younger women so that the typical male in his forties is often marrying a woman ten years his junior. Should a woman re-enter singlehood in her late thirties or beyond, she may be likely to remain single for the rest of her life. The single male population that is left further decreases the eligible men—some experts suggest as many as 14% by adding "closet queens" to the usual percentage, have poorer educations, are less well-off, least well situated occupationally and the most prone to mental and physical illness. This assessment comes from the work the New Other Woman, a research study, by Laurel Richardson out of Ohio State University. Richardson studied through interviews a number of these women. She notes that our cultural preference is still strong for men to "marry down" and for women to "marry up" in status—so strong, in fact, that any single woman over 25 with a college degree has somewhat reduced her chances of ever getting married. In 1985, for every 10 women between 40 and 49 years of age with a college education, there are only 32 single men who are older and better educated available as potential mates. For the female executive and professional, an elite class of women who have graduate training and achieved economic independence, there are very few men available. U.S. Census Bureau (1987) data suggests things may not be as bleak as suggested earlier for women up to 39 for until that year men outnumber women. One should remember many men won't marry and many are not marriable (alcoholics, mental instability, health problems and characterlogical misfits). From 40-44 there is about a million more women at 54 this is nearly double. From 19 up there are 28.7 males and 36.3 females.

Richardson (Human Development Specialist) suggests that the future forecast is an increased liaison between the single women and married men because the male-female ratio is widening. The typical reasons for these alignments will be:

(1) Older, divorced women who have lived most of their lives economically dependent, have little money and ability to compete in the singles' market will welcome general economic support and/or the extras a married man can provide like meals and vacations on a live out or live in basis.

(2) Some women will want a relationship which is cool and emotionally distant, while they pursue career or educational goals or they may want a relationship that provides sex without undue commitment to or time demands from their lover.

(3) Some women, more independent and liberated, will enter such a relationship because they think it will be more egalitarian than with a single man with fewer struggles.

For whatever reasons, based upon current indicators, somewhere between half and two-thirds of married men are expected to have extramarital liaisons and most of these will be with single women. The two major groups readied for these involvements are the "old guard" and the "new recruits." The old guard are those women who have come to value their relationships with married men. And even when their past one have been far from perfect, are ready for another relationship. The "new recruits" come from two sections: the newly divorced, the single woman, for everyone over 25, because of the lack of socially approved male companionship lessen with each passing year.

Richardson (Human Development Specialist) summarizes her conclusions by stating that the emotional needs (of women) are too deep, the cultural dicta too strong, the socialization too repetitive, and the social world too organized around heterosexual couplehood for most women who are not involved with a man to feel "attractive," or "valuable," or "normal," for many to forego the temptation of being the other woman, for the options are too few for the 33 million single women in America today!

The Jennifer Syndrome

Another phenomenon less noticed and pervasive is the Jennifer Syndrome. This syndrome is described by Barbara Gordon as the liaison between the middle age man and the young girl (20-25 year olds). It may also be a 75-year-old man and a 40-year-old woman. The men involved like these women because they have a certain amount of bounce, youth and malleability and they are not scarred. They do not carry a lot of psychological baggage from past failure in jobs, in love and they don't have children. Some men when discussing this situation say the Jennifer is not judgmental, they offer blind adoration and they stimulate. Hopefully these men (and they are increasing) think it will provide a new chance to prove life hasn't passed them by or give them the impetus to do something they have always wanted to do—write a book, take a certain trip, etc. It used to be that the men involved were mainly in their 40's and 50's but now many men 65 are getting involved. Do these men marry their Jennifers? Yes. Many are very helpful in career development and other projects.

At mid-life men become less aggressive, more passive, sensual at the same time the wife has been at home and wants to experience the male part of their persona, to achieve on their own, suggests David Gutmann of Northwestern University. So the assertiveness of a man's spouse is threatening to him. What one thing that may quiet that fear and make him feel as macho and aggressive as he used to feel—a young woman who doesn't judge him. For the Janet's (those who are divorced, middle-aged, and carry a lot of bitterness and psychological baggage from yesteryear) most men will avoid them if they can. And some men will turn to Jennifers. What about a Jeffrey for women in their middlescent years? There is for some a man. A woman of 40 to 50 is at her sexual peak of responsiveness, even though she may have lost the ability to bear children (though most have not). She is experienced, young men are potent and eager to learn. It's not uncommon in France where many such liaisons exist and increasingly it's becoming more common in the United States. According to Barbara Gordon, whenever she speaks on this subject, women stand up and ask "What about getting us a Jeffrey?"—it's only fair. A few years ago I was speaking to a naval officers wives club and was interrupted by a chorus following words on Jeffrey greeted me with "We want Jeffrey," maybe it was more than the wine they were drinking.

Assessments

By the time most people have reached their forties or shortly thereafter they make an assessment of their lives. They begin by comparing their present life—in all areas, their body changes, their home, their marriage and economic circumstance—and relate it to their future prospects. There might not be enough time to re-tread sufficiently to realize their earlier dreams. The despair for man may be more acute for he is judged by "having made it" through his job and the kind of living it affords. Most women in the past have been considered successful, at least to society, if they have managed to stay married and cared for children. Over the several decades this has been changing. There is increased pressure for a woman to succeed in a career beyond that of being a housewife. Unfortunately, stress and pressure to succeed will be an accompaniment in this attempt.

The success of the housewife will be easily judged for she typically has no earned money to show though she may be worth her weight in gold. The glory of the middleaged woman is found in the success of her children and in particular the homage of her sons. Wives are not usually as upset about the husband's career or job as he may be, if they have not suffered real hardship, but a wife will worry when her husband is unhappy. But as children leave the home, couples have to rely more on each other for companionship, company and ego support. If they find little common ground to support these needs and the growth demand that come from cultural and personal expectations, then the marriage is dead. It is believed that only one of four marriages grow into more effective ones from the twenties to the fifties. Others stay together by force of habit, fear of failure alone, cultural taboo and children, in many divorces occurs.

According to Roger Gould, as long as marriage is seen as a static arrangement two unchanging people, any substantial change in either person must initially be perceived as a violation of the original contract. It was not supposed to change in any substantial way. Demands from the wife to pursue new direction in keeping with the mastery motivation is though to be a break in the contract agreed to at the marriage beginning. There are others, yes many women who argue via the Bible, fundamentalism, tradition, etc., that woman's place is to be subservient to the man and she would do everything he desires (Total Woman no less) but not a competitor or free agent in life or marriage. Many women who march to protest abortion or for ecological concerns are not able to face the challenge of their own internal definition. Who am I? What should I do for myself? When they do redefine themselves and set out on the journey to find in the consciousness-raising stage of personal emancipation, as Roger Gould calls it, they will have to educate their men, learn new skills, and channel their aggressiveness away from anger directed to a man/men (who took all those years away from me) and work out their own salvation. We remember Charles Kingsley's lines—"Ay, marriage is the life-long miracle. The self-begetting wonder, daily fresh."

What To Look For In Marriage

Most advice falls on deaf ears whether about marriage or otherwise or if not then, since our perceptions of the intent and quality in people varies so widely, it defies being a science, so even advice taken is often inappropriate. Most of us are aware of the usual field of eligibility of males and females that exists. Aside from the fact that choice favors the male, for unfortunately the number of women in middle age are more numerous than men, and that women are said as they age to "rot" rather than mature as men supposedly do. Besides this, our choices have limitations for there exists the usual factors: endogamy—the marrying of homefolk; exogamy—marrying those outside our family; homogamy—marrying those like us, that is in our class; and finally proximity—we marry those who are near. Like most automobile accidents, which happen within 25 miles of our homes, marriages operate the same way. The fantasy marriage with Tom Cruise or Nicole Kidman will not happen, or with an other desirable with prestige, because of this principle. In our mobile society, we can do something about this circumstance. If we live in a small town with few opportunities to meet eligible men, then we can move to a city. When I was a school principal in a small community some years ago, a 39 year old woman biology teacher came to me about going to another community—she would like to get married but little chance seemed to exist in our town, and although she liked her work, she asked for my advice. I had to tell the lady in her own interest to go to another location. Several years later in the new community she had met a man and married him. In a smaller community one is usually handicapped for beyond the lack of choice the widowed or divorced has much less chance to socialize. A man isn't as handicapped but even so he may find little choice in the rural community or small town to make a suitable marriage.

This is no longer true although ads for a partner in magazines, etc., have been around for over fifty years, through the use of computers possibilities of attracting some one are endless. Thousands of couples in the past decade and the numbers are increasing have been brought together via the computers. It offers opportunity to present yourself to a variety of interested persons. Protection is afforded by use of pseudonyms, use of a code, etc. and careful investigation. If a person is selected to correspond with you, you still can hide your identity and if continued liking to meet the person you can arrange a meeting at a neutral place with protected conditions and location. It is not fool proof. Unfortunately in many cases of fraud have been unearthed. Flimflam artists are always about looking to practice aggrandizement on you and separate you from your money. Agencies abound for coupling up people. Typically videotapes are utilized to introduce yourself in which you talk about your self—schooling, work, likes and dislikes, personality and wish for friendships. These companies charge fees and some times bring successful union together. TV shows like the Dating Game and others of more recent origin stimulate this approach to meeting people.

Types of Marriage

Most social and behavioral scientists believe that two general varieties of marriage exist. *Traditional* marriages are those in which the spouses allocate roles and responsibilities on the basis of sex. The husband's role encompasses traditional "male" activities and traits. For example, he controls the economic aspects of family life and has the authority to make decisions for the entire family. The wife's role encompasses traditional "female" activities and traits. For example, she is responsible for domestic tasks, including management of the house and children. Traditional relationships often involve little direct or overt expression of emotion between the spouses. Rather, each partner relies some on relatives and same-sex friends for companionship and affection (Peplau, 1983). Today the traditional marriage does incorporate emotional expression between husband and wife and compromise on some issues and work distribution. Television "sitcoms" that were popular during the late 1950s through the 1970s showcased this type of marriage. *The Donna Reed Show, Father Knows Best, I Love Lucy, All in the Family*, which shows marriages in which the husband worked outside the home and functioned as the sole "breadwinner," primary disciplinarian, and decision maker for the family, whereas the wife stayed at home, raised the children, and took care of domestic tasks such as cooking the family meals, shopping, and cleaning.

A second type of marriage, and one that is increasingly common, is the *Egalitarian, peer, or equal-status* marriage. Unlike traditional relationships, in which tasks and roles are divided along gender lines, egalitarian marriages are characterized by shared roles and responsibility in all aspects of married life. Both the husband and the wife are assumed to be capable of displaying—and expected to contribute to the relationship—social support and caregiving, affection and emotion, sexuality, financial resources, parenting skills, and domestic labor. Television highlighted this kind of union in 1980s programs such as *The Cosby Show* and *Roseanne.* Sociologists Pepper Schwartz and Virginia Rutter (1998) noted that true peer marriages are relatively rare: "The potential for power sharing, obligation sharing, and resource sharing in marriage is there, though not commonly acted upon. Pairs with the ambition of egalitarianism often fall short, into the 'near peer' category." For instance many women who share economic help with the husband still find they do more housework than the husband and looking after children, usually arrange for child care and do most of the taking of children to doctors offices, school programs, shopping and recreation. These "near peer" marriages usually involve a husband who helps with child care and household labor, and a wife who provides financial resources and makes economic decisions, to a greater degree than would be expected in traditional marriages. Although truly egalitarian marriages may still be relatively uncommon, there is some evidence that partners who achieve them experience high levels of companionship and mutual respect as well as low levels of anger and conflict. In sum, "equity has its rewards."

Regardless of the type of marriage all people start with certain ideas about the person they would like to marry. The following lists from research by Regan and Berscheid (1997) provide the rank order of characteristics desire in a partner. Both list intelligence number four on the list while on honesty and trustworthiness men list this second while women put it first. Easygoing nature is categorized number ten by both sexes. Interesting men place attractive appearance third while women put it ninth. External attributes are ranked higher by men than women, for instance appearance and health.

Top 10 Desired Characteristics in a Marriage Partner

Men	*Women*
Good overall personality	Honesty and trustworthiness
Honesty and trustworthiness	Kindness and compassion
Attractive appearance	Good overall personality
Intelligence	Intelligence
Good health	Attentive to one's partner
Kindness and compassion	Good sense of humor
Good sense of humor	Self-confidence
Self-confidence	Good health
Attentive to one's partner	Attractive appearance
Easygoing nature	Easygoing nature

Signs of Non-love in People in Marriage

1. Giving little time to the partner.
2. Does not listen to partner's discussion of problems.
3. Attracted to another man or woman.
4. Mistrusts the spouse.
5. Has little or no sex.
6. Personality problems (Cf Fromme's list of these later in the chapter.)

Most everyone wishes to be loved and to love. For most this means to marry, although we see many persons in the in-between years today who never marry but carry on cohabitation. An increasing phenomenon is cohabitation especially in urban centers where men and women take up living with each other share sex, expenses, or even children. A kind of marriage which means they may live apart but do most things together, go on trips, even pool resources and in general look after the interest of the other person. Many men and women who divorce feel utterly devastated so that they launch themselves into a number of sexual adventures, many because they have been deprived in the last months or years of good sexual activity so can hardly contain the pressure. Particularly for women, since the double standard still lingers, they will not find it to their advantage to sleep around. This is cul-de-sac with AIDS about. For this often keeps a good prospect for remarriage from approaching the woman—the grapevine works swiftly and accurately and takes its toll. Maybe you say "damn the torpedoes full speed ahead." Many men have a partially erroneous idea that the divorcee and the widow to some extent are in great need for sex; many mistake this attention for something deeper only to find play time is over in a hurry and they are worse off than before. Many women overlook good prospects through bypassing older men. Their notions of their physical and social status frequently get in the way of even allowing themselves to become friend with men 15 to 20 years older. Marlon Brando is quoted as having said that for a woman, her best sexual partner may be the 50-year-old healthy man. This has been echoed by some experts, for he is more mature, therefore responds to more needs, is slower to arousal, therefore gives greater attention to the woman. However, once aroused the androgen stimulation is sufficient to continue an erection for a considerable time usually longer than his younger counterpart.

I have a friend of long standing, as young men we participated in athletics together and as adults we both became teachers. He worked in the summer as a Camp Director while I usually taught high school classes in the summer. One summer, when he was 26, he invited me to his camp for a weekend to meet his girlfriend and introduce me to a friend of hers. I was appalled when I got there to find his girlfriend was 35. She was ancient, I told him and in no way would this last the year out. He married her a year later accepting her son by her first marriage with gusto. A few years ago, my wife and I were in Miami and we called my friend. We met for dinner, and during our meal he reminded me of what I had said 20 years earlier—I blushed and apologized profusely for being so juvenile. Although he bragged of having less gray hair than I, the real show was the woman. She had changed very little over the years, that marriage had done wonders for her—for both of them. This story suggests aside from age factors in marriage that we should not make a decision on whom we should go out with and certainly whom we should marry solely on the advice of others. We ourselves are the best judges. Many women who are older—40 to 50 years of age and beyond have attracted and married younger men. We are knowledgeable enough by now to know we should usually marry within our social and economic classes. Love will not conquer all despite its pervasive ring. Beyond this however most persons contemplating marriage wish to talk it over with a confidante.

Allan Fromme lists five signs of non-love. Regardless of the fit, these should be considered when looking at a prospect for marriage. These signs are:

1. The person does not have many friends or very few. It can be rationalized that they work all the time, are committed to the care of a mother or father hence stay close by, and after all he loves you and pours out adulation. Maybe you feel he is the victim of his or her environment. Caution suggests that the one who has great capacity

for love spreads it over many people. He or she is loving in general. One who has few or nor friends or only finds one person interesting is not likely to have a well-developed ability to love.

2. The person has the feeling that "nobody loves me" or "nobody understands me." The individual who feels unloved is usually one who is not loving and is not giving love. The psychological mechanism is one of the defense known as projection. We project on to other people our unpleasant selves which we do not like to face. Often in an argument a man feels rage rising in him and shouts at his opponent, "What are you getting so mad about?" Yet this man has been doing all the talking and others cannot get any words into the conversation. A good tactic sometimes but not rational. Suffice it to say, the projection here suggests, if I feel nobody loves me, the probability is that I am not loving toward anybody.

3. Excessive ambition in a person pre-empts ability to love. The inability to love is seen in persons who are possessed by a drive to get ahead or reach some pinnacle in the world. This person has a "love" and has no room for another like the man who spends all his time with his business in the pursuit of making a million. Or the woman whose passion is wrapped up in real estate or selling of stocks and bonds has found her love. If ambition is excessive, we usually can be sure that there is little emotion left over for other people or enough to sustain a healthy marriage relationship. This is especially crucial in the middle-aged person for it smacks of neuroticism serving to blind one's inner fear of failure and providing a routine which allows one to keep from flying to pieces.

4. The inability to say no is another important sign of non-love. Genuine love grows from respecting the other person and ourselves. Those who can't say no appear to be very loving but in truth may be just the opposite. This type of person who is driving compulsively to please everyone does it to gain favor. It is as though she has to please because she feels down deep that she is unworthy of love otherwise. This is very damaging to ability to love.

5. The person who is the perfectionist. Avoid this individual like the plague. For if you marry, you'll be uncomfortable in a very brief time. For loving by this person is conditioned upon the fact of your performance—for he says, I will love you if you will do this or do that. This person cannot tolerate our foibles, in fact, cannot abide people generally for he is perfect. Most of us are human and make many

> mistakes and faux pas. The female perfectionist makes an excellent secretary or research assistant because she has to do it right. When the perfect housewife can't control every situation and dirt gets on the rug all hell breaks loose. This kind of person—be it man or woman, will be extremely difficult to live with; they are usually inflexible and humorless generally.

We must recognize that love has strings attached to it. We are brought up to understand this—"If you don't stop hitting your sister, I won't love you." So we learn in childhood under certain conditions we are loved. The brave middlescent like the spirited child will risk much on occasions for adventure but the vulnerable child will watch his step. The middlescent who feels insecure and the need to be loved, with an object to lay their love upon, might be inclined to risk little in fear of not finding a partner. This can be shortsighted but many women and some men think they can change their partners. This is unlikely. Although we have talked about growth and change in marriage and a person forty years of age certainly can adjust, learning new ways, but the structure of personality will not be entirely reversed.

You say to me the value of having a mate overrides other considerations. I know that there are swap-offs and that couples rarely join in marriage on equal terms, even though this is the ideal. I remember a lady speaking to me about her possible marriage; she had four girls, the prospective man had six children. She was college educated; he was not. He did have a good income. The question of suitability, given affection and love, involved around would she be willing to undertake to care for his children in return for love and being a good provider. The answer came after the introduction of their children to each other in a short-term family-like situation. They did not get married. The lady did marry a minister (Episcopal) even though she was divorced and had four children. In this instance the children may have been the catalysts in the marriage, in addition to love.

Most men will however steer clear of a woman with several young children. With the wealthy this may be of less concern. It seems to be difficult to make a suitable arrangement when two people also bring their children with them to a union. The children, particularly between the ages of 10–16, in many cases they resent the intrusion of the new man and eventually this lead to friction between the couple. Some men will entertain the idea of taking a woman into marriage who has small children if there are no more than two of them. Frequently the negotiation in these cases involves a woman of relative youth with the older man's financial ability. The children get a father, the wife and children support. There are instances where usually the woman does not work at a career. In many cases the combining efforts by both partners working makes for greater advantages in their lives—more affluence, more clothes, vacations, larger homes and cultural advantages. One thing is true, those who marry in middle age do not have to consider pleasing families of the mates we chose or to justify our lifestyle; we take for granted that at 40 or 50 we are our own person. We are never going to be able to guarantee our love or the love of other people will be perfect. Our ability to love has been influenced by the earlier loves of our childhood. Adult love is frequently imperfect because childhood love was faulty. There are many points at which learning to love takes a wrong turn and all in the normal process of growing up. Growing up itself is an obstacle course filled with booby traps. Everything struggles to grow—young animals, tender plants and sensitive human beings. The most important thing in most of our lives is love—love with a special person or persons. That our love lives are filled with hazards is understandable for the thing that is so important we can't control—that is, another person. So we learn to adjust, to give and take, and to be hopeful. Remarriages are often superior to first ones because the illusions of youth are gone, couples try infinitely more to be successful, have fewer expectations and they understand more of the totality of life. Nevertheless the figures show that divorce rate are just about as high for the second marriage as in first marriage.

For second wives and husbands, to some degree, there is some expected foreknowledge and consideration necessary before entering into marriage. In the first place, most men do remarry, usually three out of four, within a year to three year period of being divorced or widowed. Ninety percent of all remarried men who were divorced say that their second marriage is better. Research shows about the same percent divorce rate in this group. The divorced man marries in 2.7 years and the widowed in 3.5 years. There are many men who marry within a year but fewer women. Women who remarry do so at a smaller percentage rate. Men remarry for a variety of reasons—to escape loneliness, the discomfort of eating out or fixing meals, business purpose where wives are required, sexual relations, to regain the status marriage conferred, younger men wish to have children and older ones to have a place for his children to visit. Jean Baer in her book *The Second Wife* suggests some less valid reasons for marrying; marriage on the rebound, that is to show the former wife he can do what she does, because of sadistic-masochistic traits, extreme dependence of always having had a woman in his life, and he may marry out of passivity, that is some woman wishes to marry him so he does without much thought one way or the other. There are some important items one should go over while assessing the possibility of marriage. These apply for men and women.

1. Has the divorce or death experience been growth experience for the prospective partner? Where depression and passivity is chronic, caution is advised.
2. Does the intention to marry relate to social and status climbing? Sometimes one will accept this as part of a negotiation.
3. In the case of the man, has he been a good provider? Or in the case of the woman, has she been a good mother?
4. Is he or she still in love with the ex-spouse? This needs to be known or it will color the life thereafter in important ways.
5. How many times have they been married? Three or four times in marriage adds up to your being the next loser.
6. Is he or she remarriageable? Sometimes the romantic notions may not correspond to your timing. He or she having survived a divorce may want time to play the field or if you are the first attraction after divorce you might receive the brunt of the sad saga of the first marriage. Dr. Albert Ellis, noted New York psychologist, says that "many individuals especially those who have been married or lost their mates thrive on living alone for the rest of their lives—but also thrive on intermittent and even permanent love affairs along with their domestic privacy."

Jean Baer gives advice for the prospective second wives during courtship that should be considered seriously. Many persons marry in haste only to think about what they have done in leisure. Perhaps doubt will be the lot of all of us in the pre-marriage situation but some can be relieved by foreknowledge before we make the final step.

1. You should find out all you can about the previous marriage, why it broke up, get a three-dimensional picture, do not take the word of the man solely for many will hide important aspects of the circumstance. Remember the divorce settlements are public record and can be examined in the Register of Deeds or Document Department Offices. Remember also that this information covers up real problems of a marriage to facilitate a divorce. Often a false charge is admitted to such as constructive deception that may be a cover for adultery. In no fault divorce this may not matter. Nevertheless the records about divorce are usually accurate.

2. Love him openly, warmly, constantly.
3. See as much of him as you can in a variety of situations.
4. Talk over every aspect of the financial situation—alimony, loans, taxes, obligations, wills, and insurance, etc. The matter of middlescent property, holdings of stocks and bonds and what will be the disposal made of them need to be settled in advance. Many couples will wish their estates to go principally to their children; attendance to this removes a large hurdle.
5. Examine your basic ideas about lifestyles.
6. Make sure you are sexually compatible—you're not children, you can talk over these matters, if sex was good or bad before you should know it. Some people demand sex under less than normal conditions—they need to be beaten or tied up or they need to inflict pain on you before release or satisfaction is obtained.
7. After a man is 35, you may get change in his life, but don't expect it. Don't carp about his leisure pursuits, be it football, fishing, or what he does in his work life, if he's 45 this is fairly well set.
8. Make life exciting for your prospective husband—be generous at the appropriate times with gifts, introduce him to new friends and places. He will think life with you is going to be exciting.
9. Remember, children of your spouse will resent you even if you have no children, and if this is the case it will complicate matters for you. The children will not wish to share their parents with a strange brood. Children, in loyalty to their absent parent, will not want you to take up with a "new" father. My brother and sister and I all resisted any special attention by a man to our mother following our father's death. We were 15, 17 and 19. This was a mistake, for mother never married although she was only 43 when widowed and was an attractive and healthy woman.

There are some pitfalls in courtship. Don't overestimate how much you care for his children and if you don't like them, forget about pursuing this courtship idea. You should be scrupulously honest about your life, your health, your life with your former spouse or friends. If you fabricate tales about yourself or ex-mate, they sometimes come back to haunt you and frequently if they chance to meet your ex-husband he may be liked by your present boyfriend. So believing horror stories about him will fall on deaf ears! Your courtship shouldn't last forever if you intend to marry, for males are frequently procrastinators and will offer a variety of excuses—wait until the children are out of school or until my former wife remarries. Of course, if you don't wish to marry but have a steady friend, then fair enough, this is no great concern.

Remarriage can serve as a healing balm, it can also be very trying. You will have to control your desire to express differences between the former and present life. If children are involved no matter how good they appear to be, you will have some problems—the natural parents do and so will you. Try not to compete with his children for affection. You will have, in some instances, to expect irritation from an ex-wife, sometimes this comes from an ex-husband. Trust your husband even if your former one was a rat, and try to keep romance alive and when life's demands are hard on you tell your husband some adjustments are needed. Establish a pattern of talking out problems or over things from the very beginning.

OPEN AND CLOSED MARRIAGES

This leads up to the topic of open and closed marriages. These are styles of marriage that are classified and peer type of marriages. An open marriage may sound exciting to the couple who has begun to find life a drag. But few people, in my opinion, can stand the emotional stresses involved in intimacy given to others than the partners (typically marriage gives exclusive right to sex forbidding those outside) which is sometimes found in these arrangements. These are people like the O'Neills who are professional on this subject contrasting open and closed marriages are anthropologists, their data comes from interviewing 400 couples who concluded that human relationships are the focal point in marriage difficulties. The O'Neills say closed marriage represents the stagnant, rigid pattern of marriage often seen in middle-age marriages and inevitably ends in separation. The assumptions of the closed marriage are as follows: Marriage will last forever, it means total commitment, it will bring happiness, it will give comfort and security, the mates will always be true to each other and we will never be lonely again. All problems can be solved in marriage by sex and love. Also, it means the ultimate goal in marriage is having a child; sacrifice is the measure of true love, that any change will come gradually with the maturity of age; that any other kind of change is disruptive and means a loss of love and finally, that the person you marry can fulfill all your needs, economic, physical, sexual, intellectual and emotional. Such is this credo.

On the other hand, the O'Neills say that the "open" marriage begets growth, intimacy, personal development, and vitality. This type of marriage is characterized by:

1. That you will share most but not everything.
2. That each partner will change, and that change can occur through conflict as well as through gradual development.
3. That each will accept responsibility for himself and grant it to his mate.
4. That each partner will be different in needs, capacities, values, and expectations because he is a different person, not because they are husband and wife.
5. That the mutual goal is the relationship, not status, or the house on the hill.
6. That children are not needed as proof of your love for each other.
7. That should you choose to have children, you undertake the role of parents knowingly and willingly as the greatest responsibility in life.
8. That liking and loving will grow because of the mutual respect that your open relationship engenders.

There is much to be said for this type of marriage. There are, however, many that interpret from their religious and social heritage a view that marriage means the man is the head of the family, the center of family activity, and the subservient role belonging to the wife is ordained of God. This type of marriage can be satisfying given the acceptance of the principles entailed with it and acknowledging that adult life is a plateau with little change. Most marriages, however labeled, will usually have some elements of both of types of relationships. One can use the above for a check-up on the conditions that exist in a marriage and set some realistic goals for change. This means recognizing that the ability to make some change will facilitate future change with less difficulty. Men and women should be considered equal, the childbearing function does not relegate the woman to an inferior status nor does the fact that women live longer suggest they are the necessarily superior sex as is presently bandied about by some. When stress and pressure to succeed in the business world of commerce and art evens out life expectancies may also balance out and perhaps the lesser affliction of disease in the middle years of woman will not be thought of as just a function of the uterus.

Dr. Clyde Veder, sociologist, said that he believed that over half of the divorces could be circumvented in America if both parties went to see a marriage counselor. And he says that even a third could be saved if only one had counseling. The power, if continued a few years, is such that in the United States over 10,000 divorced persons remarry their former spouse every year. I know several couples who divorced still cohabitated with the former spouse then after several years remarried. Evidently, the discord between them was less destructive than the alternative disruption of new arrangements. Although we are talking about divorce here, it should be mentioned that many marriages that are in difficulty could be modified without resorting to divorce. Increasingly, numbers of persons who marry have had premarital counseling service offered by some church ministries, community agencies, or through college courses as marriage and the family or related ones in psychology and these help solve problemed marriages. Many divorced persons give pause to reflect, what went wrong with my marriage? The demands of marriage are so elevated and often unrealistic that the goals are impossible to reach, differential growth rates pose a problem and most people do not try to impose the discipline on themselves that is necessary for marriage to be successful. When marriages are first made, the expectancy exists that the couple will grow together; even though this may take place, they may grow in different directions or rates than the other. Some marriages can thrive on this if it is a part of agreed-upon freedom. In some cases there is simply no growth for one of the partners. Uncorrected difficulties in a marriage eventually come attached to strong emotions often developing deep hostility toward the partner who is unwilling to change when the other partner's demands grow and change has taken place in them. Before couples become deadlocked emotionally, counseling should be sought about the marriage. It may do nothing substantial to save the marriage but it will clear the air somewhat and ultimately prepare the way for a less emotional separation and divorce. It will also have the effect of softening the blow for children, and if they are older provide insight into the marriage problems. Children also know that an attempt to reconcile differences is being made and that they are not the cause of the divorce but that it is caused by problems beyond them. Being realistic, the second divorce is sometimes due to children where the families cannot intermesh and be compatible.

There are a few things that a counselor can do for the couple who has reached an impasse. If a couple is left alone, things usually go from bad to worse. Under the pressure of hurt feelings and disappointment, they lash out at each other, or withdraw from each other. This creates more injury—most people can stand some argument but not the silent treatment. As disappointment builds up, so do the barriers to communication and hopes for settling differences become almost nil. With our basic needs unfulfilled—to love, to be comforted, to be understood and have a confidante—it is only a matter of time before we turn to other sources of help and solace. The new support or interest may come from a new love and sex interest, our children, our careers, the security of our parents, or in alcohol or drugs. David Mace, the well-known writer and authority on marriage, says that something that could have been good turns out bad. He suggests it is like a child who received a building kit and tries to make a model plane. In his lack of know-how, he cannot put it together. In increasing exasperation, he uses unnecessary force to place it together only to break it. With patience exhausted and control gone, he smashes the pieces that he looked forward to completing. Yet with the help of a cooperative parent, the child might have been made the model airplane which he would have been proud of. Where the situation is analogous, the help of a marriage counselor might affect a cure for an ailing marriage. A certified marriage counselor can serve to mediate between a man and wife, help to clarify the issues involved; in short, he or she can serve an interpreter. Competent counselors have training in fields of guidance and counseling, human relations, and come from professionals in psychiatry, social, work, ministry and psychology or education. Although, unfortunately, in many states marriage counselors are not required to be licensed members of a recognized professional organization as the American Association of Marriage and Family Counselors, these licensed counselors are competent to deal with problems between husband and wife; also the family in general. Counseling will not save all marriages from dissolving, but if a couple is honest in attempting to find a solution, which may finally be divorce, a certified marriage counselor can help. The counselor is most effective in working with a man and wife when they bring the marital problems to him as early as possible. When a marriage is emotionally deadlocked, the relationship falls apart rapidly. When a wife and husband are no longer working together talking it over but begin to work against each other or they inflict injuries on each other, which cools their affection and builds up hostility and resentment; under tension things are often said with the couple becoming cruel to each other in their attitudes and actions. Often the things they do to each other under stress become greater causes of conflict between them than the original disagreement that started it all. Of course, minor problems should be worked through by husband and wife, lover's irritations and tiffs are minor things. Quarrels are natural to marriage, also some shouting and ventilation of anger; these can usually be worked out by the couple. When there is no way out of a logger-head situation, then it is time to seek help.

Another condition which assists the counselor if both woman and man will cooperate fully in the process of counseling. Where only one partner cooperates, it is difficult to assist as usually the airing of a problem requires a recitation of both partners to allow the counselor to have a reasonable view of the situation. The wife of a physician came to me for counseling and, at my suggestion, brought her husband in also. I subsequently had their life histories and a clear view of their problems. The cooperation of the physician was excellent until we got to the point where some moves to compromise the positions of the parties was in the offing. He refused to see any obstacles his life gave his wife, the revelation of his "extra" life was painful to the wife but she wanted him to come home early one day a week to spend with the four daughters. I then suggested nothing more could be done by me. I was convinced that there were characterological problems with the physician although I could discover little tangible evidenced from any psychological testing but his wife was to me obviously suffering from depression. Despite the difficulties the wife hung on to the marriage, apparently she loved her husband and she also had four children of varying young ages under her care. I recommended to her she get a physical examination for any problems and see if minerals and vitamins were sufficient in her diet.

A final necessary element in successful counseling is that the marriage partners should be willing to continue with therapy sessions for a reasonable length of time. Certainly the expenditure of time, money and effort is tiresome. In some instances the mates feel relief as soon s they have gotten the problem expressed to someone and then often cut-off seeing the counselor. This is a mistake most of the time, for usually only superficial matters have been altered. The effect of counseling has a greater impact—it aims to be a process through which the growth of personality is advanced and which will avoid the recurrence of the type of problem they had before. Marriage counseling can be expensive—from one hundred fifty dollars to two hundred dollars a session, although many of these counseling centers sometimes adjust the fee to the financial circumstances of the family. There are also some services that are provided free of charge offered by United Fund Agencies. You can look in the local phone book for the number of mental health agencies and Social Welfare for assistance along these lines.

Despite the fact that life represents a continuation of problems and solutions, there remains for the middlescent couple the promise of the good life. It can be a time for new intimacy, with children gone a renewed interest in each other that existed in the earlier years of marriage can be resumed. Planning to do things together, being alone to share moments of tenderness not allowed for some time now is possible and doing things for each other often forgotten in the heat of child raising is also realizable. Husband and wife by the middle years have learned to intermingle their roles. Sharp divisions of function highlighted by certain assumptions of society will increasingly be changed. Husbands become more nurturant of wives and their parents in the in-between years, he helps do more chores formerly reserved only for you and in general is more understanding. He will support your drive for mastery or engaging in a new enterprise. Maybe you garden together or work in the yard or paint your house, the cooperation that can now be felt is delicious thought to cherish, lifting life together to a new and higher level.

A new relationship with children that are grown or near grown can occur as children begin to see the wisdom of earlier parental guidance. The mid-life person has learned not to give (hopefully) advice unless it is sought. Children have accomplished the task of becoming independent and now have no fear you will overwhelm their egos and control their lives. Their response to us can be adult to adult who enhances life for them and us. Deeper relationships with friends can become a reality with time for socialization that heretofore existed only sandwiched in get-togethers between hurry-hurry schedules of children and parents. Time is now afforded to seek companionship with people we would like to cultivate and to improve our rapport with those we already know. Finally, there is the opportunity to devote energies to new community service, which we would like. Most persons in their earlier adult years volunteered for work or most likely were "drafted" to do jobs for agencies like the United Fund, relief organizations, church fund raising and school activity. Now the luxury exists for you to choose. The enrichment that comes from doing some needed work because we want to do it colors our whole life. Certainly it is true, as spoken by the ancient and venerable prophet, Hillel, "If you are not for yourself, who is and if only for yourself, what are you; and if not now when?"

CHAPTER IX

DIVORCE AND AFTERWARDS

"After the Party is Over"

Voltaire wrote "divorce dates from just about the same time as marriage; I think that marriage is a few weeks the more ancient." This is like saying death is present at birth. It is undoubtedly true that the seeds of divorce are present at the outset of marriage. The fact that of every two marriages one ends in divorce has been true since 1985. The question is whether this trend will finally be reversed when enough couples, mainly young ones, base their marriages on growth principles or will serial marriage prophesized by Toffler some years ago in his *Future Shock* mark the direction in coupling and uncoupling remains to be seen. It is easy to account for a number of uncouplings from marriage by the fact that they were mismatches in the beginning. In western society with an emphasis on material success, the sensual gratification of every need breeds unrealistic goals for people. The fact of increasing longevity also affects the divorce rates. In our mobile society the initial bonding takes place with little formality, with little background experience in making choices among people and virtually no restriction as, with whom; only one question is raised, do I love him or her.

It is a wonder that as many marriages last as long as they do for the factors which are involved are so overwhelming that the number of inappropriate marriages to begin with are astronomical. Another problem is that in a period of transition like we now find ourselves, the typical traditional marriage is being severely tested. The feminist movement, rights' movement existential philosophies and the concept of "open" marriage trend to cohabitation proclaim that marriage rests upon the assumption that the growth of partners in a marriage to their highest potential is the ideal. The shackles of suppression of women's roles have been broken—release that accounts for millions of women seeking their own identities—and for many the "new fulfilled person" demands separation from their spouse. The more divorces there are, the easier it is for others to seek them. The former taboos are nearly erased except in a few enclaves involving some religious ethnic groups, and small towns and rural communities. Today it is often possible for a Protestant minister to be divorced and maintain his pastorate or marry a divorced woman.

The theories about divorce suggest the changing family roles in society account for increasing divorce rates. The family was once responsible for religious experience of their offspring, their general education, recreation and leisure; discipline, medical attention and employment too were part of the total integrated family enterprise. Outside agencies have taken over many of these functions and those that remain are largely by-products of the family—the socialization of children, companionship and happiness. Changing roles of the partners in a marriage has contributed to divorce—mothers earning a living or a good part of it outside of the home makes it possible to separate from a marriage which is less than satisfactory. The women's liberation movement credo suggests that less rigidity in marriage roles should replace the ones generally held to that separation of many of the functions in traditional marriage are erased. In this situation, where both can play a variety of roles or parts in the drama of life, if one leaves the marriage it makes less difference than before when the lines were fixed. In the notion of romantic love is inbedded the seed-bed for divorce for when the period of "I could eat you up" is over and the love-object has been eaten up frequently regurgitation follows. This shallow basis for many marriages leaves only a stale taste in one's mouth. The breakup of the nuclear family brought about by the "musical chairs" game occasioned by the demand of companies, employment opportunities and by our general mobility, often means leaving the extended family behind, placing people in an environment where the support and control through family mores and customs is lacking. This then becomes the harbinger of many marriage downfalls. Many marriage problems one must, recognize and relate to immaturity of the spouses, unequal status, sexual incompatibility and lack of motivation for improvement.

The reasons why almost half of all marriages will end in divorce, when in 1900 only one marriage in fourteen culminated in this fashion, can be summarized as: (1) the change from rural to urban way of life; (2) change in the status of women; (3) grounds for divorce change for instance use of particularly the no-contest rule provided in the statutes of many states "no fault" divorce. The erosion of economic blackmail and continuance of "dead marriages" forwarded under the adversarial system; and (4) loss of values which reinforced the principle of life-long monogamy. The nature of divorce is complex and does not occur overnight. Many factors interact as seen in what G. Levinger calls those aspects, which bear upon the stability of marriage. There are two features to this scheme, on one hand, external support and internal attractions which tend to keep marriage together and external attractions which work against marriage. If the supports are indeed commanding enough in terms of the internal attraction (comfort, companionship, status, personality needs, love), then marriage will be healthy. If the internal attractions are insufficient, then the marriage may stay together based upon external supports due to such things as legal barriers, religious commitment, family ties, children or career needs. When the external attractions to escape marriage become strong enough, then the emotional tie to marriage will be broken. The impetus—the attraction of another man or woman, growth opportunities, freedom from responsibility, then divorce is inevitable. Divorce is rarely a simple matter, the emotional and adjustment aspects are at the least very trying and energy sapping.

EFFECTS OF DIVORCE

The effects of divorce are pervasive and its impact is great upon the nuclear family and to a lesser extent the wider kinship group; in addition, it has a relationship with economics, status, adjustment in living and social arrangements and our psychological equilibrium.

The question arises, is divorce helpful or harmful? There are some basic principles upon which to draw some conclusions; however, besides these it depends upon individuals and the circumstances. In the case of adversarial (court contested) these are more likely to be the case and much less likely in a mediated or no-fault divorce.

(1) Usually divorce, no matter how amiable or how much desired is like the loss of a loved-one in death. Compounding loneliness and lost status is the feeling expressed by many a divorced person of being a fifth wheel.

(2) It is sometimes difficult for many women to adjust to a single status and to assume responsibility for economic matters is overwhelming to many—women may find that getting credit, banking and investing is not so easy even if they are used to holding down a job.

(3) Some of these same difficulties haunt the divorcing man who usually moves out of the home to less satisfactory surroundings where he

becomes responsible for his meals, laundry and countless little things unnoticed before. Even if the man is desirous of divorce he frequently finds the demands made on his finances resources limits him from launching his new freedom with anything near affluence.

(4) The effect on family and children, let alone friends, brings guilt and suffering regardless of who is the alleged victim or villain beyond pre-calculation and as is frequently suggested, one can divorce a spouse but never a child.

And, most experts in marriage attribute the majority of breakups to both parties, not solely the one awarded a decree if it be via the courts. There are some positive things about divorce.

(1) Many persons bonded in marriage in unequal situations such as being immature, educational levels, mental health, social and economic backgrounds, frequently profit by divorce. The years of trauma bring no healing of the difficulties hence bring about formal separation. Divorce is often devastating on children, but it is not essential that a child have two parents certainly when they are a warring father and mother. The important thing is the quality of the one parent relationship; hopefully both parents will continue to be responsible to the children for that is crucial to their mental health.

(2) Divorced persons, both men and women, have higher rates of remarriage than single and widowed of similar ages. And at the present rate of 80-90 percent of men divorced marry again and 75 percent of women do. Two out of five of these will end in divorce.

(3) The divorced person is given the opportunity to reconstruct his or her life, construct a new view of self and independence, take on new responsibility of their choosing, get an education denied by early marriage and develop into a responsible self-directing person.

Some guidelines for divorcing parents are: Don't try to isolate the child from the difficulties prior to the breakup; he or she can sense trouble, it is better to know than not to know. Give him or her simple, honest explanations on a level he or she can understand without loading your problems on them. Make it clear he or she is not the blame. Don't ask the young child to decide which parent he is to live with, older children should be consulted about their feelings in this matter. Reassure the child or children that both parents will continue to love and care for them. Hopefully this will be the case. Reaffirm your love to them.

Effect on Children

Paul Friggens suggests a number of things, which serve to augment what was discussed above about dealing with the child in the divorce situation. Over a million children a year are involved in divorce, less than 40% live to be 18 in an intact family! The trauma felt by the child is devastating; it will be considerably less if the divorce is amicable. It may also be that many parents are divorcing with sheer joy for one or both are going to new "loves" so that the implication for them is not death dealing. If it is multiple, the more difficult for the child, for he or she has to adjust to two new important people in his life. Dissolvement of a marriage for many often is much like death; the child like the adult not only feels guilt but beyond this attributes the breakup to himself or herself. Friggen says:

(1) Let your child know that you are parents forever. Divorce is not the end of your responsibility as parents—your children need ongoing affection, interest, and concern from each parent. This is particularly true for very young children. There should be no divorce before children are six or seven, but unfortunately this is the optimal for when a marriage is broken up, the child's home is gone, he loses trust and confidence in himself. Many mothers go to work following a separation and the child senses therefore an additional loss. The age of 6-12 are no doubt crucial ones too, for children are just beginning to see, understand parental problems, but they remain only bystanders. If at all possible, it would be better to avoid abruptly uprooting the child from his accustomed pattern of life. An effort should be made, at least for a time, to keep the same house, the same school and companions for the children. Don't get rid of the playthings—old teddy bears, dog-eared books or toys. The child often feels singly alone, after a divorce, for sometimes the little girl or boy goes with mother and the older brothers and sometimes sisters go with their father and move, many times some distance away. Many younger middlescent divorcees go back for a time to their parents' home taking children far from the spouse and possibly other children. Children desperately need stability provided by both parents and the grandparents also.

(2) Consider the trauma inflicted upon the child. Divorce may be next to death in its pain, inducing grief, hate, despair and depression. Children are often left out when parents turn their anguish on themselves. Of course, in the child the hope of the re-uniting of their parents is held out as a promise. Children often feel they are unloved and

will be abandoned by their parents and reason, if you loved me you would stay together—or "if you leave Daddy, you can leave me." I recently observed a little boy of five united with his stepfather after a six-months separation period (the father and mother had divorced) proclaim over and over "I love you, daddy, I love you, daddy." At five years of age he has suffered two losses of fathers, the second father (step) decided he should see the boy on a regular basis so this will take some of the fear and unhappiness out of his life. But prognosis for happiness is slight for the boy who is already nervous, fearful, talks incessantly and is hyperkinetic. Children, like this one, grow up and marry but many of them are not able to love, for they lose the sense of being loved and worthwhileness, therefore, cannot confer trust and genuine affection upon another person. Even natural separations are hard for children. Early this summer I met a small girl (6 or 7) at a beach gathering, her absent father was a naval officer stationed abroad. I picked her up and sat her on my lap. I asked her a number of questions about herself and before she left me, she kissed me. Later we went down to the water's edge, she took my hand and wanted me when we entered the ocean to hold her above the waves. Before we left the surf, she asked me if she could call me daddy. "Certainly," I said as I wondered about the life of this little girl.

(3) Your ability to cope will transfer to the child or children. Children react to the difficulties involved in a divorce much the same way we do. If we take the route of nurturing bitterness and the turning of our children against our former spouse it leads to being non-productive. Some time we need help from outsiders in making our way. Consider the case of Evelyn Porter who was deserted by her husband after thirteen years of marriage; she was the mother of three children, none old enough to hold a job. She had been, as she described it, "just a housewife," with little education and no kin people to help. She was frightened and bitter. The children were seriously affected by their mother's struggle and despair. They became rebellious and were often in trouble at school. To survive she went on welfare. Evelyn's case was referred to the courts (conciliation); she was introduced to counselors who encouraged her to enroll in an office training course; having done so she was able to land a civil service position as a clerk. She found her self-confidence increasing each step of the way in developing a new life. Her mental health improved and her children were doing better in school. Trying to hold in your spitefulness is dif-

ficult but reciting the bad things about your former spouse, particularly to your children, does not help. In any event we should try to be fair with the children about our divorce—simply tell them why we are divorcing and remember they need both parents. A number of good books written for young children are available in Waldenbooks stores or like stores which explain divorce very well in suitable language. Do not help your spouse divorce the children also. If we blast their mother or father, we aid in programming them for fear and failure in their lives—the bottom line suggests to them, who can you be sure of—mom, dad or me?

(4) The child should not be used as a pawn. Often in an attempt to get back at the former spouse, the child is used as the agent. One husband had his child spy on his former wife to confirm suspicions he had about her. In the long run the child refused to continue this activity and as a consequence felt guilty of betraying both parents. Even after our marriages have broken up, we should try to be reasonable in our treatment of our children, their desire for visitation, vacations, and in regard to gifts, that is, not overdoing giving at the expense of the other parent. Children should not be tempted to play one parent against another—they frequently do this anyway with little encouragement. Parents vying for affection of the child can get them started in this game. The sting of separation felt by children from one parent or the other can be relieved considerably by making visitation with us, if we do not have custody, a happy time. We should plan things which the child will enjoy, although visits should not just be fun and buying trips for this has the effect of setting up invidious comparisons between parents, also of spoiling the child. This tendency is difficult to suppress for we feel responsible for the child's changed world and wish to compensate for it. And we should keep appointments for visitation with the child or children for this engenders trust and love. If there are things we must do while visitation is in progress we should do it, explaining why it is necessary. For very young children this should be prevented for if they have to be left in the charge of a strange person, it can be very traumatic for them. Appointments or work at the office you need to do can be shared by taking them along. In fact, if there is work to be done at home, the yard or the store, let them assist you where possible. This has the effect of helping them understand you and what you do, and eventually they will see how it relates to them. We should make them feel

that they are loved and have two homes to be welcomed into—yours and your spouse's.

There does not seem to be an appropriate time for divorce for children short of adulthood. Even then it has some effect on them. But during the early formative years, most children have difficulties. In a study by Wallerstein and Kelly, of 121 children (ages 2½ to 18 years) of divorced parents, they found the following behavior situations to exist.

(1) Children 2½ to 3½—

Many had lost their toilet training, cried, had been fearful, and trouble sleeping, sucked their thumbs, were more aggressive, had thrown tantrums; showed patterns called by psychologists as regression—a return to earlier childhood behavior. Where mothers were absorbed in their own hurt, children were more troubled a year after the divorce; these children were depressed. Others under more normal emotional conditions were over the tendencies noted above.

(2) Children 3¾ to 5—

These children were less likely to regress but still were apt to whine, be irritable and to cry. These children were painfully bewildered by their father's absence. They felt responsible for their fathers leaving and in general were worse off than at the time of the divorce—more inhibited, less self-esteem, sadness and need.

(3) Children 5 to 6—

These children, like those younger, were more anxious and aggressive toward others than usual at the time of divorce; they were restless, cried sometimes, tended to be irritable and were moody. For some they were worse after a year but for the most part understood what divorce changes meant. They could discuss their fathers or mothers absence. About half of the children in this study were worse off than before. One surprising result was that some fathers improved their relations with their children after separation but this didn't' affect the decline in stability among half.

(4) Children ages 7 to 8—

These youngsters showed considerable sadness about the divorce and unlike younger children did not get relief from fantasizing like 4 or 5 year olds who often dreamed of getting their parents back together. With no way to relieve their pain, they cried a lot. They supposed themselves to be deprived and wanted reassurances brought by, in many cases, asking for toys or bicycles. Many of these children became compulsive and insatiable eaters. Children in these ages apparently did not feel responsible for the divorces but more stronger than younger children in wanting a father image and to visit often with their fathers. Some of the boys in this age wanted their mothers to marry so they could have a father. Many children in these years expressed anger toward the mother for being responsible for, as they thought, driving the father from home. At the same time they were fearful of mother's power for she had generally taken a greater role in the matters of discipline before the separation. Children of this age obviously had great conflicts and will take sides, but after a year most have come to grips with the reality of the situation and become more adjusted. However, one of every four do not become psychologically adjusted after a year of the divorce.

(5) Children 9 to 11—

It was found that children in this age have utilized two approaches to adjustment. One an outward acceptance with intensified activities which serves to shield them from reality. The other response was one of extreme anger and weakness. These children, at least many of them, developed headaches, stomach problems, many did poorly in school. Torn between the parents, sometimes they "helped" and sometimes "hurt" their parents as if to punish them for their tug of war dilemmas. These children by this time (10-11) had learned to feel sympathy for their parents and often comforted them. After a year things had improved for these, though many still felt anger toward the parent they didn't live with, therefore mainly fathers.

(6) Adolescents—

These children like those in the age brackets preceding it felt no responsibility for the divorce of their parents but the degree of pain found among these seemingly callous youth was greater than anticipated. Many were negative about the idea of their marriage, we worried about their future, education, jobs, etc. The divorce served in many adolescents to accelerate the recognition of differences in parents and the process of disengagement from one parent was speeded up, although the knowledge of parents' sexual needs often caused anxiety. Sometimes the adolescents were capable of standing aloof from their parents when they found themselves in a war for their allegiance. Some of the youth reported in the Wallerstein and Kelly

> study had psychological problems—some engaged in wanton sex, drinking and drug taking. Most had adjusted fairly well after a year. Many adolescents could see the breakup coming for some months even years because of the chronic conflict. Some adolescents even benefited from the divorce by gaining an understanding of themselves and their development. The researchers in the thought those youth who did the best were those able to establish some distance from the parental crisis and where their parents one way or the other permitted this. These cases are probably rare.

A way of summarizing the research the usual case takes children a year to settle the basic hurt, the conflict and anger for the typical child or adolescent. Tied to the duration of maladjustment of the child or children is the length of the continued argument, hostility, and emotion generated between the parents themselves. The final negative effect on children is still to be discovered, but we should remember that it does not turn our children into homosexuals, deviates, etc. It should be noted, one positive effect on some children is that in the case where there are many children in the family particularly the young, who are likely to receive less attention by their parents, in dividing the family they are likely to receive more. In fact they may be the only child left with a parent or one of two that are with a parent.

Many fathers do not tell their children about divorce but leave it to the mother. We believe this is a mistake. We also suggest the following things be told by the father to the child or children concerning divorce.

1. <u>Tell the truth</u>—children are remarkably perceptive; telling them will help them cope with the problem.
2. <u>Spare the grim details</u>—limits should be set; the bedroom problems or extra bedroom ones should be omitted.
3. <u>Be clear in what you say and say it when divorce is definite</u>—language should be appropriate to the age level and don't shock children with last-minute revelations that you're leaving. It is hard to decide the right time but in giving reaction time to the children and a chance to question, they can better absorb the psychological jolt. Remember, do not apologize for if this was all that was needed in the first place there would be no need to separate.
4. <u>Allow children to ventilate their feelings</u>—yes, even to having small children hitting you, cursing you, throwing tantrums and inconsolable crying, will allow a degree of calm and the beginning of acceptance.

5. Assure your child or children by telling them of your love and outline the future for them—where they will live, their schooling, expectation of your visits and care. Your children need to be reassured about their security, even older ones will worry about clothes, spending money, camp or college. Don't use this session to win loyalty to yourself either.
6. The children should know that the decision to divorce is final—reconciliation might take place but holding out false promises continues the anguish and feeling of insecurity with the children.

For single parents the following guidelines are offered as adapted from Oken and Haynes (1993)

1. Accept responsibilities and challenges. Maintain a positive attitude and the feeling that solutions are possible.
2. Give the parental role high priority. Successful single parents are willing to sacrifice time, money, and energy to meet their children's needs.
3. Use consistent, non-punitive discipline.
4. Emphasize open communication. Encourage trust and the open expression of feelings.
5. Foster individuality within a supportive family unit.
6. Recognize the need for self-nurturance. Parents must understand the need to have children understand the situation and be able to help their children with this matter.

The Effects of Divorce on Men

Most men experience "separation shock" even those who felt escape from the marriage was desirable. This shock can produce intense emotional and physical reactions in men. The following scenario is true mainly of the adversarial divorcement much less true with mediated divorces although usually one spouse will suffer the marriage ending. Many feel absolutely lost, for in many cases the children are gone and as a new single he is faced with finding a new set of friends, look after his clothes, meals and the cleaning of his new quarters. Many of your former friends and associates, with whom you previously socialized, will no longer welcome you as a singleton, and indeed many where the divorce has been pending or in the offing, have taken sides. More often than not, the wife's side for she has determined the family's social life and if she did not work out of the home, she usually has had time to be well-acquainted in the home neighborhood, whereas a man may know only a few of your neighbors. This all ads up to the feeling of anomie—not unlike death. There is, if the marriage has lasted for some time, the continuing attachment to your former life. At one time you were the king in your castle and now you're alone, remembering your former life—your wife, your children and all the wonderful memories one usually has built-up over the years. The responses of anger, jealousy, fear of the future, guilt, self-blame and sickness all well up in you. You have diarrhea, headaches, insomnia, hives, palpitations of the heart, muscle twitching, and chronic colds. For almost all men it will take something like two years to get over this though for some a longer period is required. Men get over the immediate effects, then when the final decree time comes the symptoms often recur all over again. Nevertheless a part of man's life is gone, he feels inadequate to cope with life, his ego status is nearly zero, and he feels he will be rejected by all women. For a few who have a woman they are going to live with, this is another matter. A number of men have told me that they feel so guilty they give much more in a divorce settlement than was necessary. And many are overwhelmed by the fact that their families frequently take the side of the daughter-in-law. Be sure you tell your side of the story for otherwise you and your children many hear how terrible you were, how you manhandled your wife, ran out with other women and were in short a Scrooge. The hypocrisy in society is much greater than the inexperienced person would ever believe. I know both men and women who eventually withdrew from their churches because of the post-divorce atmosphere toward them. There is a lot of heartache for men who have not really thought about some aspects that go along with the divorced life. In fact, some who were titillated by women before, some of them married women, will find that they flee from you when you are single—the married women consider their games of stolen moments, glances, handholding, heavy hugging at dances and tete-a-tetes safe when you were married but a no-no if you are single. The single women frequently don't want to be put on the spot (are not interested in marriage) nor do they want to hear the tale of woe and will not be put on the spot if their playmate is married. Even so the bon vivant who goes out gadding about every night is a myth. For the middlescent man, a shock of another type might be experienced, the demand of some women will give him claustrophobia in the genital area.

The first several months are the most difficult ones, although according to Robert Weiss, a divorce expert, normalcy isn't reached until two to four years have passed. You do get over the feeling of wanting to die somehow, you muddle through. Now the following advice has helped quite a few people during these times.

1. Tell your side of the story, tell your friends and kinspeople. Family who will help to look after the children should know right away.
2. Be prepared for a range of responses from outright condemnation of you to withholding of comment. Some will offer help while others dig for details.
3. Be discreet about broadcasting your divorce at work for many would be put in jeopardy by this announcement. In some cases this suggests if the guy can't keep his personal life together he makes a poor representative for us. Other bosses might take the view that home entertainment for our clients is out now. In any event, many people believe that divorced persons can't be as effective as before they were divorced. You should nevertheless explain the circumstances to your immediate superior and let him know you think the effects of the divorce, at least the worst part, will be over soon. Your co-workers need know little of the details but tell them the simple facts briefly.
4. Try extra hard to keep up with your work even though you won't feel like working and will be distressed. On the other hand don't use your work as an escape; it does help to have a regular routine both at work and away. Overtime work may work against you when support payments are decided upon by the judge.
5. Don't be afraid to ask for help. Some of the best use of money may be in counseling—men usually resist this, but if it helps to set your head straight and assists you in making a better decision, it will be more than worth the time and money you invested. In selection of a counselor, get a trained person and/or one recommended by the Mental Health Agency or some other reliable group. Avoid the far-out guru type. Mel Kranzler, authority on divorce, says that seeking professional help is one way to avoid the pain you need not suffer and it's a good sign of mental health.
6. One should not give way to believing you are a victim. Think about what you can do for yourself. A new suit, haircut, learn something about child care or how to cook several dishes; if you are out of shape, start running. Most of all we need to consider what have we learned from our divorce. Krantzler in his *Creative Divorce* says we need to set realistic goals for ourselves; despite the problems that hassle us, still life presents alternative choices to us—face the unpleasant

circumstances, then take stock of your credits and move positively forward. Be sure to look at yourself in terms of how you act toward others, your view of women and relationship with your children. No matter how painful this should be a beginning of a new you.

The Effect of Divorce on Women

Much of what has been said of men can be said of women. They are more likely to have the custody of children than the husband. In many cases the burden of going it alone, particularly if they are housewives only, can cause a complete emotional collapse. But women are not usually afraid to ask for help and they almost always have a network of friends they can tell their troubles to and help and advice they can expect. The traditional roles played in society by women allow them more easily to ventilate their feeling and receive attention from varied sources, than men. This can be of help, nevertheless some will undergo extreme depression and need the assistance of a counselor or psychiatrist. Many times the minister of your church has had special training in this area and will be glad to have you contact him. Frequently women feel the need to get a person (of the opposite sex) that they do not know to listen to them as an aid in talking out their difficulties. Expressing one's feelings to an empathetic listener works wonders!! If the husband has initiated the divorce, the woman in all probability reacts in anger, and if she asked for the divorce, the likelihood of feeling guilty is there. Usually there is an ambivalence about divorce which shifts from euphoria to depression—many women greet divorce with elation then give way to despair, feelings of regret and inadequacy develop in time. As a woman has to fit herself into a new role—that of a divorced woman—there is no clear, generally accepted model for such a woman in our society. The decisions, if she doesn't plan to stay with the home, are legion. Does she move to another town, go home to mother? What name should she use, what work do you do, and how to use your time? All of these call for answers! And if you are a woman trying to look after five young children, you have real difficulty. Remarriage as a prospect is virtually nil, and unless general financial help is coming, your immediate life prospects are grim indeed!

The role of the divorced woman is especially difficult in other ways. She has to remake her social life at the same time she is coping with the work-a-day world. Women friends and relatives who rallied around her at first soon go back to their former concerns or they may see a possible rival in her. They may resent the younger middlescent woman acting like an adolescent and the woman herself might in turn find it difficult to act as an eligible woman, at the same time looking after her children. The problem of children enters the picture also—what do you tell them about the new man? Dr. Robert Weiss, Harvard sociologist, says that divorce is like influenza rather than unemployment. If everybody is unemployed, it makes it a little easier. If everyone has the flu, you still feel sick. But then flue is rarely fatal and most people recover with amazing resiliency. Middle and older middlescent women will find it more difficult to get back to normal. For with a marriage of twenty years or more dissolving, the prospects of another is not as likely as it is for men in the same age range. But many women with twenty-five, even thirty years of marriage behind them nevertheless in this day walk out on their men fearlessly saying they have had it. The runaway spouse in 1973 was about 300 men to 1 woman; by 1977 it was 2 to 1 and today it is even. researchers say these women range between very immature and the very mature who thought life would be a partnership of equals. In these cases the relief is greater than the alternatives—fear of lack of money, loneliness and condemnation.

For many women who divorce, the picture is not all bleak at least in one city. In a study by the sociologist William Goode, found as a result of questioning 425 divorced women in Detroit that 37 percent had not suffered seriously after separation. Only 30 percent felt they had been discriminated against as divorcees, more than half reported that they had been able to keep their old friends, and most of the others said that they had been successful in making new friends. These women seem to be a special group though many women find not much trouble and considered help, not the typical and this study does not reflect current views.

For most women extreme loneliness is their lot, at least for some months despite Goode's survey the results of which suggest that many women would put a brave face on the events in public or in an interview which possibly belie the actual private circumstance. Women undergoing hormonal changes, cessation of the menses, etc., have compounded problems and may therefore seek solace in eating and drinking, becoming for the first time overweight or even obese. This further militates against their self image. Their children frequently are put upon by a lonely mother who makes outrageous emotional demands, particularly on small children.

The needs of a woman can be overwhelming and for that reason it is easy to understand the emotional support they feel they need to elicit from their children. Most women divorcees have several months of frequent crying sessions where the young daughter and sons get involved in the crying spells. This has an ulterior effect on the children. Divorced women need companionship, that is, adult friends, and a sexual partner. Modern research indicates that sexual urges do not ordinarily slacken off to zero, whatever the age of the divorced person. Many divorced women and particularly widows, according to William Masters "have this incredible need to be with men, and they do something about it." In many instances the man is married. Women who would not consider cheating in their marriage, once that marriage is terminated, don't feel so strongly about that any more. Paul Gebbard of the Indiana Institute for Sex reports that most widows who find new sexual partners do so in the first year of widowhood, and he adds, "there is no lack of men willing to give solace to a new widow." Divorced women find men also but not with the same ease or as often as does the younger widow. Much of this has been tempered by the advent of herpes and particularly AIDS. Unfortunately divorce, New York psychiatrist Alvin Goldfarb notes, drives many women to excessive eating, drinking, taking of reckless chances, and in cities cause women to promote attacks on themselves by actively resisting muggers. As for opportunity to remarry, divorced women, and for that matter men also, have greater chances to marry than those never married. Divorced women according to statistics a decade or so ago (Glick), remarry at the rate of 135 per 1000 while their widowed sisters only 10 per 1000. This has changed somewhat today but the same differences exist. Religious views of many and the views of the church, although altered somewhat in the past decade, pose a problem to many who divorce or are facing it; the early Christian church forbade divorce on any grounds. Monsignor Stephen J. Kelleher, a former Judge of the Marriage Tribunal of the Archdiocese of New York, published a book called *Divorce and Remarriage for Catholics?* In this work he maintains that conflict among marriage partners prevents human growth and suggests that not everyone should be expected to live up to doctrinal principles of the indissolution of marriage. Though the Catholic Church is generally firm on the issue, certain segments (Italian women have the right to divorce and keep their own names even if married) of the church do not inveigh against it. We must remember that no matter how much we might have wished that things would have turned out differently for us, we could not control all the factors and conditions working to cause a marital breakdown.

There are things women can keep in mind to help them during the transition from divorce to afterwards.

1. One must not accept the view that this is the end of the world. Sure one party is over! But another can be planned and enjoyed. Today is the beginning day of my second life.

2. One needs help from a variety of sources—our families, friends, a professional counselor perhaps, and usually our physician. The latter can understand our need to control our emotional lives, therefore can prescribe what we need and give advice about our health matters. One should not increase the number of tranquilizers, i.e., Valium, Xanax, Librium, Donatal, Meprobamate, etc. on her own ideas. Diet needs should be looked after also.
3. Get involved in a regular routine which allows little time for moping around or being by yourself. This will help you from becoming engrossed in self pity and ego crucifixion. If you don't have a routine, get one which provides time daily for self-improvement; that is, some reading, rest, taking care of your personal matters, dress and bathe each day—put on lipstick; don't overdo this and make up when you go out for this telegraphs your problem or advertises you in a way you really don't want. Make yourself eat breakfast and if you do not exercise, start this as a set thing. Walk or run or work in the yard, but if possible make it vigorous exercise. Eat out often, if it can only be McDonald's or the corner Drug Store. Take in movies, plays, and enroll in a course at a college or university. They have non-credit and credit courses on everything. The idea is to keep yourself occupied constructively. Go to the beauty shop and get a new hairstyle. You'll get compliments and attention.
4. Force yourself to reconstruct your life and thereby improve your mental health. This will give you self-respect. There is something to be learned from divorce. If you haven't worked outside of the home, get a job, go back to school if necessary to train yourself. If children keep you tied closely to the house, you can arrange some time for part-time work or college. In the chapter on money, there are references dealing with what can be done at home to make money if working away from home is out of the question.
5. We must finally realize that it is our lives and precious few people will care whether we succeed or fail. Success of failure will be largely due to our efforts; we are the catalysts in this enterprise, be certain of that—now, chin up, chest out, full speed ahead!

GETTING A DIVORCE

There are a number of things we should be aware of in a divorce case. At the outset one should get competent advice. This is much more difficult than it seems. If there is any chance of reconciliation, do not go to a lawyer for your initial help unless he is trained in mediation and reconciliation. Unfortunately, many lawyers take the adversary position and are intent upon legally separating you from your spouse with the least amount of effort and for the maximum amount of money and they are often slow to get the divorce finalized. Go to a marriage counselor first; the answer may still be divorce but he or she will not set about to untie you. The ethics of the average lawyer would chill you if you didn't already know something about this. One bright young lawyer in an eastern seaboard state told me that many lawyers love the divorce case, particularly where they are defending a young attractive middlescent woman with whom they provide hands-on therapy in addition to extracting a large fee. Of course, a few women meet their next husbands this way. A little foreknowledge will be of inestimable help. One such bit of knowledge is that there are states in which you can arrange for your own divorce. Guides for doing this are constantly being revised, so check in your state for a guide; some states for whom guides have been made are: Maine, Illinois, California, Massachusetts, Maryland, Virginia and the District of Columbia. (Cf. the reference near the end of this chapter.)

Many men seek a lawyer only after their wives have filed for divorce. One man thinking that he would talk it over with his wife's lawyer hoping that reconciliation was in the offing admitted to the lawyer that he had been a poor husband in many regards but that he loved his wife and wished to remain married. Unfortunately he said too much and what he said he later found written in the bill of particulars against him. Men are wary of lawyers who say they practice family law for they are viewed by many as only a grade above the accident-indemnity lawyer. This is probably unfair and many men may expect too much from the lawyer; nonetheless, to be cautious is important. In seeking a lawyer, one should not get a kinsman; in my family we have been bitten twice, in other than divorce matters, by this error. Check for a divorce lawyer, not for one who doesn't specialize in divorce, for this may create problems for you when there are complex money problems and fine point considerations. The Martindale-Hubbell Law Directory is a start, which will enable you to find the specialization you want, and some names of lawyers. The local bar association usually has referral service. Some men's and women's groups have referral service as a part of their membership fee. Once you have several names, (NOW, YWCA) it would be worth it to interview several of them. Bar associations who refer legal counsel to you are lawyers who generally expect to get $100-$350 an hour for their services.

You should gather material in an approach to an interview. Information bearing on the problem would include: your case, family facts, your financial situation and be prepared to state your objectives. If, for example, you refuse to pay alimony (there may be no way around it) or must have the better of two cars because of your work, tell the prospective lawyer. Where you will compromise is also important, like trading a share of the home for the wife's share of the business. If you are a woman and have little knowledge of your husband's financial circumstances, it becomes important to find out if possible, or at least alert the lawyer to the possibilities. Here are some things you should discuss with the prospective lawyer: (1) personal information (including your assets) but do not give details of sexual activities for those are beyond what is necessary; (2) support needed particularly for the woman, what monies do both make, what prospects considering age for the future; (3) custody of children and visitation rights (who pays what for travel expenses involved in visitation), this is important for women too as men today are receiving custody of children; (4) child's support and education; (5) medical and dental costs; (6) life insurance, property, stocks and bonds; (7) tax matters, wills, trusts, debts and obligations; and (8) fees for lawyers, expenses, etc. You suggest this is too much for just deciding on a lawyer, perhaps, but this usually is a one time thing and in preparing for this will make you conversant with the ramifications of divorce; in addition the interview itself will clarify things for you and provide some information that is important. Now, beyond this, inquire as to the experience of the lawyer, his record of handling such matters, get neutral opinions on him and if possible the names of two people who have used his or her services. Will he be available at a time of emergency and is he trustworthy? I know a friend who engaged a "name lawyer" who compromised him with the wife's lawyer by agreeing to let the wife go into the home which she had deserted, while he was out of town and get the pick of the furniture although an agreement (This is malpractice.) had been reached that both parties would be present and the disposition of the furniture following the previously made accord. A good bet for both men and women may be a woman lawyer, and don't overlook a minority one (only a few are available outside urban centers) for frequently these people will work harder for justice and have reasonable fees. At best, unfortunately, it is a hazardous undertaking and unfortunately at a time when you are most vulnerable to any kind of help offered. But be assured this process of selecting from several lawyers will save you money and satisfaction in the end.

Remember in all of this, when you do choose a lawyer, level with him no matter how hurtful it is and draw up an agreement simply stating what he has agreed to as to payment of fees, time to be given (some lawyers usually provide their services in terms of half or whole hours—typically $100-$350 an hour or more!). Then, if you have the money, send him a retainer—usually $300-$400 some will want more, will suffice. If, having secured a lawyer, you feel he has done nothing for you, he refused to move the case along or has cheated you, fire him and get some other legal counsel. If the lawyer has abused you, report it to the Bar Association's Ethics Committee in your area. One man I know whose wife's lawyer called him at odd hours (midnight), etc., effecting a change in voice and identity, threatened him in order to scare him from making such a grievance petition. He reported this to his own lawyer for advice and was surprised that it was passed off as "just bizarre behavior." If you're on the receiving end of this, it's more than bizarre, but lawyers frequently, like other professionals, stick together. However, this kind of behavior should be reported to local ethics committees.

No-Fault Divorce

No-fault divorce is designed to minimize blame and the adversarial incentive that exists in a divorce case. This type of divorce is the most common type in some states. California instituted the first law (1972) abolishing any requirement of fault as a basis for marriage dissolvement. No-fault divorce laws, though they vary in the different states, is allowed in all fifty states. The California law, though, perhaps the most liberal, began as a conservative attempt to reduce the number of divorces, stipulates the following:

1. No grounds are needed to obtain a divorce.
2. Proof of fault or guilt is unnecessary to obtain a decree.
3. One spouse can decide to get a divorce without the consent or agreement of the other.
4. New standards for alimony and property awards seek to treat men and women equally annulling former sex based traditions.
5. Financial awards are no longer linked to fault, rather they are based upon current financial needs and resources available to meet those needs. However, in Florida and some other states, fault is relevant in deciding alimony.
6. The new protocol is designed to create a social and psychological climate, which will foster amiable divorce rather than adversarial procedures.

No-fault has affected property division, alimony, child support, and custody decisions in and out of the courts. The court's main legal guidelines are based on what is fair and equitable between the parties. Courts are devising child support and spousal tables to make their rulings more consistent. Actuarial tables are developed according to income and local cost of living and should be available at most courthouses in counties and cities, also in public libraries. No-fault is a breakthrough toward creating more humane and effective divorce procedures. Many states have simplified divorce laws allowing couples to do their own divorce. Divorce manuals abound for couples, these usually outline, step by step, the procedures. *How to do Your Own Divorce in California* published by the Nolo Press has sold over a million copies. One work in the 5th Edition, *How to File Your Own Divorce*" by Haman is used by many. Many other manuals exist representing specific states individual requirements and may be found in bookstores and stationary shops. The practical result of "no-fault" divorce has for older women who have been principally homemaker has been to drastically reduced settlements they have received. Adjustment maintenance increasingly adds a plus to this situation for women.

Negotiated Settlements

This divorce is a resolution of the issues between the couple out-of-court. The better divorce lawyers handle most of their cases in this fashion. When the parties are not after revenue or airing their grievances this method allows them to cooperate and satisfy each other's needs. Little time is wasted nor is money thrown away on legal warfare. Cooperation between the couple can provide:

1. Child-care scheduling thereby reducing expenses for this service.
2. When business is involved this provides a negotiation or a mediation opportunity allowing the business to prosper whereas the contentious might destroy the business.
3. Tax savings approach can be effected by cooperative tax planning, allowing both to have more cash. For instance, if a parent in a low income bracket is receiving both alimony and child support while the payee parent is in a high tax category both can have more money if they call the payment family support which combines alimony and child support. This is fully deductible.

Mediated (Cooperative Divorce) Settlement

This is a method whereby couples can have a third party mediate their differences relative to property divisions, child custody, payments of support and the like without the damaging adversarial approach allowing for a more humane way to end a marital relationship. The third party may be a mental health professional or a counselor and some are lawyers who have committed themselves to this philosophy. Joan Blades, an authority on Marriage Dissolution through Mediation, suggest these benefits from mediation:

1. Parents develop richer and more rewarding relationships with their children after divorce particularly fathers who spend more time with their children after a divorce than before.
2. Individual spouses recover old skills and strengths that were dormant and discover new ones. Traditional gender roles are expanded upon by learning new skills of the other sex—car repair, bookkeeping, carpentry for the woman, for the man—cooking, child care and shopping, etc.
3. Divorce is a catalyst for reassessment of ones life resulting in change of work, going back to school, moving, getting a new perspective.
4. Damaging and nonfunctional communication patterns that existed between the partners is terminated and if noticed then corrected in future relationships.

There are typically five steps in mediation—introduction and commitment stage, the definition stage, negotiation stage, the agreement stage and the contracting stage. The process allows time to become comfortable with the process, reduce emotional agitation and perhaps resistance to the mediation itself. The focus of mediation is an attempt to get the couple to forecast their lives after the final separation. The mediators have access to the necessary legal or attorney's information and forms to conclude the settlement or brochures. The final settlement is reviewed by a judge. Mediation is required in contested divorces certainly where children re involved. Many mediators provide all kinds of guidelines for the couple "Parents When the Other Parent is Angry" to "Successful Partnership for Parenting." Generally the cost of mediation is less than traditional divorces and studies such as Stephen Bahr's indicate children adjust better following this method than in the adversarial one, also there is more likelihood that the agreement will be honored and that more cooperation will exist after the divorce, spouses will have greater self-determination and self respect after mediation, less money is spent by the couple and the state and, on the whole, mediating couples tend to be more satisfied with the outcome of the divorce. They are both better able to begin building their new lives emotionally and better able to take care of child custody disputes before any court appearance. It should be noted that California in 1981, the first state to require mediation economically. Some forms that are typical relating to the mediation process are given below.

CONTRACT & CONFIDENTIAL QUESTIONNAIRE

CONTRACT TO PARTICIPATE IN MEDIATION

We, ______________________________ agree to abide by the Rules
(clients)
of the Northwest Mediation Service which we have received and read. We agree to pay the sum of $__________ per hour for the services of the mediators when the services of the mediators when the services are performed, plus a $25.00 set up fee. This will be paid by:

(1) the clients in equal shares: (2) all by ____________________________; (3) the clients in these proportions:

____

____

We, __________________________, agree to abide by the Rules of the
(mediators)
Northwest Mediation Service and to use our utmost effort in helping the clients reach a mutual agreement on the issues before them.

DATED: ________________________________

______________________________	______________________________
Client	Mediator
______________________________	______________________________
Client	Mediator

CONFIDENTIAL
QUESTIONNAIRE FOR CLIENTS
CONTEMPLATING MARITAL TERMINATION

This questionnaire has been designed to aid our legal staff in advising you of your legal rights and obligations with respect to a marital termination. All information is covered by attorney-client privilege and will, therefore, be kept in strictest confidence.

Please do your best in filling this form out based upon your knowledge at this time.

Name of Person Filling in Questionnaire ______________________________
Name of Client if Different ______________________________
Date of Completion ______________________________

Note that unless otherwise agreed at the commencement of the consultation, your initial consultation will be charged at the attorney's normal hourly rate and payment must be made at the end of the consultation.

A. INFORMATION ABOUT YOU

1. Name: ______________________________
2. (a) Telephone: Home—() ________ (b) May we phone you at work? ______
   Work—() ________ May we leave a message? ________
   Other—() __________
   (c) Note any telephone or mail restrictions with regard to your home or your place of employment:
   ____
   ____
3. (a) In what county do you reside? ____________ How long? __________
   (b) Mailing address: ______________________________
   (c) Residence address (if different from above) :______________________
4. Birthdate: ______________________________
5. (a) Former name(s): ______________________________
   (b) Do you wish your former name restored? ____ Now? _____ Later? ____
   Think about it? __________ (c) If yes, which name? ________________
6. Social Security Number: ______________________________
7. (a) Employer: ______________________________
   (b) Location address: ______________________________
   (c) Days/Hours at work: ______________________________
   (d) Pay: Approximate monthly net from employment: ________________
   Other monthly net income: ______________________________

(Note: There are 4 1/3 weeks per month; to determine "net pay" deduct only SDI, FICA, withholding tax, mandatory retirement contributions. Do not deduct credit union payments stock or savings plan, etc. Other net income includes that after taxes from investments, rentals, savings, or business.)

(e) Do you have medical and/or dental coverage through your employer? ___
(g) At what cost to you? ______________________________
(f) How long have you worked at this play of employment? ______________

8. Do you have any health problems for which special attention is required?
____

If so, describe briefly: ______________________________

9. What is the cost of childcare enabling you to work? __________________

10. Are you contemplating remarriage at present? ______________________

11. If you are currently residing with anyone (other than your spouse or children) state: Name:
__________________ Age: _________ Relationship to you: ____________

12. Also, please describe the monetary arrangements between you and the above person, if any:
____

B. <u>GENERAL INFORMATION ABOUT YOUR PRESENT MARRIAGE</u>

1. Your name: ______________________________

2, Your spouse's name: ______________________________

3. Date of marriage: ______________________________

4. Place of marriage: (City) ______________________ (State) ____________

5. How long have you lived in Santa Clara County _____________
California _____________
Your spouse: ______________________________
____

6. If you have been served with divorce-related papers, date served: _________

7. Which of the parties wishes the dissolution? ______________________

8. Do you desire reconciliation? ___________ If so, are you interested in marital counscling?
_______________________ Has there been marital counseling in the past?
____
With whom? ______________________________

9. Describe any violence which has recently occurred between you and your spouse or which your spouse might allege has occurred.________________
____

B. SUPPORT ARRANGEMENTS BETWEEN YOU AND SPOUSE

1. If you have already separated or discussed separating, detail the financial arrangements you have made:

(a) Periodic payments (how much, how often, etc.)

____

____

____

____

(b) Direct payment of living expenses (monthly and other) such as mortgages (list items, amounts, and how often paid):

____

____

____

____

(c) Other:

____

____

____

____

2. Is there an agreement in writing covering support arrangements? __________

____

3. What support arrangement do you believe would be fair? __________

____

No Divorce Approach

A number of sociologists have reported a phenomena as growing and occurring among very young adults and the young middlescence 35-45 that should be observed. This is the situation which has existed for sometime, namely that of not getting a divorce—just separating. This situation is hazardous to property rights of the parties in years to come. This approach was mainly one utilized by the lower and lower middle class persons in yesteryear. Today thousands of couples leave each other by moving out and/or in cohabitation with a new partner without any inclination to affirm a divorce by legal means. How much this will grow or be problematic is unknown but where remarriage and children are involved most couples will legally divorce and I believe they should! For the poor many certainly couldn't pay for it.

Grounds for Divorce

Before we look at some of the problems of divorce such as custody of children, support payments, money division, and property, let us examine the grounds for divorce and the legal procedure of the court system. Grounds for divorce in the past in the United States have been very restrictive as evidenced by the fact that several decades ago adultery was the only basis for divorce. Now varieties of reasons are allowed in most states, as is the right to divorce without blaming either of the partners. Courts permit termination of a marriage only for valid reasons. It is not enough that the middle aged couple have grown tired of each other, for many middlescent people have fantasies about divorce, envisioning unbridled freedom and bliss through divorce (many find once done they really didn't need or want it). In Virginia living apart and separate with or without cohaitation of one year before filing is sufficient grounds for divorce. Grounds for the divorce in her past occurred by petition under the following grievances:

1. Cruelty, mental or physical—this involves the regular abuse and attack on the partner's emotional well-being and physical body. Not all states allow "cruelty" in general but allow repeated strikings and beating as a ground.
2. Desertion—in most instances, one year in an abandoned state is sufficient for divorce though some states require more. If support (financial) is given, then this alters the situation to some degree.
3. Chronic Drunkenness or Narcotic Drug Abuse—some states spell out the time; New Hampshire says two years, others longer. Testimony of several witnesses who know the subjects is usually sufficient.
4. Adultery is a universal ground either through admission or proof, it is less used today because of the difficulty of securing documentation and in past times it was often a sham entered into by officials—judges, etc., since it was the only escape from marriage. Most states require an independent witness to corroborate the testimony of the complainant.
5. Imprisonment of the spouse—usually some significant period of being incarcerated is involved. Also it relates many times to lack of support which is a ground for divorce itself.
6. Lack of support—the chronic gamble, reckless spender and drunk provides a prospect for relief to those using this approach. These ele-

ments usually accompany the grievance; just being unemployed is generally not enough evidence as they can get welfare assistance.

7. Insanity—provisions are made for divorce under this circumstance in at least half of the states. Most states require three to five years of incurable insanity which means that in most cases this will be judged by their being institutionalized.
8. Idiocy—this can be a matter of annulment as a fact not known previous to marriage (false pretense for instance) or development following venereal disease and chronic drunkenness, or being a moron.
9. Sexual deviations—Impotence, or syphilitic disease, unnatural sexual acts, like sodomy, corruption—prostitution of one's daughter or the wife being one.

Getting a Lawyer

It is better to obtain the services of a lawyer than do it yourself. The maize of information required, the procedures involved, and general support you get will be worth the money spent. However, the legal field is full of charlatans ready to take your money and do little for you, many lawyers are dilatory only working on your case when you push them. Be sure you get lawyer who is sympathetic for you and your divorce. Check the Lawyer's Local Association that deals with ethics and adequacy of your attorney. The Martindale-Hubbell Law Directory could be a help. Get the names of clients who have used a prospective lawyer and listen to what they say, also get information from others who might know a good law firm or person to handle your case. This is extremely important. I have friends who have told me their lawyer didn't seem to like them for one reason or the other. Your lawyer should be highly motivated to do his best for you. Do more than look in the yellow pages for a counselor to assist you. Client's rights are listed here followed by client's responsibilities. Those listed below are universal.

RESIDENCY REQUIREMENTS

STATEMENT OF CLIENT'S RIGHTS

Your Attorney is providing you with this document to inform you of what you, as a client, are entitled to by law or by custom. To help prevent any misunderstanding between you and your attorney please read this document carefully.

If you ever have any questions about these rights, or about the way your case is being handled, do not hesitate to ask your attorney. He or she should be readily available to represent your best interests and keep you informed about your case.

An attorney may not refuse to represent you on the basis of race, creed, color, sex, sexual orientation, age, national origin or disability.

You are entitled to an attorney who will be capable of handling your case; show you courtesy and consideration at all times; represent you zealously; and preserve your confidences and secrets that are revealed in the course of the relationship.

You are entitled to a written retainer agreement which must set forth, in plain language, the nature of the relationship and the details of the fee arrangement. At your request, and before you sign the agreement, you are entitled to have your attorney clarify in writing any of its terms, or include additional provisions.

You are entitled to fully understand the proposed rates and retainer fee before you sign a retainer agreement, as in any other contract.

You may refuse to enter into any fee arrangement that you find unsatisfactory.

Your attorney may not request a fee that is contingent on the securing of a divorce or on the amount of money or property that may be obtained.

Your attorney may not request a retainer fee that is nonrefundable. That is, should you discharge your attorney, or should your attorney withdraw from the case, before the retainer is used up, he or she is entitled to be paid commensurate with the work performed on your case and any expenses, but must return the balance of the retainer to you. However, your attorney may enter into a minimum fee arrangement with you that provides for the payment of a specific amount below which the fee will not fall based upon the handling of the case to its conclusion.

You are entitled to know the approximate number of attorneys and other legal staff members who will be working your case at any given time and what you will be charged for the services of each.

You are entitled to know in advance how you will be asked to pay legal fees and expenses, and how the retainer, if any, will be spent.

At your request, and after your attorney has had a reasonable opportunity to investigate your case, you are entitled to be given an estimate of approximate future costs of your case, which estimate shall be made in good faith but may be subject to change due to facts and circumstances affecting the case.

You are entitled to receive a written, itemized bill on a regular basis, at least every 60 days.

You are expected to review the itemized bills sent by counsel, and to raise any objections of errors in a timely manner. Time spent in discussion or explanation of bills will not be charged to you.

You are expected to be truthful in all discussions with your attorney, and to provide all relevant information and documentation to enable him or her to competently prepare your case.

You are entitled to be kept informed of the status of your case, and to be provided with copies of correspondence and documents prepared on your behalf or received from the court or your adversary.

You have the right to be present in court at the time that conferences are held.

You are entitled to make the ultimate decision on the objectives to be pursued in your case, and to make the final decision regarding the settlement of your case.

Your attorney's written retainer agreement must specify under what circumstances he or she might seek to withdraw as your attorney for non-payment of legal fees. If an action or proceeding is pending, the court may give your attorney a "charging lien," which entitles your attorney to payment for services already rendered at the end of the case out of the proceeds of the final order or judgement.

You are under no legal obligation to sign a confession of judgment or promissory note, or to agree to a lien or mortgage on your home to cover legal fees. Your attorney's written retainer agreement must specify whether, and under what circumstances, such security may be requested. In no event may such security interest be obtained by your attorney without prior court approval and notice to your adversary. An attorney's security interest in the marital residence cannot be foreclosed against you.

You are entitled to have your attorney's best efforts exerted on your behalf, but no particular results can be guaranteed.

If you entrust money with an attorney for an escrow deposit in your case, the attorney must safeguard the escrow in a special bank account. You are entitled to a written escrow agreement, a written receipt, and a complete record concerning the escrow. When the terms of the escrow agreement have been performed, the attorney must promptly make payment of the escrow to all persons who are entitled to it.

In the event of a fee dispute, you may have the right to seek arbitration. Your attorney will provide you with the necessary information regarding arbitration in the event of a fee dispute, or upon your request.

Date: ________________

Receipt Acknowledged:

By: ____________________________________

Signature Line—Attorney

By: ____________________________________

Signature Line—Client

Source: Adapted from New York State Unified Court System

STATEMENT OF CLIENT'S RESPONSIBILITIES

Reciprocal trust, courtesy and respect are the hallmarks of the attorney-client relationship. Within that relationship, the client looks to the attorney for expertise, education, sound judgment, protection, advocacy and representation. These expectations can be achieved only if the client fulfills the following responsibilities.

1. The client is expected to treat the lawyer and the lawyer's staff with courtesy and consideration.

2. The client's relationship with the lawyer must be one of complete candor and the lawyer must be apprised of all facts or circumstances of the matter being handled by the lawyer even if the client believes that those facts may be detrimental to the client's cause.

3. The client must honor the fee arrangement as agreed to with the lawyer, in accordance with law.

4. All bills for services rendered which are tendered to the client pursuant to the agreed upon fee arrangement should be paid promptly.

5. The client may withdraw from the attorney-client relationship, subject to financial commitments under the agreed to fee arrangement, and, in certain cases need court approval.

6. Although the client should expect that his or her correspondence, telephone calls and other communications will be answered within a reasonable time frame, the client should recognize that the lawyer has other clients equally demanding of the lawyer's time and attention.

7. The client should maintain contact with the lawyer, promptly notify the lawyer of any change in telephone number of address and respond promptly to a request by the lawyer for information and cooperation.

RESIDENCY REQUIREMENTS

A No residency time, only bona fide Residency	B State Requirements	No residency time, only bona fide residency	State Requirements
Alabama	6 months	Nevada	6 weeks
Alaska	30 days	New Hampshire	1 year[1]
Arizona	90 days	New Jersey	1 year
Arkansas	60 days[1]	New Mexico	6 months
California	6 months	New York	1 year
Colorado	90 days	North Carolina	6 months
Connecticut	1 year	North Dakota	6 months
Delaware	6 months	Ohio	6 months
Florida	6 months	Oklahoma	6 months
Georgia	6 months	Oregon	6 months[4]
Hawaii	6 months	Pennsylvania	6 months
Idaho	6 weeks	Rhode Island	1 year
Illinois	90 days	South Carolina	1 year[5]
Indiana	6 months	South Dakota	None
Iowa	1 year	Tennessee	6 months
Kansas	60 days	Texas	6 months
Kentucky	180 days	Utah	90 days
Louisiana	12 months	Vermont	6 months
Maine	6 months	Virginia	6 months
Maryland	1 year	Washington	1 year
Massachusetts	1 year[2]	West Virginia	1 year
Michigan	1 year[2]	Wisconsin	6 months
Minnesota	180 days	Wyoming	60 days
Mississippi	6 months	Washington, DC	6 months
Missouri	90 days	Puerto Rico	1 year
Montana	90 days	Virgin Islands	6 weeks
Nebraska	ear		

[1] Sixty days prior to filing and three months prior to final decree.
[2] One year, if cause arose outside of state.
[3] Cause must have arose in state.
[4] Unless married in Oregon, and one party is a resident of or domiciled in Oregon at the start of the action.
[5] Three months, if both parties are residing in South Carolina.
Source: Adapted from *American Bar Association, Family Law Section*

Annulments are usually granted for causes occurring before the marriage. Many grievances listed earlier fall in this category. Pregnancy before marriage or even lack of it, where the woman claims a man made her pregnant and coerced into a marriage; if the woman defrauded the man by falsely claiming pregnancy to induce marriage. In fact, fraud is a major ground for annulment, e.g., lack of intent to live as man and wife. Exaggeration of one's financial status is also used as a basis for annulments, as is under age for legal marriage. There are few annulments in most states. Increasingly states allow divorce under the rubric of incompatibility or irretrievable breakdown in the marriage. Constructive desertion is allowed also; this is where a spouse leaves the home under threats, bad treatment, etc. Some courts have a waiting period, and some lecture to the participants. The duration of residency requirements follows. The U.S. Supreme Court has ruled that divorce granted in one state is valid in another state providing that: (1) both parties are aware of the proceedings; (2) at least one party has established residence in the state granting the decree, and (3) either both principals are present at the hearing or the absent one is represented by an attorney. The usual divorce takes three to nine months if things go normally. But this is not the case when arguments over property, money, insurance, home equity, etc. and involved—the trial may take two years, the system involving lawyers, courts, etc., take their own sweet time. A divorce can be gotten in Las Vegas in six weeks. One member of a couple must be a resident of the state giving the decree. The residence requirement varies form six weeks in Nevada to five years in Massachusetts. Even less time for divorce is required in places like Mexico but one wants to be sure this is accepted by the state he or she lives in some cases it will not be.

Legal Steps To A Divorce

The first step to divorce is to file a petition for divorce. This is usually done with the help of a lawyer. This petition tells the court the facts of your marriage, it describes the grounds for the divorce and asks the court to grant the divorce with certain considerations. If you are a woman filing, you will be the plaintiff and your husband the defendant. The following shows the legal grounds for divorce which uniformly show no fault to be the basic approach to divorce. Even so many states have facilitated, the restrictions and the protocol involved. Judicial separation is attached the no fault in most instances. In some states living apart and having a separation for a certain length of time is sufficient like New Jersey, New York, Arkansas, Connecticut, District of Columbia, Hawaii, Illinois, Maryland, Minnesota, Missouri, Nevada, New Hampshire, Oregon, Pennsylvania, Rhode Island, South Carolina, Tennessee, Texas, Utah, Vermont, Virginia and West Virginia.

Legal Grounds for Divorce

Jurisdiction	**LEGAL GROUNDS**
Alabama	No-fault; traditional; incompatibility; living separate and apart for 2 years; judicial separation
Alaska	No-fault; traditional; incompatibility; judicial separation
Arizona	No-fault; traditional; judicial separation
Arkansas	No-fault; traditional; living separate and apart for 18 months; judicial separation
California	No-fault; judicial separation
Colorado	No-fault; judicial separation
Connecticut	No-fault; traditional; living separate and apart for 18 months; judicial separation
Delaware	No-fault; living separate and apart for 6 months
District of Columbia	No-fault; living separate and apart for 1 year; judicial separation
Florida	No-fault
Georgia	No-fault; traditional
Hawaii	No-fault; living separate and apart for 2 years; judicial separation
Idaho	No-fault; traditional; judicial separation
Illinois	No-fault; traditional; living separate and apart for 2 years; judicial separation
Indiana	No-fault; traditional; judicial separation
Iowa	No-fault; judicial separation
Kansas	No-fault; traditional; incompatibility; judicial separation

Kentucky	No-fault; living separate and apart for 60 days; judicial separation
Louisiana	No-fault; traditional; living separate and apart for 6 months; judicial separation
Maine	No-fault; traditional; judicial separation
Maryland	No-fault; traditional; living separate and apart for 2 years
Massachusetts	No-fault; traditional; judicial separation
Michigan	No-fault; judicial separation
Minnesota	No-fault; living separate and apart for 60 days; judicial separation
Mississippi	No-fault; traditional
Missouri	No-fault; traditional; living separate and apart for 1 year; judicial separation
Montana	No-fault; incompatibility; living separate and apart for 180 days; judicial separation
Nebraska	No-fault; judicial separation
Nevada	Incompatibility; living separate and apart for 1 year; judicial separation
New Hampshire	No-fault; traditional living separate and apart for 2 years
New Jersey	No-fault; traditional; living separate and apart for 18 months
New Mexico	No-fault; traditional; incompatibility; judicial separation
New York	Traditional; living separate and apart for 1 year; judicial separation
North Carolina	No-fault, living separate and apart for 1 year; judicial separation
North Dakota	No-fault; traditional; judicial separation
Ohio	No-fault; traditional; incompatibility; living separate and apart for 1 year
Oklahoma	Incompatibility; judicial separation
Oregon	No-fault; judicial separation
Pennsylvania	No-fault; traditional; living separate and apart for 2 years
Rhode Island	No-fault; traditional; living separate and apart for 3 years; judicial separation
South Carolina	no-fault; traditional; living separate and apart for 1 year; judicial separation

South Dakota	No-fault; traditional; judicial separation
Tennessee	No-fault; traditional; living separate and apart for 2 years; judicial separation
Texas	No-fault; traditional; living separate and apart for 3 years
Utah	No-fault; traditional; living separate and apart for 3 years; judicial separation
Vermont	No-fault; traditional; living separate and apart for 6 months
Virginia	No-fault; traditional; living separate and apart for 1 year, 6 months if no children; judicial separation
Washington	No-fault
West Virginia	No-fault; traditional; living separate and apart for 1 year; judicial separation
Wisconsin	No-fault; judicial separation
Wyoming	No-fault; traditional; incompatibility; judicial separation[1]

[1] Source: Adapted from American Bar Association, Family Law Section

A petition to the court follows which includes basic data and appeal to get relief of a number of issues, support, custody and protection.

IN THE CIRCUIT COURT OF ________________ COUNTY
COUNTY DEPARTMENT, DIVORCE DIVISION

Mary Smith,

Plaintiff

James Smith, No. _______________

Defendant

COMPLAINT FOR DIVORCE

What follows in the complaint is the charges connected with the divorce and plea for relief. Given here is the data relative to place of residence, children, residency time, marriage date, request for custody of children, support and to keep the domicile; finally the bill of particulars which argue for the severing of the marriage ties.

it concludes the document....

WHEREFORE plaintiff Mary Smith, prays as follows:
For a Judgment of Divorce; for temporary and permanent care, custody, control, and education of the children; for such relief as in equity may be just.

____
Mary Smith, Plaintiff

STATE OF ______________________
COUNTY OF ____________________S.S.

Mary Smith, being first duly sworn on oath, deposes and states that the contents of the aforegoing complaint are true (except to matters alleged to be on information and belief and those she believes to be true).

____
Mary Smith

Subscribed and Sworn to Before Me
this _______ day of ________________, 200

____
Notary Public

The law demands that you make a reasonable effort to notify the other party that you have filed for divorce. This is done through a summons, legal notice that the other party is suing for divorce. The summons can be gotten by appearing with the spouse at the Clerk of Court's Office or having it delivered by a third party or the Sheriff's Department to the residence. The summons and petition for divorce are published in a legal periodical; for most this means a local and/or country newspaper. A typical summons follows.

IN THE NAME OF THE PEOPLE OF THE STATE OF ________________
IN THE CIRCUIT COURT OF ________________ COUNTY _________

Mary Smith,

Plaintiff

James Smith, No. ________________

Plaintiff

SUMMONS

To each defendant:

YOU ARE SUMMONED and required to file an answer in this case, or otherwise file your appearance, in the office of the clerk of this court within ____days after notice of this summons, not counting the day of service. IF YOU FAIL TO DO SO, A JUDGMENT BY DEFAULT MAY BE TAKEN AGAINST YOU FOR THE RELIEF ASKED IN THE COMPLAINT.

To the officer:

This summons must be returned by the officer or other persons to whom it was given for service, with endorsement of service and fees, if any, immediately after service. If service cannot be made, this summons shall be returned so endorsed. This summons may not be served later than 30 days after this date.

WITNESS ________________________, 200____

Signature

____

Clerk of Court

It is usually important to ask the courts for a temporary order when you file the divorce petition. In this you ask the judge to grant certain rights until the divorce becomes final, like custody of the children, financial consideration, right to the home, and attorney's fees. In most cases the request for an order is done by the wife. In the case where one of the partners does not respond to the summons of the plaintiff, two things can happen: first, the judge can hold a hearing on the basis of a temporary order and grant everything asked or secondly, you (the plaintiff) may get the divorce granted by default. If the defendant isn't present, the divorce is granted. Sometimes this is pre-arranged; this is done to facilitate the decision making. Judges will, upon discovering collusion, fail to grant the divorce under these circumstances. In the case where the party does not default, the defendant will have (usually) a lawyer draw up the legal papers for a defense of the charges and may counter-charge (file a cross-complaint). The judge will then issue a temporary order determining what disposition in the interim is to be made of money, domiciling and custody of children, etc. If reconciliation occurs, the proceedings may be stopped.

Usually before the trial for divorce goes into court an attempt at negotiation is made. Issues are resolved hopefully on property, custody, support, etc. This is the time to gather facts—most states require extensive financial revelations to be made of debts, income, etc. Here is a typical Financial Disclosure (some are shorter) used in New York.

FINANCIAL DISCLOSURE AFFIDAVIT

F.C.A. 413-1, 424-A: Art. 5-b
D.R.L. 236-B, 2240

Form 4-17
(Financial Disclosure Affidavit)
9/99

FAMILY COURT OF THE STATE OF NEW YORK
COUNTY OF

In the Matter of a Proceeding for Support

Docket No.

(Commissioner of Social Services, Assignor,
on behalf of , Assignee)

Petitioner

S.S.# (Assignor)

FINANCIAL DISCLOSURE AFFIDAVIT

-against-

Respondent.

S.S.#

NOTICE: YOU ARE REQUIRED TO ATTACH TO THIS FORM A CURRENT AND REPRESENTATIVE PAYCHECK STUB AND A COPY OF YOUR MOST RECENTLY FILED STATE AND FEDERAL INCOME TAX RETURNS, INCLUDING A COPY OF THE W-2 WAGE AND TAX STATEMENT(S) SUBMITTED WITH THE RETURNS. YOU MAY ALSO BE REQUIRED TO PRODUCE OTHER PAYCHECK STUBS, EMPLOYMENT OR BUSINESS RECORDS AND PROOF OF CLAIMED EXPENSES. IN ADDITION, YOU ARE REQUIRED TO PROVIDE INFORMATION RELATING TO ALL GROUP HEALTH PLANS AVAILABLE TO YOU FOR THE PROVISION OF CARE OR OTHER MEDICAL BENEFITS FOR THE CHILDREN) FOR WHOM SUPPORT IS SOUGHT.

STATE OF NEW YORK)
):SS.:
COUNTY OF)

____________________________, the (Petitioner)(Respondent) here in, residing at _______
___________________________________, being duly sworn, deposes and says that the following is an accurate statement of my income from all sources, my liabilities, my assets and my net worth, from whatever sources, and whatever kind and nature, and wherever situated:

I. <u>INCOME FROM ALL SOURCES:</u> The correct amount of the child support obligation is presumed to be a percentage of income as defined by law. The percentages are set forth in Addendum A. Other pertinent information is set forth in Addenda B and C. List your income from all sources as follows:

a. <u>Wages and Salaries</u> (as reportable on Federal and State income tax returns):

1. Employer and address ______
2. Number of members in household ______
3. Number of dependents ______
4. Hours worked per week ______
5. Weekly gross salary/wages ______
6. Weekly deductions: ______
   a. Social Security (FICA) Tax ______
   b. New York State Tax ______
   c. Federal Tax ______
   d. Other payroll deductions ______
7. Income of other members of household ______

<u>NOTE:</u> ATTACH INFORMATION FOR ADDITIONAL EMPLOYERS SEPRATELY TO THIS FORM.

b. <u>Self-Employment Income</u> (Describe and list self-employment income; attach to this form the most recently filed Federal and State income tax returns, including all schedules):

______

______

______

______

c. <u>Income/Dividend Income:</u> ______

______

______

d. <u>Other income:</u>
1. Workers Compensation ______
2. Disability Benefits ______
3. Unemployment Insurance Benefits ______
4. Social Security Benefits ______
5. Veterans Benefits ______
6. Pensions and Retirement Benefits ______
7. Fellowships/Stipends/Annuities ______

e. <u>Income from other sources:</u> (List here and explain any other income including but not limited to: non-income producing assets; employment 'perks' and reimbursed expenses; fringe benefits as a result of employment; periodic income, personal injury settlements; non-reported income; and money, goods and services provided by relatives and friends) ______

______

______

II. ASSETS: The Court can consider the assets of the custodial parent and/or the non-custodial parent in its award of child support. List your assets as follows:

a. Savings account balance (Name of Bank: ______) a) $ ______
b. Checking account balance (Name of bank: ______) b) $ ______
c. Automobile(s) (Year and make: ______) c) $ ______
   Loan information ______
d. Residence owned (Address: ______) d) $ ______
e. Other real estate owned ______ e) $ ______
f. Other assets (For example: stocks, bonds, trailers, boat, etc.) ______ f) $ ______
g. Driver's, professional, recreational, sporting and other licenses and permits held (provide name of issuing agency, license number and attach a copy if possible) ______

______

______

NOTE: ATTACH TO THIS FORM ANY INFORMATION AS TO ANY ADDITIONAL ASSETS

III. DEDUCTIONS FROM INCOME: The Court allows certain deductions from income prior to applying the child support percentages. List the deductions that apply to you as follows:

a. Unreimbursed employee business expenses a) $ ____________
b. Maintenance actually paid to spouse not a part to this action* b) $ ____________
c. Maintenance actually paid to spouse who is a party to this action c) $ ____________
d. Child support actually paid on behalf of non-subject child(ren)* d) $ ____________
e. Family Assistance e) $ ____________
f. Supplemental Security Income f) $ ____________
g. NYC/Yonkers Income Tax g) $ ____________
h. FICA h) $ ____________

***Attach to this form a copy of the appropriate Court Order**

IV. HEALTH INSURANCE, UNREIMBURSED HEALTH-RELATED EXPENSES, CHILD CARE EXPENSES AND EDUCATIONAL EXPENSES: As part of the child support obligation, parents shall be directed to provide health insurance, pay a pro-rated share of unreimbursed health-related expenses, pay a pro-rated share of child care expenses and in the Court's discretion pay educational expenses. List your information as follows and cross out or delete inapplicable provisions:

a. I (have)(do not have) health insurance coverage (through employment)(privately purchased)(through the "Child Health Plus" program).

1. My coverage includes (dental)(prescription drug)(optical)(other health care services or benefits [specify]:
2. The portion of the cost of the insurance paid by my employer or through my employment is ____________. The cost of the insurance paid by me is $ ________________.
3. The person(s) covered by my insurance is/are: ________________________________
____
4. My policy number is ____________.
5. Coverage (does)(does not) presently include my child(ren). The additional cost to me to include my child(ren) would be [specify cost for each type of benefit; if benefit unavailable, so indicate]:
   Medical: $____________ per ________. Optical: $____________ per ______.
   Dental: $____________ per ________. Prescription drugs $________ per ______.
   Other Health Services or Benefits [specify]: ____________ $________ per ______.
6. The name and address of my primary (and secondary) health insurer is/are: __________
____
7. My primary (and secondary) health plan administrator is/are: (indicate name, address and telephone number of contact person for employer or organization): ______________
____
8. There are (medical)(dental)(prescription drug)(optical)(other health care benefits [specify]:) insurance benefits available to the child(ren) through an individual who is not a party to this action. This individual is [indicate name and relationship]: ____.
   These benefits cost as follows: ____.

b. My child care provider is: ________________________________. The average number of hours of child care incurred per week are: ________________________________

c. My child's educational needs and expenses are: ________________________________
____

V. VARIANCE FROM THE PERCENTAGES: The Family Court Act allows the Court to order support different from the percentages if the Court finds that the support based upon the percentages would be unjust or inappropriate due to certain factors. The factors are set forth in Addendum D. The following is/are the factor(s) that the Court should consider in this case: _____
____

VI. EXPENSES: In ordering support by the percentages the Court is not obligated to consider expenses. However, if the Court varies from the percentages, expenses may be considered. List

a. Rent or mortgage payment
b. Mortgage interest and amortization — a) $________
c. Realty taxes (if not included in mortgage payment) — b) $________
d. Insurance on realty — c) $________
e. Utilities: gas_____ electric/water____ telephone _____ cable____ — d) $________
f. Garbage collection — e) $________
g. Household repairs (specify): ____________________________ — f) $________
h. Food — g) $________
i. Charge accounts, loans, etc. 1) ____________________ — h) $________
(from section VII below) 2) ____________________ — i) $________
3) ____________________
j. Automobile expenses: gas _____ maintenance ________ insurance & fees _____ loan____________ — j) $________
k. Public transportation
l. Life insurance — k) $________
m. Health insurance — l) $________
n. Clothing: self $__________ others: $_________ (explain: ________) — m) $________
o. Laundry and dry cleaning — n) $________
p. Education and tuition (explain: ______________________________) — o) $________
q. Child care — p) $________
r. Contributions — q) $________
s. Union dues (mandatory: yes ____ no____) — r) $________
t. Entertainment — s) $________
u. Miscellaneous person expenses (specify: ___________________) — t) $________
v. Other (specify: ______________________________________) — u) $________
v) $________

VI. LIABILITIES, LOANS AND DEBTS: In ordering support by the percentages the Court is not obligated to consider liabilities, loans, and debts. However, if the Court varies from the percentages, they may be considered. List your liabilities, loans and debts as follows:

Creditor _____________	Creditor ____________	Creditor ______________
Purpose ___________	Purpose ___________	Purpose __________
Date incurred ________	Date incurred ________	Date incurred _______
Total balance due _____	Total balance due ____	Total balance due _____

NOTE: ATTACH TO THIS FORM INFORMATION REGARDING ANY ADDITIONAL DEBTS.

I. LIFE AND ACCIDENT INSURANCE: The Court may direct you to purchase and maintain life and/or accident insurance benefits or assign benefits on existing policies for the benefit of your children. List your insurance policy or policies as follows:

a. Life insurance: (Name of insurer): ____________________ $ ___________________
Beneficiary/Beneficiaries: ______________________________________

b. Accident insurance: (Name of insurer): ____________________ $ ___________________
(Name of insurer): ______________________________________
This information is current as of (specify date) __________________________.

____
(Petitioner)(Respondent)

____
Print or Type Name

____
Signature of Attorney, if any

____
Attorney's Name (Print or Type)

____
____
____
Attorney's Address and Telephone Number

I have carefully read the foregoing statement and attest to its truth and accuracy.
Sworn to before me this ____________________
day of ____________________, __________.

____
(Deputy) Clerk of the Court
Notary Public

Adapted from the New York State Court, NY

ADDENDUM A
CHILD SUPPORT PERCENTAGES

The child support percentages that shall be applied by the Court unless the Court makes a finding that the non-custodial parent's share is unjust or inappropriate are as follows: 17% for one child; 25% for two children; 29% for three children; 31% for five children; and no less than 35% for five or more children.

ADDENDUM B
COMBINED PARENTAL INCOME OVER $80,000.00

Where combined parental income exceeds $80,000.00, the Court shall determine the amount of child support for the amount of the combined parental income in excess of such dollar amount through consideration of the factors set forth in Addendum D and or the support percentage set forth in Addendum A.

ADDENDUM C
SELF-SUPPORT RESERVE

Where the annual amount of the basic child support obligation would reduce the non-custodial parent's income below the poverty income guidelines amount for a single person as reported by the federal Department of Health and Human Services, the basic child support obligation shall be twenty-five dollars per month unless the interests of justice dictate otherwise. Where the annual amount of the basic child support obligation would reduce the non-custodial parent's income below the self-support reserve but not below, the poverty income guidelines amount of a single person as reported by the federal Department of Health and Human Services, the basic child support obligation shall be fifty dollars per month or the difference between the non-custodial parent's income and the self-support reserve, whichever is greater.

ADDENDUM D
VARIANCE FROM THE PERCENTAGES

The Court has the discretion to vary from the percentages if it finds that the non-custodial parent's pro-rata share of the basic child support obligation is unjust or inappropriate. This finding shall be based upon consideration of the following factors:

1. The financial resources of the custodial and non-custodial parent, and those of the child.
2. The physical and emotional health of the child and his/her special needs and aptitudes.
3. The standard of living the child would have enjoyed had the marriage or household not been dissolved.
4. The tax consequences to the parties
5. The non-monetary contributions that the parents will make toward the care and well-being of the child.
6. The educational needs of either parent.
7. A determination that the gross income of one parent is substantially less than the other parent's' gross income.

8. The needs of the children of the non-custodial parent for whom the non-custodial parent is providing support who are not subject to the instant action and who support has not been deducted from income, and the financial resource of any person obligated to support such children, provided, however, that this factor may apply only if the resources available to support such children are less than the resources available to support the children who are subject to the instant action.
9. Provided that the child is not on public assistance (i) extraordinary expenses incurred by the non-custodial parent in exercising visitation, or (ii) expenses incurred by the non-custodial parent in extended visitation provided that the custodial parent's expenses are substantially reduced as a result thereof.
10. Any other factors the Court determines are relevant in each case.

NOTE: The language in the above Addenda is paraphrased from that in the statute for the purposes of simplification. For statutory language, see Family Court Act Sections 413(1) and 424-a and Domestic Relations Law Sections 236-B and 240.

If a partner is concealing something, as a wealthy woman hiding her true worth, then an order—a subpoena ordering her bank to produce a statement and also an injunction can be issued forbidding any money to be taken from the account until the matter is settled in court. You may also directly question your spouse through court permission and have a court stenographer take it down. Her lawyer can be present. You will pay the bill. During the period before the divorce trial, you may want to get witnesses to support your claim as to your business, if one claims unjustly to be involved with it, or on custody where proper parenting is an issue. Getting information by wire tapping is legal under certain situations such as on your own phone if you do the installation, but in most cases—nine of ten—are settled out of court and most states provide leeway in their statutes so this is not needed. In some states there may be other matters required in similar cases.

Uncontested Divorces

The hearing in an uncontested divorce case is routine with your lawyer asking questions from the material stated in the petition to divorce such as:

In the course of your marriage, were you a true and faithful affectionate woman?

Yes (Plaintiff)

Has your husband severely mistreated you over the last three years and harassed you, calling you vile names in public?

Yes (Plaintiff)

Finally the lawyer (Plaintiff). If the judge should grant this divorce, do you request the terms of settlement be approved by this court and be made a part of this divorce decree?

Yes (Plaintiff)

If the divorce is contested, then it will be more complicated and drawn out. The evidence will have to be specific and verified. There will be cross-examination of the statements, the presented documents, and possibly witnesses of both parties by their respective lawyers. The judge may take a hand in the procedures questioning, clarifying, etc. When this is over and the judge signs the decree, in most states you are free and considered single. In some states, however, there is a required waiting period of a few days to several months (call the interlocutory period); during this period one is still married, then the person is free to remarry. A final decree then is given awarding the divorce and stating the manner in which the finances, custody, property, etc., are to be handled.

Handling Your Own Divorce

Deciding to do your own divorce can be a saver of money but is only recommended where the couple has been married only a few years, have no children and little money or property to worry about. It is essential that both husband and wife agree on everything. If there is disagreement, then a court fight will probably ensue involving lawyers. In using the do-it-yourself divorce, you should use the kits or related books made for this purpose (the public library will have information and codes [state laws]; the librarian will also provide help to find material) and the advice of women's rights and men's rights groups. The forms for filing a petition and the summons form that are necessary can be bought at some stationery stores for about $30 (a kit). Books such as *How to File Your Own Divorce* (Edward Haman) provides information on how to file and the necessary forms. You can then fill in the blanks. Be sure to use forms accepted in your own state. Remember, too, that on file in the courthouse are copies of documents filed by other couples, so ask the clerk of the court to direct you to them and the forms their venue requires. Read a few as illustrations, then guided by the wording, do your own. Ask the clerk for help if you need it; at the least he or she can tell you whether or not you have filled it out satisfactorily. Another thing you can do is to visit the court to observe what happens in other divorces; knowing this aid in reducing your anxiety. In the court in the do-it-yourself kind, you take the part of the lawyer as outlined earlier, making your statements as clear and brief as possible. When it is over, that is, when you have finished making your presentation, your final question to the judge will be: "Your Honor, may I prepare the final decree?" If the judge says "Yes," you've won your divorce! You must then prepare the final decree using the forms supplied by the clerk in the manner agreed to by the court.

Be certain money matters, property settlement, etc., are included, for it becomes the document of record. Usually several hundred dollars or more will pay for this kind of divorce. It will take time to do this, attention to detail, but it isn't too difficult and you check the final decree for accuracy for changes are sometimes made by the judge that may not find their way into the final document of divorce. A lawyer I know has this to say about "do-it-yourself" divorce. "This is like saying that a layman can lance a boil, by consulting a medical guide." But, there are subtle points that, if missed, can result in infection and gangrene, in the medical example. I'd rather go to a doctor! In divorces, beware of such issues as jurisdiction, venue, elements of proof, wording of petition and decrees, etc. You can find a lawyer who will handle an uncontested divorce for $500-$1500, and then its his responsibility.

If one can control their emotions and maintain a calm, objective demeanor, then surely there is an advantage to the do-your-own divorce. Advantages are: (1) You save the cost of a lawyer. (2) Judges often feel more sympathetic toward a person without an attorney and give a certain amount of leeway. (3) This procedure would normally speed up the divorce also cut down frustration in trying to reach your lawyer and get movement toward concluding the divorce. (4) Selecting an attorney is not easy—many mistakes are made here. Getting a good attorney is a problem you don't need.

Children in Separation and Custody

Two out of every three divorces involve children. Up until recently in only about one in ten divorce cases was there a contest over custody; however, increasingly courts are awarding children, even young ones, to their fathers. It may not mean there will be more fights over custody, though there may be. Many experts in human development believe that young children (below 6 or 7) typically should remain with their mother. (There are exceptions depending upon the quality of the parenting.) Some boys after 6 or 7 could go with the fathers and other persons (aunt, grandparents); some girls after 8 or 9 wish to live with fathers. We find generally the middlescent (those between the early forties and upper sixties) father of forty or so is more nuturant oriented than one in his twenties or thirties and has been found in many cases to understanding parenting. Custody, nonetheless whatever disposition that is made, it is the most sensitive issue in the divorce settlement. Where parents agree on custody, the court usually concurs. If it is thought by the court that the parents are not capable of handling the situation, the custody of children is given to a foster family or grandparents. Of course, older children may be asked with whom they wish to live and occasionally agencies are asked to decide with specialists like psychologists, family specialists, social workers, etc., called upon to determine the best situation for the child. Many judges are not trained in the behavior sciences sufficiently nor have the time to investigate in order to make the decision alone and they need to seek some help in these matters. Most judges in the past have assumed that men should not (judging by the fact that in about 90% of the divorces women get custody) have the children.

Most states have joint custody laws based on the "best interests of the child" if sex neutral standard that allows the court to consider whatever it deems relevant. This does not mean joint physical custody, which usually amounts to liberal visitation rights. The joint legal custody awards give both parents the right to make decisions such as authorizing medical treatment of the child but not necessarily a split in living time between two parents.

Many men attempting to get custody often refuse to pay alimony often manage to prevail because their wives cannot afford to litigate the issue. Conversely women wanting custody some times give up alimony, some child support and/or property to get to keep the children. The men argue with their wives and sometimes get an agreement to have custody of the children by harassment—daily calls, threats of prolonging legal fights, discussions about the unfit nature of the mother, her future inability to maintain a decent life in a decent situation for the children are accustomed. These attempts usually fail, particularly in court adjudicated custody but in negotiated settlement they do somewhat better. Many men who struggle hard to get custody are attempting to punish their spouse, feeling this would affect them more than anything else.

In California (and some other states), the law makes mediation mandatory whenever custody is contested. Mediation in these cases is required before the judge hears the case. California has a joint custody preference and under their laws a judge can award custody to both when only one parent wants it or when neither parent wants it. The law puts the burden on the judge who does not order joint custody to justify in writing why he has not done so. The effect of this is to weaken or do away with the maternal presumption.

Dr. May Howell, a pediatrician and researcher at Harvard University, says that in her pediatric practice she cared for more than 3,000 children from about 1,000 families and there is a small but significant number of families in which the father was the effective primary caretaker. She goes on to say that from a study done with eighteen-month-old children, about equal proportions of toddlers are attached to their fathers only, as are attached to their mothers only, and that about two-thirds of them are attracted to both fathers and mothers. This probably is not typical and the number of subjects in the sample small. Of the two biological differences, breast feeding is of minor importance, and the rough and tumble style of the latter is usually modified to be more gentle. Consistent affection and acceptance of children is important, as is protection from hazards both physical and psychological. Clearly men can be good parents, like most women, if they give their energy and devotion to it. Most men however recognize that women should be the principal source of mothering for very young children (1-3) and they probably would be overwhelmed if suddenly given sole responsibility.

One needs to assess one's ability to handle parenting alone—this should not be thought of as a way to hurt the spouse. Many men do not believe their wives will make the best parent so desire to have the child or children. In some cases, by agreement, the man is already supplying the major role in care taking in the marriage. Since more and more women are opting for careers, they will likely be willing to let husbands who can manage their work and the child let them have the care of them. Or if the marriage has produced several children, dividing the children may increase the adjustment prospect and provide the greatest benefit; this is a possibility. If there is a fight over custody of a child, one must get a lawyer that has this kind of legal experience. Men, when they seek lawyers to get custody for them, often are turned down. In this situation get a lawyer who agrees with you. One man I know, expecting a lot of women's rights arguments from his wife in a custody battle, hired an attorney competent in handling feminist issues, and he won.

Sometimes custody fights go on for years; sometimes keeping notes (meticulously) and tape recordings of conversations can provide the evidence needed to suggest the "unfit parent" not unlike the "Baby M" case. Tales of parents drinking drugging and personality problems are abrasive on children who frequently are in one fashion or the other brought into the fray. Sometimes where women have mental health problems a joint custody can be arranged where the mother won't give up control. This can have its difficulty where real joint custody is attempted, for how could a couple fighting to divorce use cooperative judgment in care taking? It tends to divide the loyalty of the child, but for practical purposes the person who maintains physical custody is in the driver's seat.

Sometimes custody changes in situations where the couple have other responsibilities which have to be considered in caring for children, such as new jobs requiring a change in location or the death of a parent or their sickness which demands consideration. Where the wife has gotten custody of the children but finds she has to help aging or sick parents, it frequently means giving up a child or children to the husband, and a former husband who is transferred across the country may necessitate his former spouse keeping the child temporarily. Many cases where this is "temporary" it turns out to be permanent.

Forcing the Issue of Custody

Some parents have used "child taking" as a method of getting custody. Sometimes cases, which are decided in two states, custody in one instance, will be given to the man and in another to the woman. The taking of one's child is no violation in a few states. All states have adopted the Uniform Child Custody Jurisdiction Act. The state whose courts have the most pertinent information have jurisdiction and will honor a decree initiated in another state but it will violate state law in these places if the child is taken.

The hiring of parents of a "Mean Gene" to get their child is nearly over. Mean Gene may have referenced Eugene Austin from Coley, Missouri, who had been employed by parents in over 500 cases where they have legal custody order or the custody matter is in dispute in the courts. Austin required that the parent accompany him in his theft, otherwise he would not do the kidnapping. About one-third of his clients were women. Others are in this business in nearly every state. Being taken (kidnapped), however, must be a traumatic experience for the child, particularly if the child has lived with the parent for any length of time. In some instances he would probably wish to live with the parent who arranged for him to be stolen. Any parent—man or woman—needs to consider seriously the effect upon the child before he takes him or her from the home of the other parent. One can conceive of an instance where it might be the wisest thing to do but I don't believe there will be many such situations. In any case The Parental Kidnapping Prevention Act of 1980 (P.L. 96-611) was passed designed to deter child snatching. when it occurs authorities can use the Federal Parent Locater to find those on child support. The Fugitive Felon Act will apply allowing a search for kidnapping parents. Suffice it to say today because of the Uniform Child Custody Act a parent cannot begin a custody determination de nova (all over again). They must return the case to and defer to the state of original jurisdiction. Many states also provide actual and punitive damages to be assessed against a parent who tries to circumvent a custody decree.

Alimony

The problem of money and alimony is the second most important concern to custody with divorcing couples. A North Carolina man said all he was left with was some old clothes and the dogs. Alimony is a bad word for men—it still exists in some states but since no fault divorce, alimony is being replaced by the term maintenance support for the spouse during and following dissolution proceedings. Increasingly women are paying maintenance to men because of greater earning ability, etc. However where alimony is given in twenty-eight states law states marital fault is relevant. Desertion, abandonment of children, taking up with another man or woman, etc., will annul alimony in many cases. In the past several years alimony has been granted in only about 1 of 7 cases (15%). The concept of alimony has changed in most states, it is now called maintenance or spousal support. Maintenance or support is provided to the woman or man on the basis of custodial support, Transitional support (adjust to new life situation—work, housing, etc.) and the state of one's earning capacity. An additional element is new that is demanding attention as a financial consideration—sharing partnership assets. Helping the husband get through law school, supporting his career, etc. are the type of things to be considered. By 1988, 23 states made provisions for the conversion of insurance on divorce. Most states have legislation requiring consideration of spousal contribution in professional degrees. In short marriages less than five years only very few were awarded alimony. Permanent alimony is given in only a small percent of the cases. Where the wife is in her early (35-45) or middlescent (45-55) years, support money is awarded to help care for children which may continue until they are eighteen unless otherwise agreed upon, but that given to the wife if marriage was between 5 to 10 years but will usually be adjusted downward until she is able to get back into the work market. If she is already working, she may get no support for herself. The median award in 1984 was approximately $4,000; where given today is much higher. Increasing alimony when given to men, or cash settlements are made to take care of joint ownership of property that went with the marriage and because women made more than men in their job. Up until recently (it still exists in many states) alimony was given typically for a total of half the years of a marriage, so that a man who was married for twenty years gave alimony for ten years. Alimony in cases of marriages of twenty years and over was usually made permanent. Newer alimony approaches, like the one adopted in Florida, gives temporary support to the woman for the purpose of adjusting herself to work and possibly a new home setting. Alimony is usually based upon the money one makes and style of living one is accustomed to; if you make $80,000 a year, the court will make generous provision for your wife and support payments for children. A wife may waive the alimony and, if this is the case, men should get this into the separation agreement. If he gives her anything, however small, it opens the door to ask at a later time for more. Some states will not allow alimony if the husband gets a divorce on the basis of his wife's adultery. If there are other sources of income, as in dividing the marital property with the wife getting part of the property, a percent of the business profits, stocks and bonds, etc., she may then not get any support money for children or herself. Frequently the amount of money given as temporary, that is, until the court makes its final decision, becomes the permanent amount. The argument usually taken by the wife's attorney is, why not continue as permanent the money already given for the living conditions have not changed? Some men have fallen for this and their lawyers allowed it to go unquestioned, only to find shortly thereafter the wife goes to work, lives with her parents and needs no money excepting where there are children, may not even then. The matter of alimony should not be taken lightly but examined, argued and fought out for neither man nor woman should be the fall guy or gal. Support can change over the years. If the wife marries, she relinquishes the alimony and typically when children reach eighteen, support is no longer a legal obligation. But if the man remarries, it does not affect the money he has to pay unless his former spouse agrees to it. If the economic circumstances change, alimony and support payments are curtailed (when the court agrees to this upon the petition of one of the parties) entirely or in proportion to the reduced salary situation. Faced with installment payments for alimony, it would be well to consider a lump sum cash settlement (although many wives will not agree to this), for at least you know with a fixed sum what you will have to pay; the other could go on for years. If you agree to a lump sum settlement and your wife dies the day of the decree, you have to pay the estate. I do not subscribe to many of the ideas it presents but I read the book of Lawyer Maurice R. Franks entitled *How to Avoid Alimony* in which he says alimony is a form of slavery and violates the equal protection clause and due process clause of the Constitution. In essence his advice to men and supposedly to women also who are required to pay alimony is to file a petition with the federal, not state, courts claiming antidiscrimination clauses of the various civil rights acts as the basis for not complying. He used this approach in his second divorce, and though the Supreme Court has refused to hear the case, it is alleged he has paid no alimony. Many men cheat on their payments (now laws give the federal authorities the right to find the delinquent party); if oppressed, man or the woman should seek changes through the court. It occurs to me that a man whose wife has done a good job of caring for his children and has been a good wife for most of their life together, it certainly would not be right to just turn her out to pasture. We should not divorce our children just because custody is given to the wife, nor expect the housewife without having a job for a long period of time to make it quickly on her own. This is difficult to handle for most, but where fathers are involved I believe over the years children will certainly honor such a parent for helping the former wife and mother.

Child Support

The question of child support differs from alimony in that it is absolutely obligatory while alimony is not. The burden relative to small children falls on both parents though the man usually pays most of the bills, certainly if he is in his middlescent years. It is true that among the newly married or among those married for just a brief time, most of these current young people divorces are resolved on the basis of no-fault. Sometimes when mothers work they often receive more pay than their spouse, mothers therefore often have to provide child support. The responsibility rests fundamentally with each parent. Some men feel put upon because they are ordered to pay support and yet have difficulty in getting access to their children. I have known women under court order who do not let the father see the child or have visitation, even when it has been spelled out in the decree. I suppose they are fearful of the child leaving or being taken away. How do they avoid it, you ask, by using boni fide or otherwise excuses—the child has prior visitation with a grandparent or aunt or school trip or they are sick; to buttress this they will get collusion with a physician who will write that the child is upset or has the flu pre-empting visiting. Of course, this isn't fair, but this is war—total war!!

In the final analysis, the amount of support is based upon:

1. the needs of the child
2. the financial status & needs
3. the standard of living the child would have enjoyed had the marriage continued
4. the physical & emotional conditions of the child and his or her education needs
5. the financial resources and needs of the non-custodial parent.

In some states like Virginia that code sets out specifically how much each parent considering the income of both parties. The older the children, the most costly, a fact that may be has been lost on men who have let their wives take care of the money. Though support allotment varies, in Illinois and some other places many judges use a rule of thumb that goes like this: For one child around 30% of the father's take-home pay, for two children 40%, for three 45%, and for four 50%. This is dependent on the economic status of the father. A man's salary of $20,000 is relieved of a higher percent than a man with an $80,000 salary. This does not include alimony. Fault is not supposed to enter into support allotments but in some cases does. Fathers are obligated to pay for a variety of "extras" but they are only legally obligated to pay for whatever is spelled out—like $400-800 per month and hospitalization are usually always included. Other things may be written in the legal obligation like summer camp, insurance, piano lessons, private schooling and/or college education, dentist bills and braces, etc. When, however, the child becomes emancipated—marries, takes a full-time job or enters the Armed Forces, reaches his or her majority, or in the case of death, the support ceases. A few states—like Virginia does, require a court order stating the obligation is ended to discontinue the support. You should note that support, if you marry a person with a child, is included in a subsequent divorce settlement regardless of kinship. Though not in all states in a common law marriage—living together constitutes—a binding of interest occurs and sharing of property is sometimes judged mandatory when brought to the attention of the court. The term palimony developed out of a living together suit brought against Lee Marvin and since then many others. Taking care of children growing out of this long-term relationship is also the responsibility of both parties. Not all states recognize a common law marriage.

Court Ordered Support

All states have statutes that allow wage assignments or income deductions from the court ordered payers of child support. A majority of the states have long-arm statues and discretion to make payment directly to the court officer. Others like Mississippi to the Human Resources Agency.

Lenore Weitzman, expert on divorce says, "no matter what his income level a divorced man is rarely ordered to part with more than one-third of his net income." This is not true today. She says that some judges set the ultimate limit of one-half of the net income. In practice usually less is given. Some judges emphasize that you shouldn't touch the goose that lays the golden egg, meaning you need to protect the father's motivation to earn. If he is overwhelmed by the burden of payment some men will quit and/or flee. Most men (80% according to a Michigan and Canadian study) when fully complying with a court ordered support will still live comfortably. More recent research indicates many less than 80% live comfortably. In recent days—several years ago—93% of the women if they lived on the support in California (probably true for most states) allotted to them by the court would be below the poverty level. This has changed due to studies like those done in Maryland in Maryland in Montgomery County which revealed most women two years after divorce (no fault) were less well off than before. If a man makes or woman makes as much as $80,000 per year then most judges will award 35% of the total for five children (28,000), for three about 25% and one less. Usually most married couples do not have enough income to live separate or apart.

A related problem to child support is inflation that has eroded the value of the dollar. The court rarely considers a built-in cost of living adjustment. Non-compliance is another issue. The U.S. Census Bureau in a study conducted several years ago found less than half received the support ordered by the court, one-third received partial payments and the other third received nothing. Compliance with alimony awards is said to be improving according to Weitzman, probably, she says because alimony tends to be awarded only in higher-income families but also tracking systems are catching the non-compliance offenders. As of 1985 thirty states gave judges the discretionary power to have child support payments made directly to the court. Most states allow 60 to 90 days grace before attaching the salaries of men or women in the arrears with support payments. Some men send the payments just before the deadline as a harassment tactic. Many women get discouraged or are in a Catch 22 situation (they do not have the funds to pursue men failing to pay) by the problems of bringing charges. They often make only one or two attempts to force payment before they quit trying. Others fail to file a complaint at all. A college librarian was an example of this. Her husband worked in the same college. Her first attempt was thwarted in bringing results. She was embarrassed by it and upset over the cost and never attempted to get the money due her even though she and her former husband worked on the same campus.

Property Division and Money Matters

As we have discussed earlier, payment for child allotment and alimony are considered support payments. Property allocation relates to the distributing of everything a wife and a husband owns. This matter is settled after one has filed for divorce or separation and before either has been decided by the court. The period between filing and the final settlement is a difficult one, for in anger one or both parties can use the personal possession of the other or jointly held items, credit, destroy gifts, misuse equipment, take important papers and treasured items. One can suffer severe loss in credit rating in a brief time during this period. A Norfolk, Virginia man's wife prior to the divorce ran up vast bills for clothing for which he was responsible. Although he had taken some precautions telling various businesses, banks, etc., he would not be responsible for the wife's debts, he nevertheless got stung for when he told a service station manager to no longer give his wife credit under this name, however, the manager continued to provide credit. Later the manager demanded payment that was not forthcoming so he turned his name into the local credit agency. One result, before this was settled, was to be rejected for a bank loan as a poor risk. The loan was to pay college tuition for a son. One cannot take the money of another, even that's shared, but it frequently happens. It is wise for a person to get an injunction (through your lawyer), if there is uncertainty as to what the spouse will attempt to do, from the court forbidding withdrawal from checking accounts, savings and loan, etc. All joint credit cards should be collected and one should write to the companies involved requesting issuance of new individual cards—that is, one for you. If a couple can trust each other, they could go down to the bank, draw out the savings and checking account funds and divide them on the spot.

Property comes in two categories—real and personal. Land and buildings are real property; everything else is personal property—furnishings, cars, money, sporting goods, jewelry, etc. Most of the problems over property come from decisions about the home, the car, furniture, and monies. Not all persons concerned have homes and real estate, and this reduces the friction between the parties making a settlement. The individual usually keeps the property brought into a marriage, other things are divided; if you are in a "community property" state (Arizona, California, Idaho, Louisiana, Nevada, New Mexico, Texas, and Washington) the things you both accrued together are community property except gifts or inheritance. The other forty-two states have equitable distribution of marital property provisions.

No-Fault Law Revisited

The law in California instructs the court to divide the community assets and liabilities equally. This action notably New York has influenced other states. Equitable division does not mean 50-50 in these states. Lack of certainty in property division makes for more litigation unfortunately also as a result the homes are ordered sold. Mothers with children or men with children are displaced often with traumatic results. Settlements in California under no-fault (1977) and fault (1978) find men getting higher awards in the division of assets as follows: the single family car, family business, and community property debts. Women receive the majority of assets that deal with family having household furnishings and money, stocks, and bonds. Most of the states have laws decreeing that the distribution of real property be as the "courts deem just and reasonable." However, in a community property state that recognizes fault, the supposition of equitable distribution bends to often favor the "innocent" party. In a number of states, property is considered as alimony. If the wife, for instance, suffers due to this, the court might award larger amounts of alimony to compensate for this loss. There are a few states that give only a third of the real property to the wife and considering the circumstances (if they are at fault) less than his or none. Dower's rights (that portion or interest in the real estate of a deceased husband which the law gives for life to his widow) are barred by divorce in many states, though the property of each is not affected.

Many authorities suggest in divorcing that you stay in your home if you can. It looks better for the person who maintains the house. Most judges thinking the home is most valuable to the women tend to award it to them. If one gets the home, then this should usually be offset by concessions on the other side. In one case, a San Francisco woman agreed to allow her husband to sell the home as part of the settlement. He sold the home to a friend and gave the wife her share of the equity. He then bought the home back at the same price which, in effect, amounted to a swindle, for the home was worth much more. Do not use this approach, and it should be mentioned that wives have used this one also. This is usually avoided because of the great suspicion that one partner has of the other, a lawyer's advice and the determination supported by the advice of friends and relatives "don't get burned" and "stick it to them." Usually an agreement is made on an appraiser or one is assigned by a judge to place a value on the home, it is then advertised and sold with the money divided; but if the home is not sold, whoever keeps the home usually gives half of the equity to the former spouse or some consideration.

It may be cheaper for a man to let his wife live in the home if there are a large number of children and a small mortgage payment, than to pay the extra support needed to give them another place to live. A man also might give the house to his wife until she marries and in some cases agreement may be reached on mortgage payments and the upkeep. This condition exists where the man can control the home disposition.

Nearly half of the states require conversion of a few insurance policies upon divorce and it would have relevance in most of the other states if presented with the argument over property (assets). Insurance is considered by most people as a career asset and refers to benefits a worker receives in the form of health, accident, and life insurance. This is sometimes called "new property and realistically should be considered for division upon divorce. It is overlooked or put aside obviously when many women according to the Older Women's League has called women without health insurance the "no-woman's land between menopause and Medicare." There were four million women in this category several years ago. There may be more now.

Some men think that wives should have everything in view of the fact that they stayed at home, raised the children, and provided for their comfort. They deserve consideration but should not have everything. Some men also think they can hide their worth by putting the family business or their savings in another person's name. Most women often have a fair idea of what their husbands are worth and the reverse is also true. Anyway this usually comes out and it's not worthwhile to lie and risk the charge of perjury; although this advice will fall on some deaf ears, it is still good advice.

Unfortunately when a couple with children divorce, it is probably that the man will become single but the woman will become a single parent. Poverty for many women begins with single parenthood. More than half of the poor families in the United States are headed by a single mother after divorce. Men go on in their occupations with their careers expanding and their salaries growing. The courts have generally treated men via the "golden egg syndrome" benignly. Some changes are being effected via insurance divisions, share in building a career or business, spousal contributions to professional degrees, pensions, but much more needs to be done for the newly poor.

Debts are often an area of controversy, particularly among younger middlescents for they have obligations many times beyond the divorcing middle age couple of 50 and upward, for these usually have unpaid mortgages, car payments, the second home, a boat and trailer, college education, operations, dental work and even clothing—furs, etc. A man in most cases is not required to assume the entire responsibility in absolving the debt both incurred. If a man pays the debts, the woman should expect less from the equity in property—real and personal—like automobiles. If a woman pays the lion's share of the debt, she should be accorded reciprocity. An agreement among the parties concerning the property is usually more satisfactory than having the court do it for you. The things you each wish should be written down as memorandum, reviewed by the attorneys, agreed upon and carried out fairly. I know of a man who continued to have his daughter go into his former wife's home to purloin certain items, even though an extensive list of items was drawn up in advance and an agreement made. The battle for property, changes in alimony and support go on after the divorce is final, hence discretion is constantly advised.

DIVORCE STATUTES—SPOUSAL SUPPORT FACTORS

JURISDICTION	FACTORS CONSIDERED
Alabama	Standard of living; marital fault relevant
Alaska	Statutory list; standard of living; marital fault not considered
Arizona	Statutory list; standard of living; status as custodial parent; marit fault not considered
Arkansas	Marital fault not considered
California	Statutory list; standard of living; marital fault not considered
Colorado	Statutory list; standard of living; status as custodial parent; marit fault not considered
Connecticut	Statutory list; standard of living; status as custodial parent; marit fault relevant
Delaware	Statutory list; standard of living; status as custodial parent; marit fault not considered
District of Columbia	Standard of living; marital fault relevant
Florida	Statutory list; standard of living; marital fault relevant
Georgia	Statutory list; standard of living; marital fault relevant
Hawaii	Statutory list; standard of living; status as custodial parent; marit fault not considered
Idaho	Statutory list; marital fault relevant
Illinois	Statutory list; standard of living; status as custodial parent; marit fault not considered
Indiana	Statutory list; standard of living; status as custodial parent; marit fault not considered
Iowa	Statutory list; standard of living; status as custodial parent; marit fault not considered
Kansas	Marital fault not considered
Kentucky	Statutory list; standard of living; marital fault relevant
Louisiana	Statutory list; status as custodial parent; marital fault relevant
Maine	Statutory list; marital fault not considered
Maryland	Statutory list; standard of living; marital fault relevant
Massachusetts	Statutory list; standard of living; marital fault relevant
Michigan	Standard of living; marital fault relevant
Minnesota	Statutory list; standard of living; status as custodial parent; marit fault not considered
Mississippi	Marital fault relevant
Missouri	Statutory list; standard of living; status as custodial parent; marit fault relevant

Montana	Statutory list; standard of living; status as custodial parent; marit fault not considered
Nebraska	Statutory list; standard of living; status as custodial parent; marit fault not considered
Nevada	Standard of living; status as custodial parent; marital fault relevant
New Hampshire	Statutory list; standard of living; status as custodial parent; marit fault relevant
New Jersey	Marital Property
New Mexico	Statutory list; standard of living; marital fault not considered
New York	Statutory list; standard of living; marital fault not considered
North Carolina	Statutory list; standard of living; marital fault relevant
North Dakota	Standard of living; marital fault relevant
Ohio	Statutory list; marital fault not considered
Oklahoma	Standard of living; status as custodial parent; marital fault not considered
Oregon	Statutory list; standard of living; status as custodial parent; marit fault not considered
Pennsylvania	Statutory list; standard of living; marital fault relevant
Rhode Island	Statutory list; standard of living; status as custodial parent; marit fault relevant
South Carolina	Statutory list; standard of living; status as custodial parent; marit fault relevant
South Dakota	Standard of living; marital fault relevant
Tennessee	Statutory list; standard of living; status as custodial parent; marit fault relevant
Texas	Statutory list; standard of living; status as custodial parent; marit fault relevant
Utah	Statutory list; standard of living; marital fault relevant
Vermont	Statutory list; standard of living; status as custodial parent; marit fault not considered
Virginia	Statutory list; standard of living; marital fault relevant
Washington	Statutory list; standard of living; marital fault not considered
West Virginia	Statutory list; status as custodial parent; marital fault relevant
Wisconsin	Statutory list; standard of living; status as custodial parent
Wyoming	Marital fault relevant[1]

[1] Source: American Bar Association, Family Law Section

Tax Planning in Divorce and Separation

A good start with the issue of tax in divorce is to secure and read the IRS Publication 504 (2004) Information for Divorced or Separated Individuals free at any IRS Office. Community property defined is found in Publication 555. The principal questions as it relates to divorce and tax are alimony, custody and exemptions and the cost of getting a divorce. Alimony payments are deductible, the persons receiving alimony must list it as income. The person giving the alimony has to supply the recipient's Social Security number on their tax return. Alimony and separate maintenance payments are monies received on behalf of a spouse or former spouse under a divorce or separation instrument if all of the following requirements are met.

1. The payment is in case (money order, check, etc.).
2. The parties do not designate that the payment is not alimony.
3. If under a decree of divorce or separate maintenance the parties are not sharing the same household.
4. If under the state or terms of the divorce or separation no liability to make any payment after the death of the recipient spouse.
5. The payment is not treated as child support.
6. The parties do not file a joint return for the year in which the qualifying payments were made.

Under the Tax Reform Act of 1986 the parties to dissolution of marriage filing separate should file alike that is both itemize or take the standard deductions. A caution here—filing separate may demand a higher tax. You generally cannot take credit for child and dependency care expenses, you cannot take earned income credit and you cannot take credit for the elderly or the permanently disabled. And you may have to include one half of any social security benefits. Support of children is allowed if over half of the total year's expenses were paid by you over a six-month period. Support includes Armed Forces Dependency allotments. Typically exemptions are allowed to one parent with custody or if both parents are given care responsibilities a trade-off is arranged. If considerable alimony is given often the payer is given the exemption whether or not he or she has custody. Exemptions to one part or the other is only allowable to legally separated or divorced persons.

Large alimony payments (Front-loaded Payments) have been limited as deductions; for instance it worked like this if a first post-separation year payment of $25,000 is made and the 2nd and 3rd years is of $4,000 each an average of these years is $4,000. This is subtracted from the $25,000 which was paid the first year leaving $21,000. The recapture rule requires subtractions of $15,000 from this $21,000 leaving $6,000. This is to be added to the payees' tax the third year. This amount can be deducted by the receiver of the alimony via the recapture rule stated above. Under the recapture rule, payments made in the second post-separation year (defined below) will be recaptured if the payments made in their post-separation year by more than $15,000. Payments regularly made in the first post-separation year will be recaptured if those payments exceed the average of the alimony or separate maintenance payments made in the second post-separation year (not including the payments recaptured as described above) and the post-separation year by more than $15,000. The excess amounts for both the first and second post-separation years will be recaptured only in the third post-separation year. A recent book by Gayle Smith (2004) in her work covers "everything you need to know" about *Divorce and Money*. It provides many examples and covers almost every category where money relates to divorce.

Joint Returns

The use of this return requires both parties use the same period, though the accounting method may be different, however, each spouse must include all of their income, exemptions, and deductions on your joint return. Each of the spouses is usually responsible jointly and individually for the tax and any interest or penalty due on your return. One spouse may be responsible for all the tax due even though the other spouse earned all the income.

Tax Help with The Cost of Divorce

You may not deduct legal fees and court costs from your tax. You may, however, deduct fees for tax advice in connection with a divorce and legal fees to get alimony. If you itemize deductions claim them on Schedule A (Form 1040) as a miscellaneous deduction subject to the 2% of adjusted gross income. You may include fees appraisers, actuaries and accountants for services in determining your correct tax or in getting alimony. You may not deduct the costs of personal advice, counseling, and legal action in a divorce. For more information see IRS Publication 529, Miscellaneous Deductions.

It should be noted that wives who receive custody following divorce and who set up a household can file as head of household. Using Rate Schedule 2, rates below that of a single person or a married person filing a separate return. Recently the Tax Reform Act also allowed the parent with custody of the children to claim a tax credit of $1,000 or so for each dependent child under age 19 or a student. For those making the standard deduction, this could be of considerable help. If you hire a tax expert or tax lawyer to help you with finances, this is also deductible. However, your other divorce costs as mentioned earlier are not items for deduction.

What we have been trying to point out is that despite the anguish and difficulty because of the divorce (some have lost or never had the emotional aspect), you must try to effect some judgment. By way of summary, realize that in most divorces something is different, therefore you must be diligent to check everything you can under the following lists. Write them out even if you have a lawyer; he is often in a hurry and will forget items that later become important.

1. List Your Personal Information and all your assets along with information of the marriage—length, problems in, date of, location of, and children.
2. Items under your support, expectations for support, how to be given, does it include automatic increases for cost of living raise, benefits at spouse's death, etc.
3. Real and Personal Property—what do I have and want, make an inventory list, what debts exist on the house, the car(s), for education? What property is deeded to me, what are my belongings, how will a division be made, discover every obligation and write it down. Are there liens on anything, your house and/or business?
4. Life Insurance and Medical Policies—what provisions for medical care for children or yourself. What disposition is to be made of policies, who can borrow on them, who pays the premiums, etc.
5. Child Support, Custody and Visitation—who will have custody of the children, who makes the decisions about education of the children, what about visitation, who arbitrates in case of a dispute, is notice to be provided when a child is sick or hospitalized: How much contribution is to be made for each child by each parent? Who pays for special things: Camps, music lessons, band instruments, etc., and insurance to cover in the event of the father's or mother's death, college attendance or professional training.
6. Obligations, Taxes and Debts—how much does each party owe, how is the indebtedness to be treated? Is there any litigation involved with a business, etc.? What monies can be saved through special features like giving money for alimony rather than specifically for child support? Do you file jointly for any year before the divorce is finalized or the year of the final decree: Are there other considerations?
7. Wills, Fees and Other Matters—does a will require modification, probably in most cases, is each part waiving their claims on the other's estate? What obligations for the husband to leave children and/or wife certain sums of money or property? In joint enterprises who acts for the children? Who pays for the attorney's fees, what about title searches, audits, appraisals, how can the billing aid in pay-

ment of taxes? How to arbitrate when agreements can't be reached: Is the separation agreement to be made part of the decree or independent of the decree? Where protection is desired, do you draw up a memorandum of separation permitted in some states listing obligations and settlement of property. Filing separately keeps this from being universal knowledge.

The matter of a divorce as indicated is complex and cannot be done without some trouble and attention to detail. We have not covered all the contingencies here; one should secure help and read some of the references at the end of this chapter. We should have mentioned cost of attorneys and fees. This is a recognized hazard due to inflation, which, for the years after this, add 10% for advancing cost. These figures ranging from low (usually in small towns and rural settings) to higher (usually found in large cities) and are typical divorce costs. Remember you cannot deduct legal fees and court costs legal fees on your taxes.

Filing Fees—$60-$80 paid when the petition is submitted.

Summons Fee—Around $12 but in some locations double this amount, plus mileage for serving the papers by a deputy in a Sheriff's office. Fee is $5 by some Sheriff's offices.

Court Reporter—$100-$125 (half or day hearing) per hour of court time, or $10 to $15 per page.

Depositions—$100-$500 plus expenses if your lawyer has to go out of town for these "proofs," or $10 to $15 per page per deposition in some states.

Copy of the Final Decree—$60-$80; none for self-filing divorcing procedures.

If you appeal to an appellate court, the transcriptions of your case could cost four to five hundred dollars plus other costs incidental to an appeal. The cost of an attorney will vary widely, for those new in the profession much less will be charged, in the typical small town or city, $250 to $300 for uncontested divorces. Older and more experienced lawyers will charge $3,000 to $5,000 for the non-contested cases. The fee in contested circumstances involving custody fights and money issues could go as high as $25,000, and for the very rich, much more, though even these kinds in the typical city and town under 100,000 population range from $2,000 to $5,000. On an hourly basis some lawyers will agree to $50-$70 an hour in a rural area to $500-$1,000 for a high class New York lawyer. The usual cost will be something in the order of $50 to $100 an hour. Whether you get an attorney by the hour or the case, be sure you get the arrangement in written form and an understanding what constitutes time. Remember most lawyers are willing to work out arrangements for payment over a period of time if needed. This also is an avenue for some but one should know the lawyer or have good recommendations that he or she has integrity and is competent.

DIVORCE
(uncontested)
$250 + COSTS
SEPARATION AGREEMENT $110.00
• ALL CONSULTATIONS FREE
• ALL PHONE INQUIRIES WELCOME
HARRY SMITH
Attorney at Law
688-2194
Main and 8th
Jacksonville, FL 33277

If you cannot afford legal advice, you can go to the Legal Aid Society in your locality, which can be found in the telephone book. You will have to submit a detailed report on your financial status. You will be, if you qualify, assigned a lawyer, usually a neophyte who may not do as well as a lawyer having practiced a number of years but he will help you. If you have questions but no office number to contact, call the county or state bar association and they will direct you to a source or provide information themselves.

Our life will suffer because of divorce in most cases. Where people are removing shackles—they are now free to go to a possible new love, they have been mismatched or terribly treated, then divorce is a jubilee time! For most of us who felt unsure, guilty, inadequate and a pervasive sense of loss, it is a tragedy! Recognized, noted and absorbed, but it is not the end of life. If we learn lessons from divorce, it provides "open sesame" to a new life, a time for personal growth and increased self-awareness. Although the upheaval is great and for many traumatic, Norman Levy, noted New York psychiatrist says, "those who have grown through their personal experiences, tragedies, and pain find it gives them a new dimension as well as appreciation and understanding." We learn from our shortcomings, we learn what the needs of others are and to more effectively meet them, and we learn the fragile nature of human being—and give and take that forwards the best of life and the value to be placed on friendship. Take time to look back to the chapter on Love, Sex and Marriage, for if you marry again, many second marriages are better than the first; we find more complementary mates and have the maturity to make it succeed. Happy hunting!

CHAPTER X

DEATH AND MIDDLESCENCE

"Aloha"

Dying is a more difficult emotional experience than it was generations ago. Natural death, unlike violent death with which the media bombards us, is removed from our awareness. Relatives and friends die separate from us, in hospitals and nursing homes where we can see them only at specified times. We are such a mobile society that often even our friends die away from where we live in their second homes and retreats .. one of my best professional friends died last year 500 miles from my home. Some of us were planning to see him in the hospital; upon investigating the most suitable time to come, we were shocked to hear he had died and that the funeral would be the next day. As it turned out, our schedule preempted our even attending the services. We organized a scholarship fund in his memory. Even under other circumstances we often do not know what the dying person really feels and wants or what is expected of us. We are afraid and confused by this event that should be seen as natural and inevitable.

Death was not such a stranger for our great-grandparents. Then people were not taken off to the hospitals but died at home surrounded by those they had known and loved all their lives. My grandparents died under these conditions. Death, especially from contagious diseases, caused the demise of those from all ages, children to the elderly. In fact over a hundred years ago during plague or national disaster, death rates reached 40%, in addition one third of all babies died in infancy. Half of all children died before their tenth birthday. To the young and to adults, death was not a remote event at all. When older people died from natural causes, their children and grandchildren who often lived in the same house or close by, were associated directly with death in the family. Now death rates are typically below 9% and infant mortality only around 1%. Association with death is fewer and farther between times.

Dying with dignity, near to people who care, is an ideal and to anyone's lifetime. It is what we can help make possible for others and eventually for ourselves. Death is a topic which must be a concern for those of us in the in-between years for some time in this period there will be a vital involvement in the arrangements of caring for the dying spouse, parent or kinsman and perhaps facing the prospect of death at close hand ourselves. Unpleasant, morbid perhaps but part of life, yes, but life lived to the fullest takes the sting out of death as Nikos Kanantzakis write in his *Report to Greco*—"For this was my greatest ambition; to leave nothing for death to take—nothing but a few bones."

It has been said that nothing is certain but death and taxes. One may wonder, if only facetiously, whether taxes are not at least the more obvious of the two. For until middle age, we usually see little of death! The taboo, however, against discussing death is itself dying. A questionnaire some years ago in *Psychology Today* on Death drew 30,000 replies from their readers—setting a record for the magazine at that time for it topped by 10,000 the response to an earlier questionnaire of theirs on sex. Dr. Edwin Shneidman, author on death, commenting on this phenomenon said it was as though those thousands of persons had been waiting for legitimate occasion to unburden themselves about death and felt cleansed thereby. "Love Story," the film about a young woman who knew she was dying and about her husband's support to the end was the sensation of the early seventies. The theme song was a best seller!

On the *Psychological Today* questionnaire referred to earlier, the question, "Who died in your first personal involvement with death?" Forty-three percent said their grandparents, the next larger figure was 18%—it was animals. So 61% in this poll had not experienced the death of a parent or brother or sister or even aunt or uncle. Most of the respondents were young adults 21-25 years of age.

However, for the middle age person, death's disruption of on-going life is greatest. He or she experience during the middlescence period the trauma of the death of parents, usually both. Also uncles and aunts and many contemporaries die. Occasionally a child is lost; this is perhaps the greatest loss that can be suffered. Geoffrey Gorer in his *Death, Grief, and Mourning* says that if the child is grown the grief is more distressing and long lasting for the parents. It is thought that this is an unnatural event—a child should outlive his parents.

Sociologists have given a lot of time and energy to studying the way we have ritualized our behavior. These are significant in reducing our tensions. But little until recently has been done to help the dying patient emotionally. Doctors Glaser and Strauss in their book, *Awareness of Dying*, describe the elaborate system that many hospitals used to create in order to withhold information from patients, particularly the information that they are dying. Indications were that doctors made short, infrequent visits, visits of friends and family become emotionally distant and wear make-believe masks. One study showed that nurses took twice as long to answer the rings of dying patients as they did those who were not terminally ill. Of course, from medical school onward the force of the physician is to effect extension of life, this still is the goal. A person often wants to know so this revelation will bring his loved ones in rapport with him. This has changed in the last decade or so with increased concern of medical schools with ethics and death. The growth of the Hospice movement and the presentation in the general literature (newspaper, psychology and sociological books and in education whether on TV or in college classrooms) about issues such as the right to die, euthanasia, suicide, artificial maintenance of life and healthy dying is bringing death out of the closet.

Theory of Death and Dying

Dr. Kubler-Ross contends that there are five emotional stages in dying. Frequently the spouse, parents and even children or brothers and sisters of the dying person go through some of the steps that follow.

1. Shock and denial—no, not me, this is one way the person has to ward off an overwhelming, situation and give oneself time to develop a defense. It is a healthy way of confronting the initial news, saying "I can lick it."
2. Then denial changes to "Why me?" or "Why my child?" Frequently people will scream at God or blame Him and become envious of the young and healthy. If people in this stage can express their rage without being judged, they can often feel enough release to begin the next stage.
3. In this stage, the bargaining stage, if you give me one more year I'll be a good Christian, or we ask to live until the children finish school or get married. Burt Reynolds played the part of a man in this stage in the movie, "The End," by promising God a generous tithe to let him escape from drowning as he attempted suicide. However, the nearer he got to shore, the less he was interested in sharing his money

with God. Bargaining represents the recognition that time is limited and life is finite.

4. The fourth stage is depression—realistic depression. The truth has irrevocably dawned—people need to cry and grieve for the loss of their own life. This is very normal behavior. Many times loved ones go through this stage with the dying person.
5. The Acceptance Stage—peace is made with the Self and then the final moment of death is neither frightening nor painful. When I asked my personal friend and surgeon a few years ago whether or not most patients at the point of death realized it, he replied, "no, in most cases." Of course not all dying patients reach this final stage of acceptance or go through all the emotions of these stages or in the order suggested by Kubler-Ross.

Some investigators say people go through a "dying trajectory"—the interval between realization of death and death. The trajectory may be weeks or months, for the old dying trajectory is leisurely and less intense. Anxiety and use of defense mechanisms mark the usual trajectory called the acute state that is when death is near. A second aspect is the chronic stage where the person recognizes their plight but hope to get well. The final stage, the terminal, hope is given up for recovery and anxiety finally fades and the person accepts their death. The dying person is given up for recovery and anxiety finally fades and the person accepts their death. Ones cultural heritage, their environmental circumstances, gender, personality and developmental level effect the dying person. Kubler-Ross believes nearly all patients (certainly those sick for a length of time) know they are dying, including children. The clues come from doctors, nurses, and loved ones. He may even set up traps for those around and noting the contradictions and draws his own conclusions.

The Dying Child

Children who are terminally ill usually are not told they are dying. There are many professionals who have cared for dying children who believe that most children (above five or six years of age) lying in bed seriously ill are worrying about death and wish for someone to help them talk about their fear. Research by Myra Blue-Bond Langer suggests that terminally ill children are aware of the fact that they are dying and suggests that they become aware through these stages.

The Information Getting Process

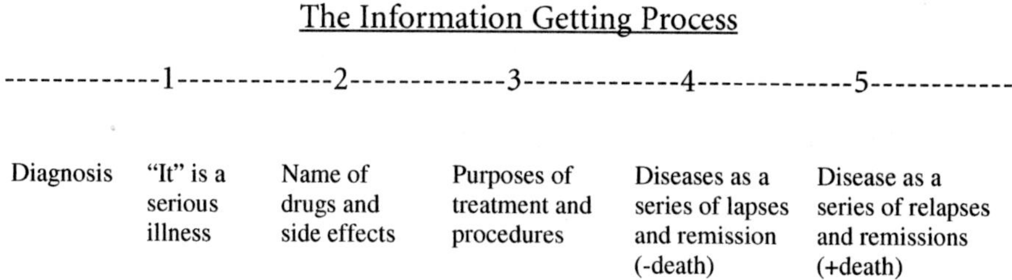

Ms. Blue-Bond Langer suggests that the leukemic child's acquisition of knowledge is a long process and even if they do not know the name of the disease, nevertheless learn its serious nature early. If another child with leukemia dies, then the child remaining changes is view of self somewhat along this line.

Self Concept Change

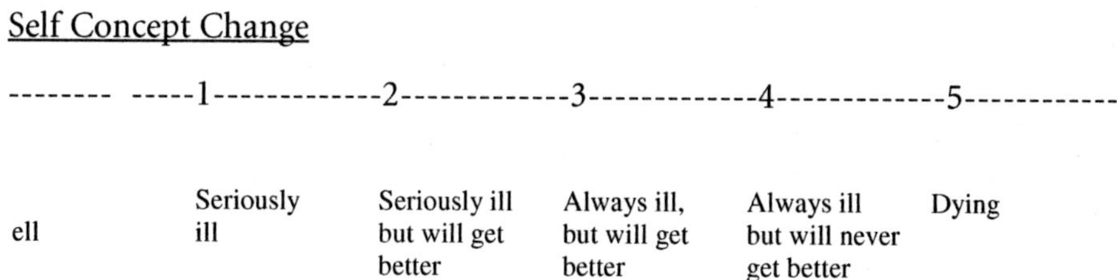

If you wonder about the maturity of the child and ability to understand you shouldn't. The intellectual ability in the child's coming to know he or she is dying is not the important element. What is significant is that the child is able to integrate and synthesize the information of his dying—this comes from ability gathered from experience, not age. According to our researcher, Blue-Bond Langer, the child passes from stage four to five in a brief time; for example, the child hears of the death of another child and quickly applies this to himself. Illustrations of this are seen in these scenarios:

Tom: Jennifer died last night. I have the same thing, don't I.

Nurse: But they are going to give you different medicine.

Tom: What happens when they run out?

Nurse: Well, maybe they will find more before then.

In the next talk the child tries to establish the cause of death by questions or stating a hypothesis and waiting for a reaction.

Jim: You know Lisa?

Mimi: (nods her head)

Jim: The one I played ball with. (pause) How did she die?

Mimi: She was sick, sicker than you.

Jim: I know that. What happened?

Mimi: Her heart stopped beating.

Jim: (Hugged Mimi and cried) I hope that that never happens to me, but…

Having established the cause of death in his own mind, the child ends the talk by comparing the deceased to himself.

There are many who feel the child goes through three stages upon recognition of dying: (1) Protest; (2) Despair; and (3) Detachment. The latter stage particularly is seen when the child if left to handle the burden and mystery of death alone and if the subject is so hush-hush, it indeed must be calamitous. In general, terminally ill children of all ages know they are dying excepting the very young. It was once thought this knowledge was only possible in children over nine years of age. These are terrifying subjects for them, but their knowledge of the finality of death based upon the most recent research confirms this.

Children from two to seven conceive of death (according to Wass) as being reversible, and that it is caused by the external and revival is possible by some means. From ages seven to eleven or twelve, death is irreversible, involves the cessation of functions, internal causation, is universal and has simple beliefs about life after death. The children above twelve years of age know of religious and philosophical theories of death, etc. One should remember that in all concepts great variability exists. Some four-year-olds have been found to understand the universality of death. Some helpful ideas for assisting the child and family with emotional aspects are offered later in this chapter.

The Dying Adolescent

At a time when young people prize their physical prowess and looks above everything, death's prospect comes as a shocking and debasing event. They are often shamed by the thought of their body being unhealthy. They are frequently highly resentful, for at a time when the struggle for independence and self-concept is most important, the growing years have come to naught. They say, "I must have been very bad to deserve this." It would not be human if they did not resent and envy the carefree, fun-filled lives of their peers. Professional health personnel have the most difficult time in dealing with dying adolescents. They have greater maturity than do younger children, hence recognize sooner their condition. The stages of dying and its emotional aspects are much like that of adults. Caretakers can facilitate the grieving process by open communication. If the process is closed then the youth cannot share their grief. In fact some try to protect their parents. One dying girl said, "Dad was upset today, I could tell. I'll try to keep a good attitude—it'll be easier on Mom and Dad." Fortunately life is safest at this time than in any other period although the toll from suicide (the third leading cause of death among adolescents) and automobile accidents is rising. In these cases there is often no forethought allowed for tomorrow.

Effect of Death on the Family

It is generally supposed that death has the least effect upon the middle-aged person. Principally this is due to the idea that they are in the prime of life (hence has strength to bear up), have some family to fill the gap of the person missing, and are experienced in death and funeralizing. Of course, this is relative to who dies and their importance in the middlescent persons' life. In the placing of stressful events and conditions on a continuum, the death of a spouse rates at the top, with a score of 100 of Life Changing Units (LCU). An investigation of Drs. Holmes and Rahe of the University of Washington found that the questioning of 5,000 subjects that they placed the death of a husband or wife at the top of the most stressful events. It is well known that of all people vulnerable to disease, those who are bereaved for some period of time have the highest risk. A study in Britain showed that the death rate for women who had been bereaved for a year or less was ten times higher than for another group of women who were similar in every respect except bereavement. Accident proneness is significant during this period; people appear to be in a daze and morose and many of them in fact are. Obviously the psyche protects by insulating the bereaved with the cloak of withdrawal putting a wall around until recovery is effected. I have seen parents who refused to admit that their son was dead—following World War II death of her young son, one mother I knew kept the gold star in her window for years claiming her son to be alive. Another mother refused to examine the body of her alleged son brought home from the war—It's not my boy! When the death of a person close to us is impending over a period of time due to a terminal illness, anticipatory grief characterizes those that will be left behind. I visited the home recently following the death of the husband of a colleague of mine to offer condolences. The lady professor embraced me as I tried to express my sorrow and offer of help. She brushed this aside instead and told and retold me—I can't cry, I just can't cry! There's no need now for you to dry, I said, for you've been grieving for years, please don't plague yourself with that. She had taken good care of her husband; undoubtedly we feel relieved after long ordeals and just a little guilty we can't cry. We can expect to have appetites vanish, insomnia to be the rule, irritability and loss of sleep characteristic of this period in our lives. We can take some comfort from the fact that mourning usually lasts for about a year after death. The sudden and unexpected loss of a loved one in an accident can cause a debilitating shock to the survivors. Recent studies of bereavement reaction show that the mourning period to last longer in these cases, often as long as three or four years where children and spouses are involved. Bereaved parents—the studies indicate—frequently showed coping difficulties including less ability to talk to relatives about their lost and they were often depressed. Bereaved spouses had even more depression, their general psychological well-being was similar to that of psychiatric out-patients—they felt less optimistic about the future and worried about bad things happening to them. Parker and Weirs call this the unexpected grief syndrome. Bereaved parents and spouses it is reported had greater tendency to change jobs and experience financial loss. Divorce is also higher among bereaved parents.

It takes time to redefine and reintegrate our lives. The greatest thing we can offer to the bereaved is to be with them, and avoid telling them what they should do. They'll ask you when they are ready for your information and help.

Rose Franblau in her work, the *Middle Generation*, says that when one member of a present-day Middle Generation couple dies, the survivor's reactions may be somewhat different than in the past. At first he may feel, typically, that he will never marry again. Then as the period of mourning approaches its end, he becomes restless and complaining. It is his way of facing the possibility that he may really want to build a new life after all. But he may fear that he will not be wanted by anyone. Finally, his mourning period over and his grief assuaged, he is ready to make a completely healthy adjustment to ongoing life. He moves out into the world again, fully prepared to take on new relationships. In a sense, by overcoming his sense of loss, he has conquered death. More and more, Ms. Franblau says, this is becoming characteristic of bereaved Middle Generation members who do not passively accept permanent widowhood as their lot while they are still young and want to build a new and different life.

My minister brother lost his wife and our mother within a month of each other. Six months later I visited him—no food was in the ice box, he was in bed (8 p.m.) and I learned from his secretary he had been ill with a variety of health problems. Fortunately, he made a miraculous recovery on the following Valentine's Day when he remarried!

This double blow is perhaps the most severe one that can exist. Sometimes there are a succession of deaths—parents, aunts and uncles, which run together. This happened to our family; the older you get the more likely that a cluster of friends and kin people will die and sometimes over a brief period of time. We start out in life far back in the pack among our family, in the middle age we reach the vanguard. Before we leave middlescence, we sometimes look around and find we are leading the parade of our people. Certainly during the middlescent years one can see forward, with a clear view, the road of life stretched out before us plainly marked.

The effect of death on both children and adolescent can be significant and revealing. According to Maria Nagy's study, there are three stages in the child's knowledge of death. Stage I—This stage is up until about age 5, the child here has not grasped the idea of finality, curiosity exists in the child about what happens to the body and why is it buried. The fact of separation between the living and the dead does not come across clearly to the child at this age. Death is also seen as very similar to sleep. In Stage II—considerable changes take place (5-9) in that the child begins to appreciate that death is final. Children tend to think of death as a person. The death-person may be a ghost, clown, or some mysterious figure that comes around at night. Another interesting feature of this period in children is that though death is final, a person who is very clever can luck out and avoid death. Death as a person is nearly universal among children; it seems to provide some sort of shield to protect the child from the full implications of the realization that death is the end—that is, final. As Nagy says, at this point death is outside us and is not general.

In Stage III death is understood in this period (9 to 10 onward) as inevitable and universal—everyone dies. A ten-year-old girl said: "It is like the flower withering away and the leaves in fall falling from the trees." Children see death in the plan and animal kingdom hence themselves. One should be cautioned against thinking that the conception of death in the final adult sense is found in every child of ten or even fifteen. The view of mental development (Piaget) and others hold is that the ability to think about thought (abstract level of ability) does not become well established until early adolescence. The point emphasized here is that children think of death differently, then too maturity and experience differ. A study of 600 mid-western children showed the following:

Children of 5-6 imagined a dead body would stay exactly as it was forever or perhaps come back in a different form.

Age 7 The body decayed

Age 8 Death as total cessation was less acceptable, increasing belief in spiritual immortality. This was true for Catholic, Protestant and Jewish children. The belief in spiritual continuation increased until the age of 13-14 when it dropped off sharply but among the Catholic children where it only dropped slightly.

The old English game of "ring around the roses" or "ashes to ashes we all fall down" is a ritual suggesting a subtle orientation to the death fact of mortality. This game played by children living in the shadow of the plague hundreds of years ago. Hide and seek was another game with a death-related origin.

When children lose their parents, sister or a brother, they may feel not only guilt and self-blame but a devastating sense of abandonment or deliberate desertion. They should be helped to understand it is not their fault nor have they been deserted. Death can be the ultimate in trauma. I witnessed a tragedy some years ago. There was a family living in an apartment where we lived, when I first began to teach in college, made up of the father and mother and two children, a girl of ten and a boy of nine. The children came from school one day to find their father dead on the kitchen floor; their mother was at work and consequently they were left to receive the shock alone. After this happened, the young son would not want to leave his mother and often he would come home from school unexcused during the day to see if his mother was there and alive. This continued until psychological therapy was suggested by the family physician. The problem, though some facets of it are undisclosed, is still plaguing the boy and his family. Significant insecurity and a feeling of aloneness apparently existed before the death of the father.

In attempting to comfort children and help them believe in personal immortality, some parents tell their children that the person who has died has gone to heaven and is extremely happy there. Nancy Doyle, a mental health writer, relates the following story and its effect. A mother painted a glowing picture of heaven to her six-year-old son about his father who had recently died being in heaven and now having the time of his life. A few weeks later the mother was stunned to find her son banging his head on a rock bursting a blood vessel. After a quick visit to the doctor, she asked why he did such a thing—the son said he wanted to join his father up in heaven having picnics and fun.

The effect of losing a parent can be so crucial that grief and its effect last long after the death. Talking to the child or adolescent in the following vein of "Well, it's been a long time since your father died, you should focus on something else," falls most often on barren ground and thwarts recovery. I knew a youngster of 15 who was so affected by his father's death (the father was 43) that he cursed God openly and literally shook his fist toward the sky. He also developed the idea he would die on the same anniversary date of his father's death the following year. He didn't die the next year; six months later he seemed to have accepted his father's death, adjusting to the reality of the situation. But it takes time, often much time.

Though death always has some laments of sadness, it often has some salutary effects upon the family. Persons in the family all bear the responsibility of caring for the incurably sick, the chronic drunkard, the drug addict, and the bed bound. For those, particularly among the very old, death is looked upon as a great release from pain and the worthlessness of life. They are ready to die having finished grieving for themselves a long time ago. The energy and economy of a caretaker taken by a desperate struggle may have stymied the development of opportunity to try new things and create new vistas. Children in a situation where the deceased formerly lived at home are given a chance to utilize the home more freely as a center of entertainment and relaxation. The death of a spouse or parent can have the effect of drawing the rest of the family together, giving them a sense of responsibility and camaraderie, which did not exist before. Another thing to remember is that many households are now presided over by one parent (nearly half in 1990) due to divorce and separation. Not to be forgotten is the fact that there is usually a legacy left (money, property, goods, equipment) from the death of parents and grandparents; if unencumbered with few or no debts, this can be a boon for the economically depressed family or a God-send to help with the children's care and future education. If this doesn't happen, still for those who have borne the labor long in care of the sick and dying, the final lifting of the load is welcomed. Neither should we exercise ourselves about what we failed to do—maybe we didn't do enough—but if we tried our best, we can take comfort in that fact. If we did nothing, then we have been rewarded already with a poisoned well of memory and poorer life.

What Will Help?

It is universally agreed that grief and a period of mourning have to be a part of the recovery usually needed to assuage the terrible feeling of loss and loneliness. Nowhere has it been expressed better than by the old bard—Shakespeare—where he wrote, "Give sorrow words," "the grief that does not speak knits up the o'erwrought heart and bids it break." The fear of being abandoned, yearning for the lost figure, and anger that this had to happen is all a part of the struggle to maintain sanity and life during our depression. Following his wife's death Booth, the great Shakespearean actor, though she was buried some distance from his performing locations, visited the grave frequently. It was said he would throw himself upon the grave and lament with oaths, which he shouted, but mainly shedding copious tears and crying for her to return. When coaxed to end "this lunacy" by kin and friends, he replied that "this is all I have left of her, my memory and grief." Though it was thought by some that his visitations related to a pathological condition and it may have been, nevertheless that the display of grief eventually helped to provide a cure. For all of us following a significant death even of famous figures—Roosevelt, Kennedy, King—a sickness unto death embrace us, we breathe slower, and melancholia engulfs us. As John Doone penned, "ask not for who the bell tolls, it tolls for thee.." no man is an island to himself.

The stages of grief have been identified by three categories—the reaction stage, disorganization and reorganization stage and reorientation and recovery stage. During the initial stage, shock is the principal characterization. Numbness and a dazed lack of feeling follow this; this reaction allows the survivor a buffer allowing them to accomplish the funeralizing details. During the second stage—disorganization and reorganization—reality sets in and disappointment that the loss cannot be recovered. Despair may leave the individual with unfocused thoughts and inability to make sense out of all activities or to be sure of themselves. They may become very dependent on others for help. The process of reorganization from such a painful emotional response is difficult because the grief-stricken person must dismantle the former structure of connectedness and activities surrounding the loved one. Feelings in this period are complicated and conflicting for to grieve is to pay respect-to give up grieving is to lose respect and probably feel guilty. To grieve is to live a tragic role; giving it up means cutting the nexus to the respect of others. Hence the feeling of loss of identity and the feeling of losing one's mind. In the final stage reorientation and recovery the person modifies the symbolic world to give the deceased a new identity outside the world of the survivors in heaven or some transcendental sphere. Funeral ceremonies, memorial services, etc., are the transitions to new perspectives on life. Grief becomes resolved when the individual is able to reintegrate with the world, interact with others, find avenues to creative living and take charge of their lives.

Learning to live without a loved one is difficult for they are a part of you and your accustomed behavior. Ways in which some people adjust are to find an explanation for the death, often this leads to a search for a scapegoat. Thought these are typically non-productive, they perhaps reduce anger and self-destructive pain. Some are mental fantasy to recapture the old patterns of the deceased. Some seek to establish communion with the dead through prayer or through mediums. A way to lessen the loss of a loved one many religious people think, is through keeping the interaction patterns intact—that is, preserving the social relationships by reuniting through spiritual references to faith in after life and promises of the Bible. Rituals and talking of the departed person through reminiscing about experiences with friends and kin are some excellent ways to mend out lives and mental health.

It is important for adults to outwardly express their feelings of grief, which are normal and give rise to ambivalent emotions of fear, loneliness, anger and guilt. During mourning this should be expressed. This great need for therapeutic talk is one of the major factors for the evolution of our funeral customs. The presence of a friend comforts a bereaved person. You don't have to feel that you must express deep philosophical thought to the bereaved person(s). Conversation with them should be natural and one should listen with empathic concern. Appropriate cards and small gifts before and after the death to loved ones are helpful. Common sense tells us that funerals are for the living. It is only recently that we have recognized, says Dr. Eric Lindemann of Harvard University, that depression, sorrow and the loss of those who belong to the supportive human environment can be equally severe hazards in a person's life.

A therapy which should not be overlooked by adults and for children is a visit for a few days or weeks to another locale during the mourning period. Even a vacation with friends or family can be a great aid in helping one sort out their lives, getting over the numbness they feel, and making a beginning on living again. Of course, one cannot run away from the environment entirely nor should they, but after the initial shock some time in another environment is helpful. Some have found that throwing themselves into a frenzy of work is good medicine—being active is certainly helpful as an aid in getting our eating and other patterns started again.

We have already mentioned how difficult it is for adults to grasp fully that someone near to them is dead and will not return. For children it is clearly much more difficult. Many children and adolescents deny the final reality and many have the expectation that the lost parent will return to their life. One only needs to remember his own childhood experience in normal separations from parents like at camp, schooling with the subsequent homesickness to confirm this. This has been found in children and adolescents who have been receiving professional therapy. A psychiatrist, M. J. Barnes, reported two nursery age children, 2½ and 4 at the time when they lost their mother, who again and again continued to express the hope and expectation that mother would return. When they were helped by the analysts and finally knew there would be no return, they reacted with panic and anger. Another therapist, M. Wolfenstein, reports on Ruth, a 15-year-old subject, who remarked some months after her mother died, "If my mother were really dead, I would be all alone…I would be terribly scared." Another time it is recalled that Ruth, in bed at night, would sometimes feel beyond control with "frustration, rage and yearning. She tore the bed clothes off the bed, rolled them into the shape of a human body, and embraced them." We should emphasize that it is immensely important that a child have available a single and permanent substitute to whom he can be or gradually become attached. Only in this circumstance can it be expected that it will ultimately be possible for the child to accept the loss as certain and then to reorganize his inner life accordingly.

Suppressing grief or denying it including anticipatory grief can have disastrous effects on anybody, especially children. Sylvia Plath in her book, *The Bell Jar*, poignantly described the harrowing mental breakdown of her young heroine and the desperate trip to her father's grave. At the grave she was overcome with convulsive grief. Years before, when her father (Plath's) was dying in the hospital, she was not permitted to see him, and even after his death she had not been allowed to attend his funeral. She didn't allow herself to cry. Her mother had never cried or shown any emotion, though she said, "What a good thing it was that the father had been spared a lot of suffering." To a young daughter, who needs and deeply loves her father, there can be no gratitude for his death. Grief is the natural response to such profound devastation. Not expressing it—or submerging it with a bunch of platitudes, eventually takes its toll on children. Author Plath's own life paralleled her story—she committed suicide at thirty. Psychoanalytic studies show tht a person who is unable to complete the grieving and mourning tasks in childhood tries to give up his or her real feelings to prevent being overwhelmed by them. Later as a result, they may be haunted by a pervasive sadness which remain unexplained and debilitating. Failure of a child to grieve fully at the loss of a parent, many psychiatrists believe, is a contributing factor in a number of suicides. Good-byes are important. The way they are said matters, of course to the dying and also even more to those who remain. How good-byes are said can reduce the lifetime scars for those left behind, especially children and adolescents who are often baffled, terrified and guilt-ridden by the experience.

A Help to Mourners

Increasingly more attention is being paid to assisting bereaved individuals to cope with their loses. Security and sense of being safe are factors facilitating reduction of tension. When the bereaved is alone a close friend or relative should come in for a few weeks, a brief visit with him or friends would be helpful to change the environment, though the home is a constant reminder of the loved one lost—it is one's best retreat and comfort. In time it will be treasured and hallowed as such. Friends and neighbors can tell the bereaved when you wish to come over for a visit when things get difficult.

Those whose only concern is expressed as pity leave the bereaved feeling weaker and less secure. Studies of statements made by caring persons to bereaved individuals that made them feel supported and understood or alienated and hurt revealed 80% of all responses made by "caring persons" could be categorized as non-helpful and low-facilitative in nature. Such statements as come with us now, it's okay to be angry with God. It must be hard to accept, tell how you're feeling and how can I be of help are facilitative (supportive). The non-facilitative is seen in sayings like: god had a purpose; I know how you feel; time heals all things; you have to keep going; he or she had a good life; it's over so let's not deal with it and you're not the only one who suffers.

Death Education

The idea of death should be presented long before a child actually encounters death as an emotion-charged event of significant loss. In this way the child at least becomes familiar with the concept of death before his first saddening personal contact with it. Younger children, Dr. Edgar Jackson in his book, *Telling A Child About Death*, says should not attend funerals, that is under three or four years of age. But at five or six this should perhaps become a part of the experience. Though some people feel that children up to eight or nine should be shielded from death, it would be a full-time and futile job to shelter a child from death in all its manifestations even in a society such as ours that has become famous for trying to keep mortality out of sight and out of mind.

Children can learn about death through pets. The significance of the death of a cat, dog or bird can make a signal impression upon a child. Some parents take this opportunity to teach about the meaning of death, by answering questions about what has happened and even having a burial and service. Some children already knowledgeable ask for a service. Children come through many ways, to find out for themselves about death, even the very young soon discover in old pictures around the house that these persons are no longer around—often they ask about them. Since in growing up children aren't separated by age in their neighborhoods playing, many four and five year olds are initiated into discussions of or listening to talk about death by older children and adolescents. Treating death as a natural process, not hiding feelings of less or on the other hand making it a way of life is recommended. The mother, we reported earlier who kept hanging the old star in the window years after her boy was reported killed, make life a burden—a burden for the young girl in the family and her husband for the ghost of the son became the focal point of living in that home; the home was organized around it.

The child and adolescent have specific needs: (1) a close loved one (the permanent substitute) or person with whom they can communicate and from whom they can receive comfort and assurance; (2) to be allowed to participate in the funeral activities (those over five); (3) to be allowed to express, act out their own grief in however long it takes. If extreme reactions are evident over a period of time, certainly professional advice from the physician first and then upon his recommendations therapy from others is suggested.

Special Circumstances of Death

The middlescent has generally in his in-between years the prospect of having some relation to special circumstances surrounding death. Many of those have to do with their parents. If one is married, then some connection with the death of four persons is not uncommon—two for you and two for your spouse. Questions arise over such subjects as euthanasia, suicide, preservation of the body in a frozen state, cremation, etc. These topics will be discussed in the following pages.

Suicide

One of the most difficult situations we can possibly have is to deal with the suicide of our spouse, parent or child. It is usually baffling, though not always, for it leaves with many unanswered questions usually, that it adds burdens far beyond the cases of those who die as the terminally ill or even suddenly if they are adults. Very few people are able to handle this with any detachment for it is not just that we have suffered a loss but that the deceased have left us the message of our ultimate failure with them or our own inadequacy in dealing with them Anthony J. La Greca says suicide by definition is the conscious intentional taking of one's life through an identifiable, discrete act. This rules out accidents although many suicides may be disguised as mishaps by the survivors.

That many sick and aged wish to die is undoubtedly true as witness the death of Nicholas A, a lonely 78 year old Polish migrant who writes a sad letter home, concluding with this paragraph:

> "I am sick and tired of the constant enemas I get, and my stomach hurts, and my left hand can't lift anything. It seems I will remain a cripple, and if with such bad health one has to suffer (and my left side hurts very much), in order not to be a burden to anyone, I decided to do away with myself." He was later found dead by a bullet discharged from a gun held in his one good hand.

The philosophical and ethical question as whether a suicide such as this always should be prevented has received comparatively little attention. There are four types of suicide presented in the book *The Suicidal Person* which our society often endorsed as being rational and in regard to which the ethics of intervention might be open to question:

1. Suicides carried out for the good of some cause such as religious, military heroism and dramatic social witness or terrorist such as the driver of the truck that crashed into an embassy in Lebanon.
2. Those carried out as a reaction to what appears to be hopeless, painful or debilitating as in terminal illness. The death of Hemingway might fall into this category.
3. Those in which circumstances are not desperate, but in which the individual is no longer receiving the pleasure from life that he wants, and so makes the decision to go through the open door away from life.
4. The so-called love pact suicide where the double death is seen as having some aesthetic value, possible being an expression of love, beauty or dedication. The "star crossed" lovers' death of Romeo and Juliet is an example.

Although the ancient Stoics of Greece and Rome upheld the right to suicide, the Christian Church beginning with the writings of St. Augustine in the *City of God* suggested suicide is never justified because, for the Christian, hope always exists. With some moderation the Church has viewed suicide thusly to this day.

Though the actual number of suicides in America was estimated to be 30,000 to 100,000 per year, less than the number killed in automobile accidents, none the less significant quality of capable persons are lost, and the potential number of suicides looms exceedingly large. In 2000 there were 40,000 suicides acknowledged adding those masked it might reach double or 80,000. This includes euthanasia, cover ups of suicide, assisted suicides by doctors and nurses through withholding air, food and medicine. This doesn't include suicide under the category of suicidal erosion or indirect suicide as in heavy smokers (two to three packs a day), drinker, reckless drivers, risk takers which when added to the others easily total beyond 100,000 a year. The lethality of method range from a 91.6 percentage effectiveness from gunshot (carbon monoxide 78%) to a 4.1% by cutting (poisons and drugs was 23%) and 11.5% respectively). It is estimated that for every completed self-instituted demise there are 10 times this number who have attempted to end their life. If we take the figure of 50,000 for a yearly toll and multiply this by the attempts, we arrive at a half of a million persons per year; in one decade this would reach 5 million persons. The presence of this vast pool in the population becomes slightly awesome.

Who are the potential suicide victims. 2003 statistics show 4 of every 100,000 are women, 11.7 for men both for all ages. The Metropolitan Life Insurance Company in a Statistical Bulletin listed the causes of suicide for a year in Detroit. Among adult women 50% related to domestic difficulties, 20% ill health, and 10% love affairs and other miscellaneous reasons. For adult men 40% ill health, 30% domestic affairs, 3% love affairs, the rest a various of causes (2003 National Center for Health Statistics). The largest age group of suicides comes from those over 65 with 31.1 of 100,000 men to only 4 of 100,000 for women, young males 15-24 17.1 for only 3 for women out of 100,000. This is down from 1980 by 1.8 of 100,000. Suicide is the eighth leading cause of death in the U.S. among people 45-64, ahead of AIDS and kidney disease ninth and tenth (nearly 9,000 in 2001) in the 45-65 group.

Models Explain Suicide

The various models attempt to explain suicide. The psychiatric and psychological models say people who kill themselves suffer from a mental or emotional disorder. Of these victims 15 to 25% are said to be alcoholics. The sociocultural models suggest suicide depends upon the individual's adjustment to the social order and its ability to influence suicide. Durkheim and advocate, states that suicide is due to the strength or weakness of the bond between an individual and social groups. Some say in Durkheim's day not much was known of psychological pathology.

The economic and political models suggest unemployment increases suicide, strikes cause a lower of suicide (creates greater integration with the group). Wars tend to unite people providing greater political integration. Suicide careers suggest some people are involved in a series of stepping stones leading to self-destruction. Researchers isolated such markers as family problems—lack of security and love when young, sexual abuse, alcoholism, illnesses, foster home problems. A study of 50 females by Stephens found two out of three had parents who did not express affection and were often relentlessly critical. One third grew up in a broken home, 3% had been sexually and physically abused, 26% were from families having mental illness and 22% from families of alcoholics. Divorce was found by Stack to relate to suicide on the magnitude that a 1 percent increase in divorce meant an additional 127 suicides.

In general suicide is usually attributed to the older person rather than the young, men rather than women, and those who have early in their lives lost a mother or father, who live alone, are depressed and in their late forties or fifties. White men have the highest rate of suicide in their 50's and 60's with black men its from 25 to 44. Black women have their highest rte 35 to 44. While white women 45 to 64. The suicide rate for American males is not as great as many countries in Europe such as Poland, Switzerland, Sweden, Denmark, Australia, Norway, etc. or Japan which has a fairly high rate. Males commit suicide 2 to 3 times more frequently than women. Women attempt suicide 3 to 5 times more frequently than males. It is said that women and the young attempt suicide and men and older people complete it.

Adolescent suicide is dramatically rising in the U.S. Any act of self-destruction whether suicidal or attempted suicide involves a complicated interplay of forces. We must recognize the risk factors. Studies of adolescents who have attempted suicide together with psychological autopsies reveal certain "risk factors." These are as follows: (1) previous attempts (the best predictor), (2) Depression, feelings of loneliness and hopelessness, (3) Psychiatric problems and antisocial personality, (4) Alcohol and drug abuse, (5) stressful life events—family turmoil, separation and divorce of parents, (6) little support and care and (7) access to firearms. Most youth suicides in the making can be observed in these risk factors hopefully by observant parents, public school and mental health organizations aid can serve to circumvent these deaths.

A mother in Meriden, Connecticut was convicted of contributing to the suicide of her 12-year old son because of the squalid conditions of her home. The filthy house with papers, debris and clothes covering the floor and the bath. The air was foul and obviously no bathing for the son. His classmates picked on him because of his bad breath and body odor drove him to kill himself. The mother, a Wal-Mart employee and part-time teacher was put on 5 years probation and remanded to community service. She showed no remorse but said she loved the boy! It represents the outcome of struggle between acceptance and rejection of life. Partly this struggle is an internal one among the conflicts of purposes, which exist within the individual. Partly it is between the individual and his immediate environment. Karl Menninger has said:

> The public is apt to jump to superficial conclusions about the motivations of suicide based on explanations which appear logical but do not explain it. The notion that the fear of poverty, a disappointment in love, a feeling of guilt about business dishonesty, and the like cause suicide, is naive and a totally inadequate assumption. People who commit suicide for these ostensible reasons have generally begun their self-destruction long before these things occur. If one takes the pains

> to investigate with patience and persistence all the circumstances internal and external, connected with the suicide one finds a very different basis for its etiology.

What about the causation of self-destruction? The sociologist Farmer suggests that the suicide probability is the function of the individual's vulnerability and the degree of certain deprivations. This varies from an earlier theory by Emile Durkheim and psychoanalytic theories because they focused mainly on vulnerability in the person. Suicides in the main are committed by psychologically damaged personalities confronted by a deprivation situation(s). The life long need of love and support of parents is demanded for their children. Persons who constantly low-rate themselves, are never optimistic about life and the future and are depressed and find little fulfillment in life, are the ones exposed to the thought of suicide. Many suicides could be prevented—unfortunately many of those thinking and talking about suicide have no one who properly interprets these signals. Chronic expressions about the hatefulness of life and extreme hopelessness are frequently clues to self-extermination.

When people talk about suicide that should be taken seriously; usually this indicates a cry for help—make me know I'm worth saving and that you care. True, many will not kill themselves that talk about it but many do and you cannot afford to take a chance. Every community of any size usually has a suicide "hot line" or "crisis line" where help and advice can be dispensed. Many ministers and social workers have special training in this area and are available for helping. We should recognize that suicide is not a crime, it was in yesteryear, and that many persons die at their own hands for good reasons as those mentioned earlier. There is no reason why the suicide should not have the same type of funeral others have and families should recognize that suicide is due to a complex origin and in which most of the time they have played only a minor role.

Euthanasia (Right to Suicide) death (thanatos). They thought man was entitled to a comfortable, painless death. In modern society the problem involved is a primary concern of medical ethics in both negative and positive ways. In the former sense it means commission of an act (putting an air bubble in a blood vessel) to terminate life, and the latter to fail to provide all that would sustain life. In the middle ages by papal authority of the Catholic Church physicians were required to tell the patient he was dying. This was done to allow time for the proper church and personal ministrations relating to the departure of the soul and good-byes to family and friends. In this situation, the person participated in his death. As late as the civil war, soldiers knowledgeable for death from wounds or impending battle gave directions about themselves and families. They also often pinned identification on coats and shirts to help the burial details, friends and kin with identity. Priests and/or chaplains were called to render last rites and to pray for them. In the hit TV mini series *Lonesome Dove*, the hero, Gus, defied the removal of a gangrenous left leg—this final loss was just too much! He stood death down!

The crux of the problem in any uniform approach to euthanasia, that is, making of laws, has been the question of homicide. The intelligent victims of painful incurable disease who desire to hasten their death are far from unreasonable. But to legislate this is impossible because it places the responsibility for mercy killing in the hands of those whose major function is to extend life. Moral, legal and social issues abound in the debate over the notion of right to suicide. The Roman Catholic Church permits an end to treatment that serves only to mean a precarious and burdensome prolongation of life. This applies only to formal medical treatment. The California case of Clarence Herbert who slipped into a coma after surgery—the doctor told the family he was clinically dead. The family allowed the doctors to terminate food and water. He subsequently died and forthwith the Los Angeles authorities prosecuted the doctor for murder. As it stands both the medical and legal professions are hesitant to take the issue of life and death out of the hands of health care deliverers and put them under control of the courts. With such legal problems on the increase right-to-suicide must contend with the possibility of having attorneys arguing over one's bedside before a judge. No problem, perhaps, until this becomes politicized as it was in Hitler's Germany when mercy killing beginnings ended as merciless killing of the Jewish and other people. The issue of sterilization of society's misanthropes has been advocated by many Americans to cure economic ills and save the race strength through pollution of its spread of "bad" genes. This was done in some institutions for the mentally retarded several decades ago, there is some indication that the U.S. government was involved. This was too much to accept but what about the right to die in a society where we hear about the right to life.

The Right to Die with Dignity or With a Struggle

Thomas Mann once said, "A man's dying is more the survivors affair than his own." In most ways this is true for we have come to view death as non-existent, institutionalized and even a product to be marketed in the western world. Philippe Aries writing in the book *Death Inside Out* tells the story of an old woman who was at first well behaved, cooperating with the doctors and the nurses in the hospital and bearing her illness courageously. One day she decided she had had enough of the struggle and the time to give up had come. She closed her eyes, never to open them again, signifying that she had withdrawn from the world and wished to await her end and to be alone. In former times this wish would have been respected and accepted as normal. But in this California hospital, it brought dismay to the medical staff, so much so that they flew in one of her sons from another city to persuade her to open her eyes on the grounds that she was "hurting everybody." Sometimes patients turn to the wall and refuse to move. We recognize in such acts one of the oldest gestures of man in the fact of death. The Jews of the Old Testament died in this fashion. Our literature hero, Tristan, did the same exclaiming that he could no longer keep hold on life. The California doctors and nurses said (of the old woman) this was only an antisocial refusal to communicate and if you will, culpable renouncing of life. Of course physicians hope that the exertion of will might affect, given time, a cure or chance for them to rectify the difficulty of disease.

There is a new model of death abroad in America today which suggests a "style of dying" which translated means an acceptable style of living while dying. What is important is that one die in a manner than can be accepted and tolerated by the survivors. The graceless style of dying is to lament one's impending death, to make a scene and outburst. Whatever he knows or feels about the condition of his health and its final decline, he must have the consideration and courage to be discreet. The view of the naturalness of death like birth is in our modern culture verboten (forbidden). Death as the natural (it is caused and clearly not natural) culmination of a long life should be the rule of things where the individual is not made a vegetable or object beyond his desire.

Jane Brody (2003) long time writer on health issues and related problems tells of her problems with her mother's death forty-five years ago. As her mother was dying the nurse slapped on the oxygen mask and asked her to hold it. She had no chance to say I love you but remembers well the "medical event." Not much has changed in the ensuing years. Rose Virani (2003) a research specialist at the City of Hope National Medical Center in California laments the loss of communication between healthcare and hospital staff when family is kept from an injured loved one like Dave Fulkerson who was hit by a car jogging with his girlfriend. In intensive care his family were not allowed to see him. After a short time he could no longer talk. They allowed one person five minutes with him every two hours. The girlfriend frustrated went home, his parents fell asleep and then awakened to hear their son had died. Communication is not the only problem in allowing peaceful deaths. In 1996,

30 healthcare groups endorsed the American Geriatric Society's important factors for quality care at the end of life. Their list follows:

(1) Alleviating physical and emotional symptoms
(2) Helping the patient maintain dignity
(3) Using treatment that reflect the patient's wishes
(4) Avoiding inappropriate aggressive care
(5) Giving the patient and family quality time together
(6) Minimizing the family's financial burden
(7) Informing patients about insurance coverage
(8) Giving the patient the best quality of life
(9) Helping the family with bereavement.

Unfortunately of review by the Geriatric Society in 2002 overwhelming disappointing results to their initiatives, Elizabeth Pitorak (2004) an end of life care expert analyzed "active dying" or total body failure, which she says, takes 10-14 days. This is the substance of what she reveals about the final days. Ms. Pitorak is Director of Hospice Institute Western Reserve, Cleveland, Ohio. "Active dying, the process of total body system failure, usually occurs over a period of 10 to 14 days, although it can take as little as 24 hours," Ms. Pitorak says.

Dying patients become dehydrated; swallowing becomes hard; and peripheral circulation decreases, resulting in perspiration and clammy skin that feels cold to the touch. This should not be a sign to pile on blankets, however, because "most dying patients can't tolerate even the slightest weight on the feet or other extremities," she wrote.

Pulmonary congestion can prompt patients to gasp for breath. But, says, supplying oxygen is not the way to relieve this "air hunger" because a dying person usually cannot benefit from it.

Rather, opening windows, using a fan, allowing space around the patient's bed and administering morphine or some other opioid are the best ways to relieve a patient's feelings of breathlessness and anxiety.

When difficulty swallowing makes eating or drinking impossible, the question of tube-feeding arises. But dying patients are usually not hungry and "the absence of hydration and nutrition may even induce an analgesic euphoria" as ketone bodies build up in the blood. Even a little sugar administered intravenously can counteract this euphoria, she noted.

Furthermore, efforts to feed a dying patient orally can result in vomiting, aspiration and a violent, rather than a peaceful, demise.

Ms. Pitorak observed that while IV fluids can help terminally ill patients who become delirious from dehydration, they can also cause swelling, nausea and pain in patients who are actively dying. But, she added, if patients on opioids have kidney failure—resulting in confusion, muscle spasms and seizures from a failure to clear the blood of the drug—hydration and less medication may help.

As someone nears the end of life, it is not unusual for them to turn inward and become less communicative, even as much as three months before death. Ms. Pitorak noted that loved ones should not confuse this withdrawal with rejection. Rather, she said, it reflects the dying person's need to leave the outer world behind and focus on inner contemplation.

Experts tell families not to wait until the last hours of life to communicate with dying loved ones. In a study of 100 terminally ill cancer patients, 56 were awake one week before they died, 44 percent were drowsy, but none were comatose. In the final six hours, however, only 8 percent were awake, 42 percent were drowsy and half were comatose, precluding any further communication.

As death approaches, oral muscles relax and secretions that accumulate in the throat or chest can result in loud, gurgling breathing sounds—the so-called death rattle—that can be disturbing. But rather than trying to suction these secretions, a process that can be discomforting and is rarely successful, Ms. Pitorak suggests repositioning the patient to one side, elevating the head and, if necessary, administering medication to reduce the secretions.

Dying patients may also moan or grunt as they breathe, but rarely is this a sign of pain, she noted. Appropriate pain relief should always be provided because a patient in pain cannot communicate effectively or die peacefully. She added that there was no evidence that pain-relieving drugs hastened death.

Patients who ask whether they are dying should be answered honestly and reassured that those left behind will be well, this is more helpful than telling patients, "You can go now."

But she warned that even when a patient can no longer respond to sights or sounds, "hearing is the last sense to leave the body, so one should never say anything near the patient that one would not want him to hear."

In the Journal of the American Medical Association two years ago, Doctor Apologists said they move away from patient as they near death leads the physician to feel guilty, insecure, frustrated and inadequate and rationalize that their time can be spent better caring for the living. But in rebuttal the doctor's absence at the period of death makes the loved ones feeling betrayed—that their departed one are not worth attention and help with bereavement. They should offer sympathy and don't abandon the family and let them be with the body as long as they wish; to do otherwise is not appropriate.

Control Over the Time and Place of Death

For the past several decades people have begun to emphasize the need to have some control over their deaths. The hospice movement was a response to this, allowing a palce where people can die gracefully. The aim of the hospice, established first some 30 years ago in England by Dame Cicely Saunders, is to provide a human, dignified environment for death. No extraordinary measures are used to prolong life—there are no blood transfusions, intravenous feedings or respirators. The hospice combines home and hospital care with hospice personnel supervising home care as long as possible. In the hospital sometimes a special separate facility, a warm homelike atmosphere is provided allowing unlimited visiting hours. Some allow patients to bring some of their own furniture; many have arrangements for cooking for the sick and serving a meal in a dining room connected. Living rooms and lounges are provided to serve the informal circumstance for friends and family. The dying patients get drugs and medication to relieve the pain but leaves him or her alert. The hospice approach takes the burden of care for the most part off the family smoothing the way for a peaceful death. Many hospices utilize volunteers and non-profit facilities thus reducing the cost, most however are connected with the regular hospital care organization.

There is a question as to what is experienced in death or whether we experience it. This aside from religious and theological views. For to experience a thing one must have a living brain and sense apparatus. In this sense, death is not part of life. Nevertheless we do experience, by thought, our future deaths and certainly no one comes to middle age without grieving and lamenting his own death countless times. From almost early childhood onward we are constantly subliminally aware of our death as well as every other man's mortality. Some interesting philosophical considerations arise here which will not be pursued; suffice it to say that we knew nothing about life before our birth, it gave us not knowing pain or suffering. On the other hand can the end of life give us concern in the same sense? We are caught in a time frame—birth to death—we do not see the boundary of our life, as the philosopher Wittgenstein in *Tractatus* says, "we cannot see beyond the boundary of our visual field; it is more correct (he says) to say that beyond the boundary of our visual field we do not see." Except through the leap of faith which the Christian and other traditions suggest we utilize, we can cross the great gulf.

Grace Craig in her *Human Development* text (1999) raises pertinent questions about the "right to die a good death." If death is a natural positive experience, do we have a right to tamper with it? Do we rob the individual of a dignified death if we artificially maintain his life systems beyond the point where he can never regain consciousness? Is there a point at which a person is meant to die, and would it be better to let nature take its course at this point? Do we prolong life because we fear death, even though the patient himself may be at peace and ready to die? These questions have been given great attention in recent times. The "Living Will" prepared by the Euthanasia Education Council appears below which has the effect of assuring the individual some control of his or her life in the last days of their lives. Patients, it is believed by most thanatologist, should be allowed to come to terms with truth of his or her condition and that they should have some control over those things that happen to him as the amount of medication he will take, even to leave the care facility and be taken home. The patient should not receive psychologically abrasive treatment, being swept along without any self-control—it's probably simpler that way but not dignified except as being orderly. This treatment may sometimes hurry death of hopelessness is acceded to in the absence of some control.

TO MY FAMILY, MY PHYSICIAN, MY LAWYER, MY CLERGYMAN
TO ANY MEDICAL FACILITY IN WHOSE CARE I HAPPEN TO BE
TO ANY INDIVIDUAL WHO MAY BECOME RESPONSIBLE FOR MY HEALTH, WELFARE OR AFFAIRS

Death is as much a reality as birth, growth, maturity and old age—it is the one certainty of life. If the time comes when I,
______________________________ can no longer take part in decisions for my own future, let this statement stand as an expression of my wishes, while I am still of sound mind.

If the situation should arise in which there is no reasonable expectation of my recovery from physical or mental disability, I request that I be allowed to die and not be kept alive by artificial means or "heroic measures". I do not fear death itself as much as the indignities of deterioration, dependence and hopeless pain. I, therefore, ask that medication be mercifully administered to me to alleviate suffering even though this may hasten the moment of death.

This request is made after careful consideration. I hope you who care for me will feel morally bound to follow its mandate. I recognize that this appears to place a heavy responsibility upon you, but it is with the intention of relieving you of such responsibility and of placing it upon myself in accordance with my strong convictions, that this statement is made.

Signed

____

Date ______________________________

Witness ______________________________

Witness ______________________________

Copies of this request have been given to

____

____

____

____

If there are other considerations in our deaths to be arranged for, they should be noted in your wills. For instance, increasingly people like to donate their bodies for medical school use (7,000 approximately per year in the United States). Thousands have donated their eyes to eye banks in the various states. This has been a project of Lions Clubs of America for years. Organ transplants if needed and approximate of ours can be bequesther. Almost always there are procedures involving legal aspects of this, the local health authorities, the coroner's office and state health officials. Precise interest in self-determination of one's body can be incorporated into the will. This requires advance foresight and action.

Cremation

The burial and services, if different, should be spelled out by the living in the last testament for often family will disregard the place of burial, etc. The desire for cremation is frequently overturned by the survivors who find it incompatible to their views. The Christian Church has often felt cremation violates the view that the body should be as it was awaiting the rapture of the coming again of Christ. Cremation is increasingly popular, particularly in California and Pacific Coast area where 14.6 were cremated while in the East South Central states only 1% (less than 5% utilize this method in the United States as a whole). For one thing it is much cheaper and the objection to not having a specific site to visit like the grave (this is possible by putting the ashes in a regular burial plot) is softened by the use of the mausoleum where the ashes are permanently deposited in an urn or receptacle. Plaques are placed in memorial rooms much like gravestones. Where not forbidden by law, the ashes can be scattered at sea or even kept at home.

Following cremation a memorial service without the body is given, with the emphasis on living and the spiritual. The type of service should be decided upon in advance. Post death events are significant in reducing prolonged grief and numbness, hence should be considered seriously and not offhandedly. Funeral directors are generally humane and helpful. They will be able to answer many of your questions putting at ease many worrisome thoughts.

Anatomical Gifts

Body donations are frequent in recent time still less than 10% in the nation give their bodies. Kinsmen and/or guardian may execute the gift usually to a medical school, work or storage facility for medical use or to a person in need of a transplant. An individual in advance of their death may execute a document for giving all or part of his body.

The American Way of Death, a former best seller by Jessica Mitford is misleading in some ways, like the suggestion that the funeral rituals are no more than a form of exploitation or the perversion of the cult of happiness paid tribute to by most Americans. The ceremonies more surely testify to the refusal of Americans to have death emptied of all meaning and a refusal to let death pass without solemnizing the occasion ritualistically in church, synagogue or chapel. It also fails to account for these services as part of grieving process—the recognition of death and beginning diminished mourning by adult children and decrease in ceremonial grief expression throughout society.

Adolescents and adults often believe that the world will end by nuclear war and that it would happen any time. Students at Brown University a few years ago requested through a petition that the administration stockpile cyanide pills for use if atomic war began. Robert Coles, psychiatrist at Harvard reported a reaction to this by blue-collar workers who said, "these spoiled rich kids—everyone else is going to die a slow death, and they want a quick way out." Death Education could, for example, deal with some topics as these: assistance to young children by care taker and teachers during a death crisis, preparing children for the shock of death through pets, etc., encourage increasing number of high schools to put units on death in health and science curriculum, providing information on the importance of grieving and ceremony in adjustment and medical and ethical issues. After all death doesn't exist in splendid isolation.

In the past ten years many persons have considered, like the psychology professor from California, preserving themselves for future time when a cure can be effected for the disease, which took their life. The packing in ice is handled in some ways like the transplant organs that sometimes are carried across the country, taking several days to reach their receptor person. The cost of this is extremely high and what are realistically offers is questionable. The Ted Williams case is a bizarre illustration of preserving the body for future use. Most scientists, at present, see little hope for reviving a person in ten years and have them live. The passage of time will, it is concluded, make irreversible changes in the cells annulling any chance for the later rebirth of life. The effect upon the brain is another problem that reduces the possibility of such occurrences at this time to bear fruit.

New Burial Approaches

In England 180 sites have been organized for Green Burial in the last 10 years. Such burial sites inter the deceased bodies as is, sometimes in wooden caskets and some without. The view according to Bishop George Russell of Huntsville, Texas of the Universal Ethician Church who has just opened an 81-acre swath of woods for family green burials. The dead he states will re-nurture the circle of life—fertilize the soil and provide a perpetual legacy to beauty. Graves at the Bishop's site must be dug with shovels instead of heavy equipment. Groups interested in this type of burial are interested both in open space preservation and alternative burials.

Bill Campbell environmental activist and small-town South Carolina physician is a great believer in simplicity to him "dust to dust" doesn't include formaldehyde injections, fancy monuments or marble—finished burial vaults. He is the motivation for a Los Angeles cemetery that is planning a nature-friendly burial ground that will be a haven for hikers as well as a final resting place. Tyler Cassity, head of the Forever Enterprize which runs Hollywood Forever Memorial Park resting place for Rudolph Valentino and Tyrone Power, has purchased San Francisco woods for green burials. No embalming, no lock step white monument so hikers will meander down woody trails. Cassidy says this would provide people a tangible way to put a permanent stop, by providing their bodies, to urban sprawl through larger natural cemeteries, preserved for the dead. You would know your death is a way of preserving a piece of this world in its natural state. With the cost of the average funeral costing $5,180, green burials offer an alternative—it also saves the mahogany trees and hardwood—also allows people to assist in furthering the universal life. Mark Musgrove of the National Cemetery Association says people prefer traditional cemeteries and he claims that if people would like to preserve space they could use cremation. Cassidy responds the green burials will cool cremation.

We can never get away from the death of significant persons in our lives—for me there have been four or five—they will never be replaced and my life has been greatly impoverished by this loss. In memory I treasure the image of a dear sister and Mother and though it has been some time, I call within myself to turn back the clock for "one more day!" I remember the words of Arnold Toynbee who said "from the middle of life onward, only he remains vitally alive who is ready to accept its ending." What we fear most of death is loss of consciousness. The story is told of a demon who promised a man eternal life if he would give up his earthly memory. After thinking about it, he turned the Devil's offer down, for he reasoned, memory is what existence means, or as the philosopher Giovanni Gentile said, "you are what you remember." Our memories lie close to selfhood.

CHAPTER XI

MONEY AND FUTURE RETIREMENT

"The Money Tree"

Money isn't everything—no, but it pays for or is connected with nearly everything we call good in life! As Mark Twain said, "it's not a disgrace to be poor but it damned is an inconvenience." Importantly, it pays for the rent and food, our medical care and part of our leisure. These things most of us will be responsible for as individuals by the typical retirement time. Women, in many cases, can expect men to look after money matters if their men survive and are married assuming, of course, their men have enough money and resources. But women increasingly need to know, even if they do not work outside the home, what is in the future for them. Many who thought their husband was arranging for their care found he hadn't or hadn't sufficiently. Increasingly, independence of men and women in their work lives and life styles demands planning for the future for oneself.

Retirement Planning

Retirement, i.e., plans for it begins today not at 62 or 65 or even 70. For the middlescent forty-five is the crucial point, that is about the point of no return; certainly at 55 relatively little can be done (Social Security and possibly a small pension) if one expects to live in the style similar at 65 as he does now. Full social security payments will required one to work until they are 67 if they are born after 1960. Even the one at 45 has typically only twenty years to retirement. My advice is to never retire in the final sense. Forty-seven percent of retirees work now, 75% of pre-retirees plan to continue working of course a number of these are under 65. One should work at something, for pay, as long as is feasible, for not only is money tied to elemental survival but to status and one's sense of worth, no matter how menial the job. Work at something even if its part time unless you are well healed or disabled.

It is true that some can find this work in volunteer work in charities, church or cause-based movements. The average person 45-year-old, we assume, has Social Security benefits building up and a retirement fund. Typically, a minimal retirement financial plan should be based upon having the mortgage paid off on a home, owning a condominium, trailer or apartment, and on having Social Security income plus an additional source of regular income—pension or annuity or other investments. In the middle years when incomes are generally at their highest (unfortunately so is the responsibility) an assessment of one's financial circumstance must be made. If, as in so many cases, finances are being handled in a haphazard fashion, much needs to be done.

<u>Successful Retirement</u>

There are three aspects we should consider in successful planning of retirement. Foremost is <u>financial security</u>, then <u>physical health</u>, and finally the <u>adjustment</u> problems involved. The first two are crucial if we are to reach a retirement time. Life expectancies tell us that people reaching 45 will survive to 76 or more. Future survival rates at given ages are, for the 40-year-old, men, 37.0 and women 41.3, a life expectancy of 39.5 years; at 50 the expectancy is 28 for men and women 32.1. (National Center for Health Statistics, 2001).

Successful planning for retirement depends upon many things including person's financial status at 35 or 45. In America the typical working man spends about sixteen years in retirement. The life expectancy for the woman at 65 is an additional 19.5 years; for man, 16.5; early retirement accounts for the discrepancy in the retirement and life span times. (National Center for Health Statistics, 2001).

> The retirement period can be those of contentment and enjoyment, but too often it is a time of uncertainty, loneliness, and anxiety, marred by increasing separation from society and the world of action and production. Many persons are not prepared for the changed status related to dropping the full-time work responsibility. Since retirement for many is mandatory at 65, thousands of healthy men and women find the imposed leisure time a booby trap not the Elysian fields they had hoped it would be. Of course, many have the option of voluntary retirement—those who are self-employed, owners of businesses, part-time workers

and the like. It is obvious that many persons reach the end of their full-time employment without much thought about it. For these, difficulties arise in adjustment. According to Simpson and McKinney of Duke University, the most reliable single predictor of success in retirement comes from the pre-retirement attitude toward completion of the work period. Those whose attitudes have been favorable to retirement prior to stopping work make the most satisfactory retirement.

Retirement is a time of adaptability. It represents a major adjustment problem to more retirees. The picture frequently presented of happy retirees in utopia-like settings is not in harmony with scientific studies bearing on adjustment. This period is often a time of uncertainty, loneliness and anxiety, affected by increasing separation from active participation in social and world affairs. Research by Simpson categorized workers into three divisions: (1) those whose work was primarily concerned with ideas—such as in teaching, writing, composers—for these retirement presented fewer problems, or (2) executives, those working with people found retirement the most difficult years of their life, and finally (3) manual workers (workers with things) who showed little evidence of new interests upon retirement, although many appeared relatively contented. This and other studies indicate that retirement difficulties tend to be greater for those whose work history involves an intense occupational culture, characteristics of college teachers and other professional groups. The underlying tone of these studies seems to be one of the quiet desperation for the continuity of some sort of meaningful work and/or escapist activity-centeredness. The emphasis is upon activity—that is as an end in itself.

There is a number of steps in successful planning for retirement. Certainly the following should be included: (1) Definition of a concept of retirement, (2) Decisions based upon fact, (3) Open mindedness in collecting retirement ideas, (4) Advanced planning, (5) Consultation with your interested kin and especially your children, (6) Realism about financial goals, (7) Carefulness in choosing the location where you should live, and (8) Advice of professionals, and the money evaluation included in this chapter, who provide ideas on money needs and trends and can assess your money status.

As mentioned earlier, essentially retirement involves three kinds of security: physical, activity, and financial. Expecting to enjoy good health at 65 or later involves making sure one has a good health regimen during the middle years. This involves when overlaid on basically good health status having a good diet—overweight is a cul de sac—one should weigh approximately what he did at thirty, say at fifty-five. Regular exercise is a must and realism in the fact of growing older, one should maintain contact with a physician and consult regularly with him or her. More persons rust away and debilitate than wear out from over use of themselves. Middle aged persons should develop a strong interest in general areas, people, hobbies, volunteer work or other kinds of part-time work which itself will later serve to help them keep up with life and remain interested in their surroundings. Community activity is a good way to invest energy in what is worthwhile and to attract new friends and provide a positive outlook in life.

One of the foremost concerns of the prospective retiree is money. One can be healthy and involved in today's living but if the source of support is considerably limited at retirement time, serious consequences are in the offering. Any list of expenditures after retirement gives housing as the major cost of living followed closely by food.

EXPENSES IN RETIREMENT

Annual expenses of an "average retired couple"

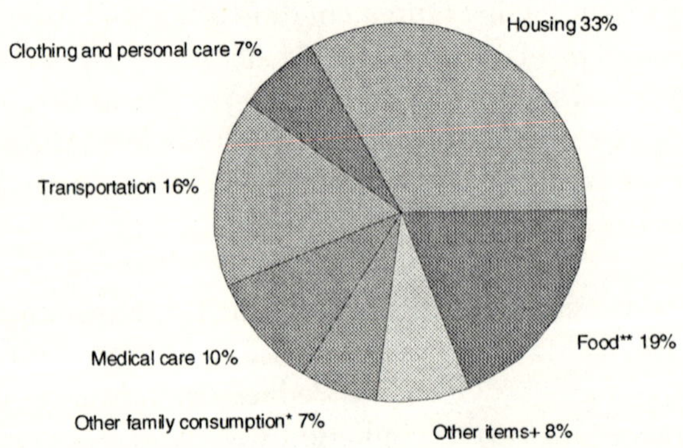

Note: The lower your income bracket, the higher the proportion of money you must spend on necessities like food and shelter, and the less you will have left for extras like travel.

*Other family consumption includes recreation, reading material, computers and cell phones, etc.

**Varies with age—less at 45-64, more afterwards—65 up.

+Other items include gifts, contributions, and life insurance.

Source: Bureau of Labor Statistics, 1999-2000

If one owns a house or apartment, the 33% for housing will be greatly reduced, however, maintenance roofing, replacement for heating/cooking, plumbing, painting and new kitchen items, i.e., stoves, refrigeration, dryers and washers plus mechanical devices for facilitating cooking and food preparation could take much of that back.

Food used to be considerably less important but with increases of staggering proportions this will be even more significant in the future due to increased proportionate cost of food and eating out. Housing and food compose some fifty-two or more per cent of one's money needs at retirement. Apartment living can be cheaper because repairs are included and yard maintenance also in the rent than home ownership usually though it is not as spacious. Typically those on Social Security can just about pay for these items if there is $800-$1000 in the monthly check. If there are no additional funds, then part-time or even full-time work usually will be a necessity. Those planning at 45 can partially circumvent the erosion that has come to those on fixed incomes (a cost of living adjustment is fixed to many retirement plans and Social Security) by adding money in safe investments (houses, land, annuities) and savings plans. It is essential that persons anticipate retirement early enough to have regular health insurance programs beyond that prospect of Medicare. One needs Medicare A & B plus another insurance source to cover what they do not, like AARP (1-800-23-5800 Ext. 13), Trigon, New York Life, Metropolitan, Blue Cross and Blue Shield or something else. In the middle years when incomes are at their highest money has to be set aside for later use. The Bureau of Labor Statistics says a person in retirement needs 70-80 percent of their final take-home pay to maintain living standards. The Certified Financial Planners say 60% to 90%. I believe the higher figure is a better yardstick. Money management skills will be needed to offset the inflation, which the table later in the chapter on money needs in retirement reveals. Since the typical retirement years for men is 16 and for women longer, it is mandatory that we think of money requirements and the investment of our resources in money accruing situations. Social Security with inflation increases and some other savings have to be effective. Good money management is essential. Your money cannot be idle, it must be used to get additional funds even though they might be small. If your company goes bankrupt or eliminates thousands of jobs like Enron, any money you can save put it in savings accounts which will earn only small amounts of interest but at least the principal will be safe there. The market is too risky to forecast in the short term. A longer-term investment (3-5 years) you could see 6-8% annual return. The major corporations' way of subversion has been copied by lessor finance offices, brokerage firms where unfortunately some brokers and others have lied about their stocks and even your holdings. One cannot begin a retirement plan at sixty and survive. If one did, he or she would need a larger windfall or short term annuities, etc. which would mature in ten years and then retirement at seventy or later is possible. Hopefully by retirement one owns a home, an apartment or condo. Unfortunately, many do not have this. Ideas about moving to Florida or Arizona must be considered carefully for the surroundings though warmer than Maine, upper New York, Minnesota or Michigan may be a cause of unhappiness. The best situation is probably one, which allows the retiree to live near some family and friends without being dependent upon them. Buying a trailer, or for those able a condominium apartment in Florida may be the answer. The hidden variable is the condo maintenance fee, which sometimes accelerate rapidly. Certainly some expenses will be less, usually in clothes, reading material, incurred entertainment and frequently tax breaks on real estate and drugs along with lodging and meals are available. Medical costs are higher along with medicines. In addition to the safeguards we have mentioned earlier, one should try to have a nest egg. If one plans to retire before the usual time, from 62-65, (average in U.S. is 62) the income needed will be at least $15,000-25,000 a year for a couple plus having the mortgage paid off on a home, a good health insurance plan and a savings of $25,000. A survey of retirement counselors produced the following list from seniors if they could do it over. 1) Plan early for severance day, 2) Be flexible, 3) Understand your social security benefits, and 4) Couples should plan and compromise together, etc.

The following questionnaire I developed for use with various groups in discussions on retirement. Many have found it helpful to pin-point needs and considerations. Put your answers down and list your resources.

REALISM AND PRE-RETIREMENT QUESTIONNAIRE

Have you thought about what retirement would be like? Yes___ No ___

Did you consider the possible adjustment problems you would have, like:

Where will I live? Yes ___ No ___

Will I have enough money to live on? Yes ___ No ___

Will I have something to do with my time? Yes ___ No ___

Should I keep on working? Yes ___ No ___

What sort of leisure pursuits will I have? Yes ___ No ___

What kind of health plan do I have? Yes ___ No ___

Am I mentally prepared for retirement? Yes ___ No ___

<u>RESOURCES FOR RETIREMENT</u>

<u>List</u>

Who are my long-term friends?
What financial resources do I have?
What hobbies and interests do I have?
What will I do to support good health?
Most people will say I'll live like I've always lived but if they aren't prepared it will not happen.
Irrespective some change will occur.

In the section that follows, you can get a picture of your financial health (your job, money habits, plans for the future, etc.). Included are some ideas on the savings and making of money that will have a decided bearing on your retirement prospects.

<u>YOUR SPENDING</u>

All too many persons spend everything they make and some spend more than they make. First, everyone should have a box or cabinet drawers in which to put bills, statements of account, record of payment, credit slips, in fact, everything that indicates money spent, even admission stubs to movies or sports events. In this way one has a record of what he is spending. Over a period of time this becomes important. Most of us, when we analyze our spending, find one of three things: (1) spending and earning are about the same; (2) we spend more than we earn; or (3) we make more than we spend. Unfortunately only ten percent of us are in the last position. In any event this latter situation means we may not have invested our money, and just to hold it is to lose it since one needs to plan on a 4 to 6 long term inflation rate as an imperative, if it's less, you make gains.

COST OF LIVING

Inflation can have an effect on everything from the cost of a home to a Big Mac at McDonald's.

EFFECTS OF 4% INFLATION		
Today	in 10 Years	in 20 Years
$30,000	$42,000	$109,556

Source: CIP, Bureau of Labor Statistics

Impact of Inflation on Your Net Worth

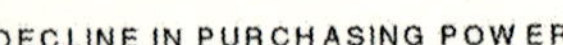

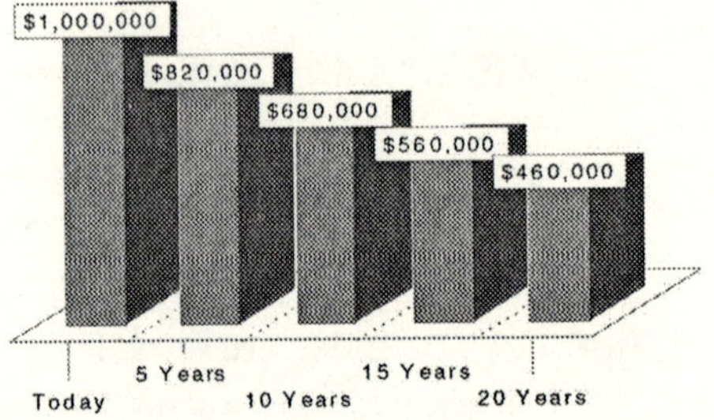

Source: From *Passport to Retirement*, Emerald Publications

What can happen to your net worth if it is unprotected from inflation?

At that same 4 percent rate of inflation, you can see how dramatically the value of your net worth could decline. With inflation at 4 percent, your money would be cut in half in 18 years. As a result, the purchasing power of a million-dollar nest egg would be reduced to $460,000 over the course of a 20-year retirement. If you had $100,000 in 20 years that would be around $46,000. Look at the following figures of the Rule of 72.

The Rule of 72

The Rule of 72 demonstrates the impact inflation can have on your purchasing power. To determine how long a given rate of inflation would take to cut the purchasing power of your money in half, divide 72 by the expected rate of inflation.

Source: From *Passport to Retirement*, Emerald Publications

6 percent inflation:

72 ÷ 6 = 12 years

4 percent inflation:

72 ÷ 4 = 18 years

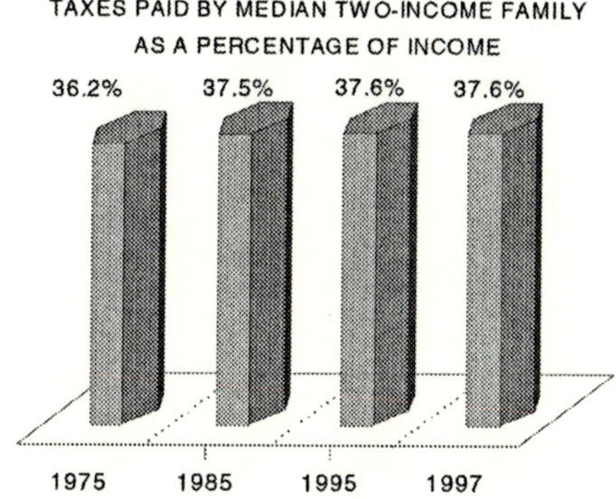

The Burden of Taxes

Another roadblock we all face is the steady burden of taxes. Where is the so-called taxpayer relief?

Despite several rounds of tax reform, Americans have paid roughly 37 cents out of each dollar to taxes for more than 20 years. And tax reform has done little to simplify the complexity and ever changing nature of the tax laws. As you can see on this chart, taxes have remained fairly steady as a percentage of household income but they could rise. Notably housing costs and taxes on them has risen dramatically in many areas of the country.

Source: Tax Foundation

INCOME TAX PROVISIONS

Current	New (with phase-in dates)
Individual Income Tax Rates (Generally) (2002)	2003-2005
15%	10%
28	15
31	25
36	28
	33
39.6	35

If you have spent more than you make and probably 20%-30% do, you are in serious trouble. In this case, the money has to come from some place it shouldn't. (That is excepting the case of emergency.) But perhaps you have been dipping into savings, borrowing money or buying too much on credit. A friend of mine used to love to make me envious by showing me all his credit cards. A severe limitation of spending resulted, even so, his wife explained, they were not out of the woods. He was a professional man with better than average resources but the mounting debt strained the marriage and made life miserable. This sort of "good life" could cost you dearly—loss of credit, pay-to-manage your funds, re-mortgaging or losing your home or car, maybe the wife or husband, etc. Anyway, to see how you stand, fill in the income and expense blanks on the following page as a start to estimate your financial health. It makes no difference if you have never done this before—start now! Include both wage earners in a household as one sum.

INCOME		EXPENSES	
Take home Pay	________	Mortgage or rent	________
Interest on bonds	________	Taxes (Property, licenses, etc.), Taxes not withheld	________
Dividends on stocks, etc.	________	Food	________
Part-time work	________	Clothing & dry cleaning	________
Bonuses	________	Utilities and fuel	________
Other	________	Loans	________
		Insurance	________
		Church & Charity	________
		Auto (gas, repair, oil, etc.)	________
		Medical bills & drugs	________
		Entertainment & Vacation	________
		Schooling/Tuition	________
		Miscellaneous	________
		Household upkeep	________
		Savings (other than deducted from salary	________
Totals	________	Difference (plus or minus)	________

If you earn between $15,000-$40,000 for a single person or $30,000-$80,000 a couple a year, your housing and food should take up over 50% of your income. This is a good gauge to judge your other expenses; remember, however, a large variable here is the number of children. In this spending scheme accounting can be kept by the month, just duplicate the various items you need. As important as spending is to get a basic fix on your finances you need to look at your debts. It is generally agreed that we ought not to owe more than 20%-30% of our yearly take home pay. Some experts suggest the debt (excluding your home and auto) we have should not exceed the amount of money we could raise immediately by raiding the savings account, piggy bank, bonds, etc. This keeps one from being overwhelmed with debt. One formula (a conservative one) for figuring a safe debt level is to multiply 10% of your take home pay by 18, the amount gives you your safe debt limit (hence 1/10 of monthly take home pay (2000) = 200. x 18 equals 3600. At $4000 a month take home pay then $7200. debt limit. This excludes mortgage payments. Though this is conservative to double invites trouble.

If you seem not to be getting anywhere with debt management, <u>pay off the old debts</u> before you take on new ones and cut expenses drastically. To estimate closely your money obligations, fill in the blanks on the following page with your debt figures.

It is encouraging to note that a Ohio State University study several years ago sponsored by the Consumer Federation of America found 26% of families with incomes from $10,000 to $25,000 had accumulated $100,000 in net assets, and 38 percent of those earning from $25,000 to $50,000 had reached the $300,000 mark.

"To our surprise, there was less of a wealth gap than we thought" in U.S. society, according to the study. They conceded that "low-six-figure" nest eggs are not enough to live on comfortably in long time retirement, but for those in their 40s and early 50s, it is a base upon which real growth can be built. The key factor is the patient building of assets over the decades. The findings not only surprised many experts, but they also illustrate how inaccurately most Americans view the wealth of their fellow citizens. Polling done in conjunction with the study shows that Americans tend to think there are far more millionaires in our society than there really are, and sharply underestimate the numbers of modestly affluent.

The general public estimates that 15 percent of all households have net assets of $1 million or more, while in reality only about 4 percent are that wealthy. On the other hand, the public estimates that only 36 percent have $100,000 or more, while the actual number is 56 percent for households headed by someone older than 45—and 42 percent for families headed by people of all ages.

	Monthly Payments		Number of Payments Left		Debt Left
Personal Loans		x		=	
Automobile		x		=	
Home Repair		x		=	
Other Installment		x		=	
Charge Accounts		x		=	
		x		=	
Credit Cards		x		=	
		x		=	
		x		=	
				=	

If your debt load is too great, a drastic turn-around is in order or for sure misery will follow—"when poverty comes in the door love flies out the window," etc. Unfortunately many pay for a car, etc., and immediately buy another when they should wait a year or two. For some help, see the appendix for "Savings on Purchase by Month."

Dealing with Debt

If you can't pay your bills, you need to act to rebuild your credit. Job loss, divorce, serious illness or poor financial management can threaten your economic security and your ability to pay your bills. And while you may be able to juggle creditors for a time, sooner or later you're apt to find yourself in dire straits. But if you have problems with debt, you're not alone. There are a number of workable ways to resolve the problem, often known as restructuring debt.

You can ask your **creditors** to rewrite your loans to extend the time you have to pay and to change the payments so that you can afford to make them. The extensions will increase your overall cost, because the creditors will charge you interest over a longer period. **Non-profit credit counselors** are available in virtually every city. For modest fees, counselors go through your debts, analyze your income and help you work out ways to handle your debts. **Loan consolidators** are private businesses that lend you money to pay off all your debts. You then owe only one creditor—them. The risk of ruining your credit is also there.

The good news is that you pay only one check a month, you can repay over a long term and you can make low monthly payments. The bad news is that the interest they charge may be very high, and you may be hit with stiff fees for paying off the loan ahead of schedule.

Preventing Debt

Credit cards can be lifesavers, most users agree. But many people who find themselves at sea financially are threatened by short-term debt, often credit card debt. According to the Federal Reserve Board, consumers on average owe more than 20% of their income, not counting what they owe in mortgages and home equity loans.

Continuing to charge can help to pull you under if you're in debt, since the interest you pay on your outstanding balances is usually higher than on most loans. Credit counselors often suggest getting rid of your credit cards, which forces you to limit what you spend. Even if you hang onto one card for emergency use, you'll find that it's probably smarter to pay mostly in cash.

Time to Repay

It takes time to repay accumulated debts, especially if you postpone confronting the problem. The National Foundation for Consumer Credit estimates that three to four years is typical for the people who come to their offices. Some other credit counselors suggest that if it's going to take five years or more, bankruptcy might be a wiser alternative though the rules for this have changed drastically.

PAYING THE CONSEQUENCES

Some of the consequences of failing to repay your debts:

- You could be assigned a bad credit rating and be unable to borrow again.
- Your wages may be garnished: a court may order your employer to pay up to 10% of your salary each pay period to people you owe.
- Lenders may sell property you put up as security.
- You could be sued and, if you lose, required to pay the legal costs of your creditors as well.

An examination of our net worth is important as we look at the future for we need to set financial goals by this. Two things are involved here—our assets and our liabilities. Make a list of your assets using the blanks. Be sure to list all your debts (for end of the month or year). The list below is the national percentages of personal debt for a sixty-year old man (salary of $50,000) nearing retirement. His wife does not work outside the home.

ASSETS		LIABILITIES	
Cash	$ 500	Debts (current)	$2,150.
Cash in bank, savings, bonds	$ 1,750.	Debts per month (Installment)	$1,000. 12,000
Borrowing amount on Insurance	$ 5,000.	Mortgage debt	$ 7,000.
Market value of house, trailer, etc.	$90,000.	Personal Loans	$ 600.
Value of lands owned	$ 8,000.	Pledge (charitable)	$ 500.
Surrender value of annuities	$12,000.	Taxes, property, etc. (Prorated per month)	$ 200.0(2,400.
Equity in pensions(s)	$60,000.	Income Tax	$ 3,600
Value of possessions, household furnishings, sports equipment, tools, jewelry, clothes, etc.	$10,000.		
Car(s)	$20,000.00 › $36,0		
Money owed to you	$ 350.		
Market value of stocks, Bonds, etc.	$ 7,500.		
IRA (CD's) money market	$16,000.		
Business interest (Equity)	$16,000. sole owı		
All other assets, (things jointly owned, etc.)	$14,000. 2 owı		
TOTAL	$251,100.00 ASSETS		$28,250.00 LIABILITIES

Difference ________________$222,850.00________________ plus
Plus or minus

(Figures represent a work sample for a married man with $50,000 year salary 60 years old.) The wife does not work outside the home.

The net worth of this couple is $222,850. They have managed their money well and their retirement plans should be realized.

As in the case of overspending which we dealt with earlier, this evaluation of your net worth can emphasize where we need to strengthen your financial structure and provide a clear picture in planning for retirement. This leads us to a brief discussion in setting goals for the future years and more leisurely times.

Most of us do not expect great wealth in our time or perhaps hereafter. With inflation, ecological energy problems, financial security is a slippery notion. But knowing our "situation"; that is—debts, liabilities and our assets, we are at a good place to move in the right direction. There are some principles—mainly in setting priorities—as listed here.

1. Having a regular income.
2. Anticipating short and long term needs.
3. Having protection against catastrophes.
4. Getting ahead some each year.
5. Setting goals and sticking with a plan.
6. Saving money every month.

Now in view of these one should decide what are absolutely essential needs and what are "wants." This latter is like a trip to Canada or Europe. The former may be a new refrigerator. If the best time to buy this is probably December and you would like to pay for all of it or a good down payment, begin to budget for it months in advance. Wants can be priority items also but they should be assigned a rank. When goals are set, the expense involved should be calculated and a plan for paying for this devised.

Your job or occupation is an important part of setting income goals unless you get lucky at the lottery or get a windfall from Uncle Joe! What follows is a scheme for rating your job. You can rate your future prospects on the job you work at now by giving 2 points for the first column (Frequently or Yes), 1 point for checking the second column (Sometimes or Maybe or Not Sure), give yourself 0 for Never or No. If you score as much a 14 you probably should stay with your job. If less, you might want to consider your situation, try to retrench or leave.

Company Status and Your Relationship

	Frequently	Sometimes	Never
1. Your supervisor calls you sometimesfor special jobs.	________	________	________
2. You receive regular pay raises which keepyou even or aheadof inflation.	________	________	________
3. You get along well with the people and supervisors with whom you work.	________	________	________
4. The supervisor asks you your opinion and suggestions about thecompany's work.	________	________	________
5. The company usually promotes its leadersfrom the inside.	________	________	________

	Yes	Maybe Not Sure	No
6. The company is well known and growing.	________	________	________
7. The company's product or service is not affected by rising prices so that operations are not reduced and employees laid off.	________	________	________

8. The pay scale and fringe benefits are equal to those of like companies.	________	________	________
9. Employee satisfaction is reasonably high, most employees have long tenure.	________	________	________
10. The company has a sizable number ofcustomers or organizations it serves.	________	________	________
Totals	________	________	________
Grand Total	________	________	________

If this gives you the idea that you're in a dead-end job or tottering company, look around for something else to do, but don't quit your job until you have another one. If your company is O.K. and you like it, try to figure out why you fail to get ahead. Government studies show the following to be good opportunities through 2008, that is, the fastest growing job markets are for professional workers and technicians, retail sales, office clerks. In terms of jobs, the best prospect is in the clerical field. The future should be bright for computer workers (in programming repair and analysis), business machine repairers, service workers, such as cosmetologists, nurses' aides, police officers, school teachers, health workers, finance officers, computer operators, cashiers, waiters and waitresses, insurance and real estate salesmen. Craftsmen and salespeople should find plenty of jobs. Opportunities for truck, bus, and taxi drivers and semi-skilled factory workers should exist in quantities. A school bus driving job is an excellent source of part-time work, motel clerk as is school teaching substitute or assistants and sales. Farm jobs will shrink, though laborers will have about the same chance as before. Colleges and universities incidentally hire hundreds of personnel as typists, clerks in warehouses, maintenance help, security, workers in cafeterias, maids in dormitories, libraries, offices, repairs (auto, plumbing, etc.), janitors, yard workers, mail delivery, security personnel and police.

Beyond this if you lack qualifications for jobs, check the local resources for training programs: high school night classes, community colleges and technical institutes, and universities (we also have non-credit courses at our college in nearly everything even bartending and bicycle repair). Correspondence courses are also a possibility. In any case you can qualify for many jobs by enrolling in a program or get information and help by asking.

INCOME NEEDED DURING RETIREMENT TO BUY $10,000 OF THE SAME GOODS & SERVICES AT THESTART OF RETIREMENT

Number of Years for the same goods & services after the start of retirement	Inflation Rate: 2%	4%	6%	8%
5	$11,041	$12,167	$13,382	$14,693
10	12,190	14,802	17,908	21,589
15	13,459	18,009	23,966	31,722
20	14,859	21,911	32,071	46,610
25	16,406	26,658	42,919	68,485

If you consider that a 1980's salary of $30,000 a year will require $36,501 in 5 years at 5% inflation, years later $44,406 will be required to equal this after ten years. In any anticipated change of job one should keep this in mind. Also remember the fringe benefits that the typical company shells out amount to an additional thirty-three percent of salary outlay. Use this as a guide in seeking new employment. The extra benefits represent money—life insurance, health insurance, pension plans and bonuses—these are items that raise your standard of living. Social Security and Workmen's Compensation is required by law and not figured with other benefits.

SOURCES OF INCOME

There are three sources of income for most people: their job, savings they accrue and investments. In many families there are two persons sharing the load of the cost of living—this requires two cars, insurance and maintenance. For many there is little left over for savings and investments. Labor Bureau figures show fewer and fewer people are investing and at the same time buying on credit and piling up debt are increasing. Before we look at income sources more closely let's examine monies that could be available for retirement. These are: pension, social security, home, Medicare A, Medicare B (to help with health expenses), investments and continued work if possible, at least on a part-time basis. These sources of retirement funds assumes one gets a pension (government workers and many in industry get pensions plus COLA—cost of living increase as do Social Security recipients) has a 401K or similar plan a person owns a home or condo and has some investments.

Most experts believe you need 80% of your current income to retire and live somewhat like you lived before. There will be changes and adjustments to make. If you have a current salary of $50,000 alone or with a spouse who works you multiply $50,000 times .80 this gives you $40,000. You may estimate Social

Security will give you about 20% (usually for this income level 21% although with $75,000 many will find Social Security pays much less than this of their retirement expenses because Social Security is taxed, some pay taxes on 50% up to 85% of their funds. (In 1996 the IRS said 7.5 million individuals paid tax on their Social Security amounting to 54.2 billion.) Annually, the Social Security Administration provides an estimate of all future benefits. (Call 1-800-772-1213). They will send you a report. Subtracting $40,000 you need from the $10,000 you need $30,000 more dollars. There is more bad news—inflation. If its fifteen years until you retire at 4% rate a year, the $30,000 funds you have if multiplied by 1.8009 the inflation factor by 30,000 finds the future additional income required is 54,027, 30,000 x 1.8009. Fortunately it has been around 2% but will rise soon. What offsets income required—pensions, 401K and assorted investments. If one does not have a pension then something like investments, rental housing, continued working will be required. If one is forty then the need to organize for saving and investment must begin now.

When you look at the additional income required (54,027) in the example and examine the table below with a 25 year life expectancy and 7% growth of investments you see 11.65 as an income generation factor x the 54,027 raise the cost of retirement to 639.609. If Social Security provides 20% that it cuts $126,000 from the need for income.

Inflation Factor

YEARS UNTIL RETIREMENT	INFLATION FACTOR	YEARS UNTIL RETIREMENT	INFLATION FACTOR	YEARS UNTIL RETIREMENT	INFLATIO FACTOR
1	1.0400	11	1.5395	21	2.3699
2	1.0816	12	1.6010	22	2.5633
3	1.1249	13	1.6651	23	2.7725
4	1.1699	14	1.7317	24	2.9987
5	1.2167	15	1.8009	25	3.2434
6	1.2653	16	1.8730	26	3.5081
7	1.2653	17	1.9479	27	3.7943
8	1.3159	18	2.0258	28	4.1039
9	1.4233	19	2.1068	29	4.4388
10	1.4802	20	2.1911	30	4.8010

Income Generation Factor (return after inflation)

EXPECTED LIFE SPAN AFTER RETIREMENT	3% RETURN	5% RETURN	7% RETURN	9% RETURN
1	0.9709	0.9524	0.9346	0.9174
2	1.9135	1.8594	1.8080	1.7591
3	2.8286	2.7232	2.6243	2.5313
4	3.7171	3.5460	3.3872	3.2397
5	4.5797	4.3295	4.1002	3.8897
6	5.4172	5.0757	4.7665	4.4859
7	6.2303	5.7864	5.3893	5.0330
8	7.0197	6.4632	5.9713	5.5348
9	7.7861	7.1078	6.5152	5.9952
10	8.50302	7.7217	7.0236	6.4177
11	9.2526	8.3064	7.4987	6.8052
12	9.9540	8.8633	8.3577	7.4869
13	10.6350	9.3936	8.7455	7.7862
14	11.2961	9.8986	9.1079	8.0607
15	11.9379	10.3797	9.1079	8.0607
20	14.8775	12.4622	10.5940	9.1285
25	17.4131	14.0939	11.6536	9.8226
30	19.6004	15.3725	12.4090	10.2737

Source: From *Passport to Retirement*, Emerald Publications

Now with a pension of 10,000 a year x 35 this would move down the income retirement need to 253,609 (126,000 + 250,000) if the pension was $35,000 a year it would generate 625 enough to take care of the problem. If you have no pension but investments such as IRA, Roth IRA, Keogh plans or annuities, these personal retirement plans offset a regular pension.

Research from Business Week (1998) indicated only 28% of pre-retirees surveyed felt very confident of having enough money for retirement. Most people think about retirement when they get about fifty. This may be too late to prepare for a suitable retirement. Even working continuously into retirement one's work is likely to change and will provide less of what is needed. The problem for many people is procrastination. The following example shows what can happen when delay occurs. Bill decides to invest $500 per month with an 8% return (a high figure in today's marketplace six percent would be more realistic). Jim waits ten years to start—the following chart reveals the difference in savings. In this illustration taxes are not considered here but taxes paid by median two-income families pay as a percentage of income since 1975 (36.2%) to 1997 (37.6%) fairly steady over the years. This tax could be reduced but the future of much less tax given the country's terrorists war is unlikely despite political talk. In any event savings are a must for every one and now is the time to begin.

INVESTMENTS

One of the ways of getting money for retirement is investments. There are many kinds and methods for doing this. Investments may through mutual funds, bonds, stocks, annuities, rental houses or condos and more safe but less productive are saving (credit) unions, bank saving, money markets currently provide small interest amounts) funds, etc. These latter types are more secure and in depression downturns that are serious one can hold on at least to the principal plus get a little more.

When one invests they may get a manager or broker to handle the purchase of stocks and bonds and other ventures. These get a percent of what they buy for you and also when you sell the stock. The fee is a percent of the amount of assets in the account (i.e., 1.5% of $100,000 = $1,500 each year). Sometimes the companies of the stocks or bonds pay some of or all of the commissions of the money manager. I lost five thousand dollars on some stock, which my broker had advised I buy, his advice netted him a commission also on the selling of the bad stock he bought for me. But many brokerage houses are connected with firms, which cover nationally with offices and have access to the latest and best information available. Nevertheless with all their ability and resources they can't always predict the market and pick sure winners. If you go this route you need to pick a company with a good tract record. Some names come to mind Wachovia Security, Edward Jones, Merrill Lynch, Smith Barney, Charles Schwab, UBS, Morgan Stanley and Olde. One can use the Internet to purchase and follow the fortune of the stock or bonds they buy and if you buy through the Internet you eliminate the commission.

Types of Investments—(1) Mutual Funds—One of the easiest ways to get into the investment arena's because small or large funds enable you to purchase mutual funds. Monies invested are pooled with other investors and the companies handling them invests in a variety of stocks, bonds or other securities. The important thing is to select the right fund—there are some 3,100 stocks on the New York Exchange but more than 10,000 mutual funds. The value of principal and return will fluctuate so when redeemed it may be worth more or less than the original cost. In today's market unlike the past fifteen years most mutual funds made good returns for people but today one must be cautious when getting into this investment. How about (2) bonds, here you are investing money as a loan to a corporation or government. A bond is an IOU certifying you have made a loan. The interest may vary going up and down but in the end of the maturity period you get back the principal plus some more usually. The information that follows is meant to apply to a stable market otherwise buyer be wary.

(3) Annuities is another kind of possible income source. There are two kinds generally of annuities—deferred and immediate ones. Deferred are designed for long-term accumulation; they postpone income to a future date. The premiums you pay have the potential to appreciate during the build-up phase on a tax-deferred basis. The money made is not taxed until they are withdrawn. Immediate annuities are designed to provide current income. Once you pay a premium you receive regular income. This method appeals to those who need to reallocate their savings for greater income. Potential increase in value on an annuity can come from a fixed return or a variable rate of return. This is true of both deferred and immediate annuities. Fixed are issued at a set rate for a specific time. The rate may be adjusted but the company involved guarantees a minimum rate set forth in the contract. Variable annuities offer differential fund opportunities according to how you chose to allocate your premiums. According to how much you think you can risk (gamble more to hopefully make more) and your objective is also involved. In the case of the variable annuities you bear the same risk as with any stock or mutual fund. They guarantee return from time of purchase. There is more expense to this. To get involved with annuities and the components, which may consist of sub-accounts, one must consult a professional—C.P.A., accountants, broker or insurance agent. Sub-accounts are those different annuities you wish to include in your portfolio. In 1997 the value of annuities have reached 87 billion dollars up from 9.3 billion in 1987 according to the National Association for Variable Annuities. Sub-accounts have increased from

175 in 1987 to more than 4,000 in 1997. Of course this is 2005 and a different situation exists so being careful in today's market is the watchword.

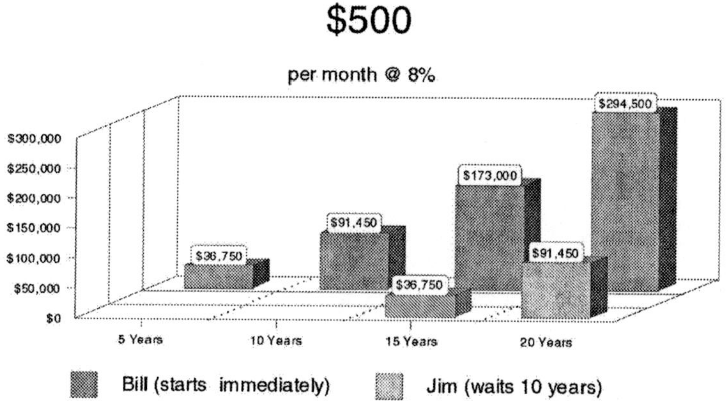

(4) The Keogh Plan is a business retirement account but difficult to set up or at least complicated. This plan involves self-employed, partnerships, and unincorporated businesses—it does allow for tax deductible contributions, one may contribute up to $41,000 per year and make tax deferred earnings.

(5) A fifth way for getting money for retirement is the IRA (Individual Retirement Accounts). If you are an active participant in an employer sponsored plan your income tax deduction may be partially or totally eliminated. Investment should be diversified, putting all your money in one account is risky—add money markets, CD's, bonds properly.

The Roth IRA created by the government to encourage people to put money aside for the later years provides for a tax favored method of saving money for their own retirement. This type of IRA features tax-free accumulation and withdrawals. Although you receive no tax deduction for contributions made to this type of IRA, qualified distributions from Roth IRA's are not included in your gross income or subject to the normal 10 percent tax penalty on early withdrawals. To help you decide look at the comparisons below and see which applies to you. Sometimes a Roth results in less retirement income if the tax bracket is lower in retirement.

IRA COMPARISON ANALYSIS

Investor Information

* Date of birth:	07/15/1954	* First year contribution:	$3,000
* Years to retirement:	15 years	* Maximizing IRA contributions:	No
* Current tax bracket:	25.0%	* Annual adjustment to IRA contributions:	N/A
* Years in retirement:	20 yrs.	* Rate of return (contributions):	9.0%
* Tax bracket in retirement:	15.0%	* Rate of return (tax savings):	9.0%
* Investing tax savings:	Yes		

	Deductible	Roth
Annual tax savings for deductible IRA	$750	N/A
Accumulated value of tax savings at retirement	$22,021	N/A
Total value at retirement	$110,103[1]	$88,083
After-tax amount if taken as lump sum at retirement	$82,578	$88,083
Annual after-tax income in retirement	$9,046	$9,649

[1]This amount includes value of tax savings.

Based upon the results above, the **ROTH IRA** would provide the greatest annual after-tax income in retirement.

IRA Comparison Analysis

Year	Annual Contributions	Annual Tax Savings for a Deductible IRA
2005	$3,000	$750
2006	$3,000	$750
2007	$3,000	$750
2008	$3,000	$750
2009	$3,000	$750
2010	$3,000	$750
2011	$3,000	$750
2012	$3,000	$750
2013	$3,000	$750
2014	$3,000	$750
2015	$3,000	$750
2016	$3,000	$750
2017	$3,000	$750
2018	$3,000	$750
2019	$3,000	$750
Total Values $45,000		$11,250

Eligibility to make deductible IRA contributions are based on plan coverage and Adjusted Gross Income. Contributions to a Roth IRA are phased out based on Adjusted Gross Income:

Married/filing jointly = $150,000—$160,000
Single = $95,000—$110,000
Married/filing sep. = $0—$10,000

This material assumes contributions and distributions are made at the end of the year. The results reflect the fact that contributions cannot be made past age 70 ½.

This calculation does not determine eligibility to make deductible or Roth IRA contributions; please refer to the IRA Deduct tool for eligibility and deductibility requirements.

CURRENT MARGINAL TAX BRACKET	ANTICIPATED INVESTMENT RETURN	YEARS UNTIL RETIREMENT							
		1	2	3	5	7	10	15	20
15%	7% 9% 11%	$ 618 $ 623 $ 628	$ 955 $ 971 $ 987	$1,311 $1,345 $1,379	$2,090 $2,181 $2,227	$2,964 $3,151 $3,351	$ 4,480 $ 4,901 $ 5,368	$ 7,670 $ 8,834 $10,201	$11,930 $14,518 $17,757
28%	7% 9% 11%	$1,148 $1,156 $1,164	$1,766 $1,791 $1,817	$2,415 $2,467 $2,520	$3,813 $3,954 $4,100	$5,355 $5,639 $5,939	$ 8,082 $ 8,599 $ 9,282	$13,291 **$14,957** $16,868	$20,093 $23,661 $27,972
31%	7% 9% 11%	$1,270 $1,279 $1,287	$1,951 $1,978 $2,005	$2,666 $2,721 $2,777	$4,199 $4,348 $4,501	$5,885 $6,183 $6,498	$ 8,730 $ 9,386 $10,097	$14,467 $16,195 $18,164	$21,729 $25,397 $29,794
36%	7% 9% 11%	$1,472 $1,481 $1,491	$2,258 $2,287 $2,316	$3,079 $3,139 $3,199	$4,834 $4,992 $5,156	$6,749 $7,065 $7,398	$ 9,955 $10,644 $11,388	$16,332 $18,123 $20,146	$24,270 $28,019 $32,453
39.6%	7% 9% 11%	$1,617 $1,627 $1,637	$2,478 $2,507 $2,537	$3,375 $3,436 $3,498	$5,284 $5,447 $5,615	$7,357 $7,682 $8,022	$10,808 $11,511 $12,267	$17,604 $19,414 $21,443	$25,963 $29,711 $34,101

ROTH PHASE OUT LIMITS

	INCOME LEVEL	CONTRIBUTION
SINGLE	Below $ 95,000	Fully eligible
	$95,000 to $110,000	Partially eligible
	Over $110,000	Not eligible
	INCOME LEVEL	CONTRIBUTION
MARRIED FILING JOINTLY	Below $150,000	Fully eligible
	$150,000 to $160,000	Partially eligible
	Over $160,000	Not eligible

To qualify for a tax-free withdrawal from a Roth IRA at retirement (age 592) a distribution must be made after a five-year holding period.

In addition, a tax-free and penalty-free distribution can be made after five years due to death or disability or a qualified first-time home purchase ($10,000 lifetime cap).

The maximum combined contribution an individual can make to traditional and Roth IRAs is $2,000 per year. At age 50, $3,000 per year; age 50+, $3,500 per year.

Source: From *Passport to Retirement*, Emerald Publications

401K Investment

Many companies have plans like the 401(k), which match contributions of their employees. If you are on such a plan you should maximize your contribution. For 2005 you are allowed to contribute up to $14,000 to a 401(k) plan and if applicable a $4000 catch-up to your account. If you are 50 or older you can make an additional "catch up" contribution, this year that amounts to $3,000. If you aren't maxing out your 401(k), at least contribute enough to qualify for your company's matching contribution. Otherwise, you're leaving free money on the table.

If your employer doesn't provide a 401(k) or similar retirement plan, then max out your contribution to an Individual Retirement Account (IRA) or other tax-qualified retirement accounts. For 2005, the contribution limit for a traditional IRA is $4,000 plus a $500 catch up. In 2006, an investment of $4,000 is allowed and a $1,000 catch up includes non-working spouses. If you are 50 or older you can contribute an additional $500. If your spouse is not working or is not covered by an employer retirement plan, he or she can still make a deductible contribution to an IRA.

If you are self-employed, do you have a retirement plan established? If not, consider setting up a SIMPLE IRA. A SIMPLE (Savings Incentive Match Plan for Employees) is designed for businesses that employ 100 or fewer people who earn at least $5,000 (this includes the self-employed). The 2005 maximum contribution is $10,000, up from $8,000 in 2003. Essentially the tax deferment goes up as the cost of living goes up. The 2005 catch up is $2,000.

If you are 50 or older, you can contribute an extra $1,500—up from $1,000 in 2003.

RETIREMENT MONEY NEEDS

The middle-aged person, within twenty to twenty-five years from retirement (at 65) needs to give serious attention to this subject. Those interested in early retirement (45-62) have undoubtedly already done this, now many are interested in a possible second career. The problem confronting us is to put together our current living standard or style into post retirement living cost. One good thing! Expenditures generally shrink. Budgets published by the Bureau of Labor Statistics show retired couples are able to maintain a similar standard of living on about half the spendable income (taxes are as much and credit over 65 more) than the typical non-retired family of four. In the rural areas the cost is somewhat less. I have suggested earlier in this chapter we should have resources of about 60 to 90 percent of our best financial years for it is difficult to estimate inflation rates or how much living costs overall for the retiring person or persons will drop. If one has a home or condominium paid for, this is an excellent start; if not and you're forty or forty-five years old, you can still take a 15-30 year mortgage on a home, or amass enough capital to rent or buy at 65.

You need to keep an eye on how your resources are growing-the social security pension funds (particularly their provisions) investments and your savings. If your employer does not have a pension plan or you are self-employed, you can start one and have your own with a tax-sheltered Individual Retirement Account. Your bank, credit union or savings and loan association or financial company such as Merrill Lynch can give you the needed information. What follows is a scheme for figuring how much will have for retirement. The monies in the brackets represent a fifty-year-old man and his wife planning (non-employed) on retiring at sixty-two. One positive note is that the cost of living is stable and the economy still runs counter to the loss of power and faith in the stock market.

MONEY ASSESSMENT FOR RETIREMENT

Regular Monies Projected (Monthly)		Additional Assets when converted to cash	
Social Security	$1,100.	Savings Accounts	($3,000.00)
Pension	500.	Investments	(3,000.00)
Annuities	350.	Stocks and Bonds	________
Others	________	Bank Certificates	________
		Other (coins, stamps)	________
		Bank Account	($2,000.00)
TOTAL	$1,950.	TOTAL	($8,000.00)

When you multiply $1,950 per month you get a yearly amount of $23,400. This is too little but of itself will grow in the ensuing years. You do have $8,000 in additional assets to use in emergencies. But this depends on a good stable market. This shows exactly what you will have and, in the event it is not enough what will have to be done. It is readily apparent that much more capital would have to be set-aside for this couple if this is the sole basis for retirement for the market is certainly not stable at the present time! As it is, a meager retirement is projected for this illustrative couple barring runaway inflation and if they own their own home. If a devastating illness costs can be handled mostly by some sort of insurance. This couple does have 12 years into which they can make some modifications. They should have an IRA and if possible participate in a thrift plan (companies often match 2-6%, the employee's share). The earnings here are untaxed until withdrawn. One should calculate the advantages of retiring at 62 rather than 65 for someone born in 1937 or earlier. If you retire at 62 you will get three additional years of money but his income will be reduced by 20 percent. If you wait to 65, you receive full benefits but you have lost three years of income, which will take 12 years of drawing to regain (based strictly on income from Social Security). You must decide if a reduced rate of Social Security will be sufficient to meet your present and future needs or if the full benefits will be necessary. Reinvestment plans are offered by 80 some large companies—Coca Cola, Xerox, Home Depot, Quaker Oats, Exxon, Electric Power companies with as little as $10 a time. The interest will accrue and when you have enough your funds will be converted to shares and they'll send you a monthly statement $10-25 a month over time can make a nice sum.

To be certain about the future plans, one should use a budget. This is a must! You can use the suggested budget form below or change it to suit yourself but should include the following major headings.

Monthly Budget

Month X Year

1. INCOME Expected ________ Actual __________

2. FIXED EXPENDITURES Expected ________ Actual __________

3. Varying Expenditures Expected ________ Actual __________

The fixed expenditure part of your budget you can have little immediate control over. Under variable expenditure there are items you can have some control over—like the water bill if it goes up greatly one month the kids may have been using too much—car washing, showering, etc. On the other hand, if the telephone bill is up or the cell phone costs too much, it may need to go maybe some body has been talking too much long distance. You might consider the telephone situation where you agree to make a minimum of calls out per month. This is sound for saving money. Perhaps clothing commands too much attention and outlay for this should be cut. In any event the beauty of a budget is it signals you that trouble is coming while you still have time to do something about it. You can cut cosmetics (God forbid!), entertainment or electricity use or smoking; how about beer and whiskey? If you'll go back to the first estimate (year) made at the beginning of this chapter, this will be a good start as a projection for the coming year. Work only a month or so in advance until you get the hang of it, then for longer periods of time. After a while, you will have a good basis for comparison of your financial situation and reach solvency if you are overextended. On the other hand, if you're doing pretty well, this will encourage you to do even better.

For those who feel they cannot handle financial problems of the future, professional counseling (financial counseling) is also a start for many mapping out retirement plans, especially where the variables—needs, inflation, money, etc., are crucial aspects. But even the younger adult needs to plan now! For the middlescent, tomorrow will be too late or as the old German proverb states, we get old too soon and smart too late!

Keeping Up the Standard of Living

You will probably need to 60 to 90% of your former pre-tax income to maintain your current lifestyle in retirement. If you made $30,000 before, you would need $18,000 (60%) to $27,000 (90%) to live as before. Many of your expenses will be reduced such as taxes, little of your social security benefits will be taxable. You also, if you are 65, will get a higher personal exemption but in general you will have less income. Work related expenses (clothes, travel, memberships, contributions) will be down or eliminated, the cost of housing reduced, or eliminated virtually (repairs and insurance remain) if the mortgage is paid. Travel is likely to be less and senior citizen discounts for lodging and meals will help with this. One should join AARP when membership is nominal but allows cheaper rates on many things like motels though questionable on insurance, i.e., car, health, etc. Also, discounts for medicine and other goods. Health and medical care will rise, those over 65 spend three times the amount of younger adults. Remember some insurance needs (personal) will be eliminated most due to the fact that children are grown and if you own your home, have some nest egg and social security, the spouse can survive. But long-term care insurance should be considered. Forty-three percent of 65ers will need home nursing or to stay at a facility average 2.5 years. A nursing home would cost $50,000-$60,000 a year at current rates.

How much do you need in retirement? There are several factors involved here as we have mentioned before. First, what resources will you have? What will you do about offsetting the inroads brought about by inflation? Do you have a plan for keeping up with the loss of purchasing power and new expenditures? If you have completed the budget form presented earlier, you know where your money is going and what is left for savings, investments—in short for retirement.

Your resources will be from the following sources: 1) Social Security, 2) Employer-sponsored retirement plans, 3) Retirement for small business owners and self-employed, 4) An IRA Account, 5) Other savings and investments. Hopefully, you have four of these five to count on for retirement or anyway three of these five. The following chart will give you a good estimate of your projected Social Security funds. The longer period of time that you pay in the maximum the higher your monthly check.

Approximation of Social Security Benefit
Starting at Age 65

Current Annual Salary	Benefit for a Working Person	Non-working Spouse Benefit
$10,000	$5,100	$2,550
15,000	6,600	3,300
20,000	8,100	4,050
25,000	9,100	4,550
30,000	9,500	4,750
35,000	9,700	4,850
40,000 or more	9,900	4,950

Now utilize the Table below for your budget. Fill in the categories in Step 1 and your supposed retirement expenses for the first year using the inflation table figure the five-year costs in retirement. Be sure to put enough in the miscellaneous space—entertainment, assistance to aging parents, or kin, repairs, gifts and contributions in total can be costly.

Having completed this you can see what you'll need in the future. To use your savings etc., for further investing. What offers the best chance to add to your financial status and increase the prospects for a continuing good life? Helpful is the Bureau of Labor data on how expenses are distributed over the past three or four years.

Younger people with several children will pay more money for housing than couples with no children. Housing goes up due to the use of nursing homes, etc., and at the same time maintaining the home also, repairs, etc.

How much will you need in retirement?

STEP I

	Current Expenses	Estimated retirement expenses
Food	______	______
Housing	______	______
Transportation	______	______
Clothing	______	______
Medical	______	______
Savings & Investments	______	______
Life insurance	______	______
Other	______	______
Total	______	______

Project for inflation

Multiply the total from Step 2 by the appropriate inflation factor from the inflation impact table at right. For example, if you are five years from retirement, you'll lose inflation factor 1.4024 to learn how much you'll actually need that first retirement year. After that, project for five years into retirement and make any other projections you think are necessary.

Your first retirement year: ______	Five years after retirement: ______	Further projections: ______

STEP II

Inflation Impact Table

(compounded at 7 percent per year)*

End of Year	Inflation factor	End of Year	Inflation factor
1	1.0700	16	2.9543
2	1.1449	17	3.1611
3	1.2250	18	3.3823
4	1.3107	19	3.6191
5	1.4024	20	3.8724
6	1.5005	21	4.1434
7	1.8055	22	4.4334
8	1.7178	23	4.7437
9	1.8380	24	5.0757
10	1.9666	25	5.4310
11	2.1042	26	5.8112
12	2.2514	27	6.2179
13	2.4117	28	6.6532
14	2.5805	29	7.1189
15	2.7611	30	7.6172

Source: Adapted from American Association of Retired Persons.

*Current inflation is not this high but allows some money leeway for retirement.

Age Group	45-54	55-64	65-75	75
Item				
Housing	22%	28%	30.5%	35.1%*
Food	13%	12%	17.8%	17.1%
Transportation	16%	15%	19.2%	12.9%
Health Care	3%	4.6%	8.4%	13.3%
Entertainment	3.1%	4.4%	3.8%	2.6%
Utilities & Public Servs.	8.4%			
Retirement Planning	7%	5.3%		
Clothing	4%	Other	20.2%	18.6%
Other	32%	23%		

*If they do not own their home.

Source: From *Passport to Retirement*, Emerald Publications

Your retirement investment strategy should be based upon generating income, minimizing risk, diversifying your investments, and having enough liquidity to get cash to satisfy needs and to counter the toll of inflation on your money. These criteria can be met by Mutual Funds, with an assist from a money company. There are funds available for investment objectives for growth, current income and keeping the principal sacrosanct. Another investment is the Zero Coupon which can help you counter inflation. The amount invested isn't touched for the period contracted for 5, 10, 15 years but if based upon municipal bonds it isn't taxed currently or later. It may be a better investment in planning for retirement or college education because the fund requires some time to general its gains but if one retires at 55 or 60 or 65, money placed in the coupons could be for five years and one could still nearly double their money in the period. Protection is absolutely guaranteed.

If you are in a higher tax bracket, you could consider tax exempt bonds from federal income taxes and sometimes from state and local income taxes, you may be able to earn more on municipals bonds than you would get after taxes on taxable investments. A tax-deferred annuity allows all you monies to accumulate for a period of time without current taxation. When the annuity payments begin, a portion of each payment is considered tax free return on principal until you recover your cost basis, after that all payments are fully taxable.

Short-term ventures provide moneymaking capabilities along with liquidity. The credit risks on those short-term (a year or less) instruments are minimal particularly where government backed such as in the case of Treasury Bills T-Bills. These bills are regularly sold at auctions and through the yields are generally lower, the investment is guaranteed if held to maturity. The Certificate of Deposit (CD) deposited in a bank or thrift institution for a specific time draws a stated amount of interest. Insured CDs can be bought backed by the federal government. The rate of yield is determined by the issuer and the purchaser and is effected by the credit quality of the issuer, their financing needs, the size of the CD being issued, the maturity of the CD and general market conditions.

In the present times caution is the key word when buying stock, in general larger companies represented by the Dow and to a less extent the NASDAQ, stock is more secure and the least secure is small company stock and those that are cheaper. This is a generality. If you have a financial advisor he would be one you trust absolutely, the same with a stockbroker; remember sometimes there are unscrupulous brokers who are motivated to make money and sometimes to make a sale they fudge giving you a stock that may not make money. They might push some stock on you that may be underwritten by some firm, which pays them to sell you a particular stock, and sometimes they ask them to guarantee the stock will not be sold for a certain period of time. Of course if we knew for certain which stocks would go up we could invest perfectly but we don't. Most investment houses Merrill Lynch, Schwab, Jones, Morgan Stanley, etc., will make suggestions about stock even urging you to buy this or that stock. It may work out but in this time of trauma like the present in the United States one must be wary. The following though not glamorous will protect your money from dwindling away as many people with varied portfolios have found. These avenues for savings and investment are the soundest of what is available. Also Credit Unions whether related to companies, the armed services, hospitals or whatever will protect your principal and make a little money for you. If you have twenty to twenty-five years to invest before retirement you can accrue a fair sum of money by IRAs and longer term CDs.

Tax-free AAA-rated Insured Municipal Bonds
2 to 4% 5 years; 4.1% 10 years
Insured as to timely payment of principal and interest.

Government-guaranteed Bonds (2004)
6 months 1.6; 10 years 4.1%
Guaranteed as to timely payment of principal and interest.

Bank-issued FDIC-insured CDs
1-year...............................**2.3%***
2-year...............................**3.15%***
3-year...............................**3.75%***
4-year...............................**3.75%***
5-year...............................**3.75%***

CDs are federally insured up to $100,000. Available from institutions nationwide. Issuer information available on request. $5,000 minimum only with a broker. Subject to availability and price change.

*Annual percentage yield. APY interest cannot remain on deposit; periodic payout of interest is required. The amount received from the sale of a CD at current market value may be the same, more or less than the amount initially invested.

U.S. Treasury Securities
1-3-years.......................**1-3.38%**
30-year.....................**1-3.85%** (As of Day/Month/Year)

There is a strong indication the U.S. government may re-issue the 30 year securities.

Guaranteed as to timely payment of principal and interest. It is expected the Feds will continue their present rates on bonds with the 10-year bond running around 10%, although, this figure could fluctuate from time to time.

Rate expressed as yield to maturity as of 2004 unless otherwise indicated. Market risk is a consideration on investments sold prior to maturity. Subject to availability and price change.

Many pre-retirees believe they will be able to count on 16 or more percent growth on their investments. Retirees know better from experience that this will not be achieved. At the present time this is impossible for most people.

Asset classes—those that have similar characteristics. There are five principal kinds of assets—cash, stocks and mutual funds based upon stocks, bonds, and bonds based upon mutual funds, fixed principal assets and tangible assets including one's home and other property. Some companies like Wachovia suggest a spread of assets in this manner—ten percent in money market accounts, 30 percent in bonds and 60 percent in stocks. Having some of each of the kinds of assets mentioned above is important since different asset classes tend to perform well at different times of the business cycle, therefore, a portfolio that is diversified over asset classes will fare a little better in periods when the market is volatile.

Nevertheless there are those that argue, at least when one approaches retirement to keep out of the stock market. Their idea is never to invest money that you will need in the next five years. That applies to money already invested. Any money in the stock market that you intend to spend in the near future should be withdrawn well before you need it. That idea applies to house down payment, college tuition, and retirement funds that you are not willing to put off if the market drops dramatically. If you are determined to spend this money put it in a safe place—that is in bonds, CDs, or money market accounts. If you intend to retire in the next five years and after you retire and are getting a pension, social security and some IRA put that money used for your retirement into five-year CDs, safe guarding your funds and making some interest at the same time.

<u>Other Options Available for Investors</u>

The present times are uncertain savings unions and money market funds save one's capital but little else. Picking a suitable alternative from stocks for you is a problem even bonds are at risk to lose value when interest rates go up, therefore, some erosion of bond prices. Some possible choices are listed below.

	Treasury notes and bonds	Savings bonds	Certificates of Deposit	State-specific municipal bond funds	Intermediate-term bond funds	GinnieMae funds
Risks	No credit risk: interest-rate and risk	No credit risk; interest-rate risk	Negligible credit risk; some interest-rate risk	Moderate credit risk and interest-rate risk	Varies depending on type and quality of bonds	Negligible credit risk; vulnerable to mortgage payment
Yields	3.30% for 5-year note; 4.37% for 10-year note	3.96% for EE bonds 2.57% for I bonds	2.74% for 22-year CDs; 4.37% for 5-year CDs	3.98% for 12 months through 6/30/02	4.98% for 12 months through 6/30/02	4.72% for 12 months through 6/30/02
Where to get them	Bureau of Public Debt, banks, brokerage firms	Bureau of Public Debt, banks	Banks, credit unions, brokerage firms	Mutual fund companies, brokerage firms	Mutual fund companies, brokerage firms	Mutual fund companies, brokerage firms
Minimum deposit or investment	$1,000	$25	$500 to $2,000	$2,500 to $3,000	$2,500 to $3,000	$2,500 to $3,000
Details to consider	Interest not taxed by states; Treasury inflation-indexed securities (TIPS) provide protection against inflation.	Interest not taxed by states	May have to pay penalty for early withdrawal; Some CDs sold by brokerage firms are callable	Interest on most muni funds isn't taxed; this raises their after-tax yield.	Fees and expenses charged by fund	Fees and expenses charged by fund
Sources of Information	Public debt. treas.gov and (800) 722-2678	Publicdebt.tr eas.gov/sav/ htm	bankrate.co m	Morningstar Inc and Morningstar.co m Lipper Inc. rating services	Morningstar Inc and Morningstar.co m Lipper Inc. rating services	Morningstar Inc and Morningstar.co m Lipper Inc. rating services

SOURCES: Historic yields for bond mutual funds adapted from Moringstar Inc.; coupon yields from Treasury notes from Bloomberg.

An investor needs to ask what are the risks? What are the costs and fees? What are the tax consequences and withdrawals? Treasury Inflation-Indexed Securities (TIPS) pay a fixed rate based upon their inflation-adjusted principal. At maturity they are redeemed at their inflation-adjusted principal or the amount paid to buy them. Series EE bonds can be deferred until the bonds cashed in that can reduce the federal tax during the years that the bonds are owned.

Bond mutual funds include various funds ranging from very conservative to ultra speculative bonds. Bond funds should be chosen over individual bonds because of the difficulty small investors have finding the prices of individual and buying the bonds at the best prices.

State specific municipal bond funds have appeal due to tax advantage. Interest income from most state specific funds is exempt from federal taxes and state taxes for residents of a particular state. This enables investors to earn an after-tax equivalent rate substantially higher than other types of bond funds would with similar risks. Ginnie Mae bond funds are issued by the government. National Mortgage offer higher yields than treasury securities. One possible problem is that Ginnie Mae bonds are backed by pools of residential mortgage loans. Meaning when interest rates drop due to prepaying their mortgage or refinance at lower rates they offer lower gains.

Divorced Women and Retirement

A special note about women who are divorced and trying to secure enough funds for the future single women have always been at greater risk than married women. In former times many who were widows had pensions and savings their husbands built up and of course some Social Security. Also many women lived with their children. Now for the first time (the late 90's) divorced women out number widows. For these women Cindy Hounsell of Women's Institute for a Secure Retirement in Washington, DC where she is Executive Director of the agency says "women should work as long as they can." The tax cut bill recently passed gives older people a chance to save more in tax sheltered retirement accounts but most women do not have enough money to take advantage of it. Women's groups are arguing as the debate over Social Security reform heats up that women should be given credit for years of home raising children. Meantime, many older women are staying on the job longer to supplement their husbands' incomes. The government should provide stipends to women who work at home with their children and many times also caring for older parents. The median weekly pay of women is 76% that of men. Many women stayed at home during a long period making the building of a large pension difficult, unlike men who never stop their jobs consequently accruing a larger pension. No fault divorce has also militated against women. A study done in Maryland (Montgomery County) (Bethesda and vicinity) looking at income of women two years after no-fault divorces found them way behind men in their financial condition even considering child care requirements. At sixty-five the income of men averages around thirty thousand dollars while that of women fifteen thousand dollars. With growing political power this will change but it will take a while. Women need to have written contracts including their husbands' pensions in the divorce settlement arrangements. This will create quite a stir but is reasonable when you consider the work of women many of whom work to help pay the bills, still look after the children and do most of the housekeeping.

New tax laws help people to invest more money without penalty for retirement and education of our children. The Economic Growth and Tax Relief Reconciliation Act of 2001 lowers income taxes, phases out estate taxes and enhances tax-deferred retirement and education savings options. Here's a brief summary of how these tax law changes can affect your retirement planning and college savings strategies:

Higher contributions to SRAs and IRAs. In 2005 under the new law, people under age 50 may be able to contribute up to $4,000 per year (over 50 another $500) to an IRA and up to $11,000 per year to an SRA. People age 50 and over may be able to contribute up to $3,500 per year to an IRA and up to $12,000 per year to an SRA. In 2006 a change for those over 50 additional $1,000.

Enhanced college savings plans. In 2004, if your adjusted gross income is $110,000 or less for a single person, $220,000 for a married couple, you can contribute up to $2,000 per year to a Coverdell Education Savings Account (previously known as an Education IRA) or some state plan. Qualified withdrawals are federal tax-free and can be used for K-12 as well as higher education expenses. See Appendix 4-1 for IRA and Retirement Plan long-term tax. The 529 American Fund allows $11,000 a year to be contributed; it must be handled through a broker such as Edward Jones.

Life insurance provides funds one can convert to cash in an emergency; it also can be used to borrow against for down payment on homes, etc. besides the obvious future money to live on if the principal or sole wage earner dies. Of course, most of the coverage you need is when children are young. When they are old and leave home, the responsibility of building their own insurance program can be theirs, thereby reducing your insurance. In the case where you have no children or dependents, a small policy to cover debts and burial expenses is sufficient. One of the best ways to save money is to combine term policies with permanent life insurance. The cheapest way to increase your coverage is to buy term, of course, the money is gone once the term period has expired. So policies allowing a conversion of term have some advantages which should be explored. A number of companies are now advertising adjusted insurance which is designed to meet the different kind of needs as life circumstances change. Terms of cash value insurance means (1) as long as you pay the premium, you are covered (2) beneficiaries get money if you die, (3) stop payment you get cash surrendered value.

One type, Variable Life Insurance, offered by Merrill Lynch and others allows you to decide the kind of investment you make on your premiums, provides a guaranteed floor of life insurance protection that doubles after ten years. This form of insurance allows you to pay that which fits your financial plan. You can borrow up to 90% of the cash value (25% during the first three years at 6%). There are no taxes to be paid while the policy is in force and the death benefit is received tax-free by the beneficiary. The underwriter for Merrill Lynch Life makes tax charges of 7% on dividends received and 15% on interest income and capital gains to cover the taxes it pays. You should examine several plans. Some variable plan will allow for better use of your money. The amount one should carry will vary according to the obligations (size of family, educational plans, etc.) and the money which will be available out of social security, pensions and savings of various kinds for sustaining life of those left. The difference should be made up through insurance.

Insurance

Many people hate to spend money for insurance. For one thing, the need of it is not easily observed (since crisis financing is a common mode) nor is its value understood. A place to live, food to eat and a car to use is another matter. Nonetheless, we have to have some kinds of insurance whether or not we like it—automobile (you could be an uninsured driver but it still costs) and homeowner's if you have a mortgage on the place you live. But at some time or the other, you will probably have to consider life, car, health and disability insurance. Let's look at these major five types.

Automobile insurance is usually required in most states and the amount of coverage varies. If you have an older car that has just about "had" it, you might consider dropping the collision clause and save the money. The tax on the old automobile may be down to nothing and worth keeping a while longer. In any event, you have to have liability insurance on your car but difference in cost of this insurance does exist between companies, so check this for savings. Remember, if you have to cover your boy and/or girl's driving that the Driver Training Course will reduce the cost. Cost and benefits vary widely but two groups that furnish insurance at a reasonable rate are Government Employee's Insurance (GEICO), State Farm Insurance and the American Association of

Retired Persons (AARP). You can join this group for a few dollars and be eligible for membership if you are fifty years old.

Homeowner's Insurance is essential as it is for renters for they need protection against fire, burglary, liability and vandalism as the owner of a home. A mortgage company will not lend money to those without a home protection policy. Unpredictable weather changes and storms are the rule rather than the exception these days, so adequate coverage is a must. Carrying $25,000 worth of insurance on a $30,000 home makes little sense or $50,000 on a $150,000 home either. Knowledge that is up-to-date on the replacement value of the home and furnishings is important.

Health insurance—Many companies underwrite employee health protection via group insurance. Some provide part of health and disability coverage, if only partly we should see to it that the entire family is covered for major medical expenses. Working members of the family should carry disability insurance if the employer does not. As one grows older the emphasis should increasingly be on disability insurance particularly after the children have become grown. Some employers such as state governments provide life insurance at very low rates. For those on Medicare (some senior groups contend it pays about 49%) a supplementary plan is necessary. The following example illustrates this: The doctor sends a bill for $100 for a stomach disorder; Medicare estimates this treatment should be $60 hence, pays only this leaving $52 for one to pay because they pay only 80% of the $60 or $48. This is why you need extra insurance. Two of the groups found by the New York Consumer Protection Board to have top rated policies—The American Association of Retired Persons and the National Council of Senior Citizens.

Ray Vicker writing on the Dow Jones culled the following pieces of advice from retired seniors. These are given here in no particular order of importance, but they summarize what I have been trying to convey to you.

Plan early for severance day.

Be flexible.

Understand your Social Security benefits.

Plan and compromise together as a couple.

Expect changes in lifestyles.

Investigate that new location thoroughly before moving.

Back Medicare with supplemental health insurance.

Watch taxes and possible IRS pitfalls.

Beware of con men after your nest eggs.

Re-evaluate your insurance needs.

Take every benefit due you.

You are younger than your children think.

Write it down.

Expect many old friends to fade into the background.

Expect new friends in every facet of your life.

Appendices

APPENDIX 1

When It Pays to Buy From the mall to the Web, saving big requires a little timing. If you can hold out, there are months of the year when discounts are traditionally deepest.

	January	February	March	April	May	June
Computers	Computer Memory	Antivirus and tax software	PDAs, laptops	Hard drives, printers	Desktops	
Electronics	Big-screen TVs, home theater systems, DVD players, CD changers		All types of TV sets	Card CD players, fax machines	Cameras, camcorders, flat-screen TVs	Cameras, DVDs, all types of TVs, headphones, car stereo systems, radios
Appliances			Washers, dryers, ovens, refrigerators, dishwashers, floor-care appliances		Small and portable appliances	TV/VCR/DVD combos, camcorders, car video equipment, CD burners
Home	Sheets, towels, furniture	Furniture			Crystal, china, silver	
House Fix-Up	Interior paint	Interior stains	Deck stains and cleaners	Exterior paint, deck stains, tools		Exterior paints
Clothing	Swimsuits, gloves, sweaters, scarves, coats, wool suits	Swimsuits	Shorts, tank tops, T-shirts	Dresses, hats, scarves, handbags	Ready-to-wear spring collections	Men's shirts, ties, golf wear
Outdoors	Golf equipment	Tennis gear, water skis	Camping gear, in-line skates	Fitness equipment racquetball gear	Basketball equipment	Volleyball equipment
Travel	Spring-summer cruises and trips to Europe, New York	Spring ski and Hawaii trips, summer Disneyland trips	Spring trips to Las Vegas, Mexico Australia	Summer cruises to Alaska, fall trips to Hawaii	Fall trips to Caribbean, Mexico	Fall and holiday trips to Europe, Caribbean
Cars	New pickup trucks and SUVs		New pickup trucks and SUVs			

PAY LESS, GET MORE

APPENDIX 2

	July	August	September	October	November	December
Computers	Hard drives, PDAs	Printer-scanner-copier combos	Digital cameras, PDAs, printers, scanners	Desktop monitors, video cards	Laptops, desk-tops, memory, games, scanners	Hard drives, PDAs
Electronics		Cordless phones, answering machines, CD boom boxes	Big-screen TVs and home theater systems	All electronics		
Appliances	Air conditioners, washers, dryers, ranges, ovens, refrigerators, dishwashers, microwave ovens					Air conditioners
Home	Sheets, towels	Furniture	Jewelry		Jewelry	
House Fix-Up		Window treatments	Interior paints, wallpaper	Interior paints, wallpaper, drapery, window treatments	Wallpaper, tools	Window treatments
Clothing	Summer apparel	Fall apparel for kids, juniors and young men		Fall and winter apparel		
Outdoors	Skis, snowboards	Cross-country skis, snow sleds	Baseball gear	Boats, canoes	Snorkeling and scuba gear, bikes	Running shoes, footballs, soccer balls
Travel		Holiday Disney trips	Winter ski trips, holiday airfares	Winter Caribbean and Mexico trips, ski trips	Last-minute European trips	Spring trips to Florida, Mexico
Cars		Previous year's models	Best month for previous year's models	Previous year's models, new minivans		New pickup trucks and SUVs

APPENDIX 3

2005 Advanced Tax Planning & Support

IRAs

CONTRIBUTION LIMITS – TRADITIONAL AND ROTH

	2002 – 2004	2005	2006 – 2007	2008
Regular	$3,000	$4,000	$4,000	$5,000
Catch-up*	500	500	1,000	1,000

*Only taxpayers age 50 and over are eligible to make catch-up contributions

ROTH IRAS

AGI Phaseout Range for Contributions to Roth IRAs:

Married Filing Jointly: $150,000 – $160,000 Single: $95,000 – $110,000

TRADITIONAL IRA DEDUCTIBILITY RULES

Filing Status	Covered by Employer's Retirement Plan?	Modified AGI 2004	Modified AGI 2005	Deductibility
Single	No	Any amount	Any amount	Full Deduction
	Yes	$44,999 or less $45,000 – $54,999 $55,000 or more	$49,999 or less $50,000 – $59,999 $60,000 or more	Full Deduction Partial Deduction No Deduction
Married Filing Jointly	Neither spouse	Any amount	Any amount	Full Deduction
	Both spouses covered	$64,999 or less $65,000 – $74,999 $75,000 or more	$69,999 or less $70,000 – $79,999 $80,000 or more	Full Deduction Partial Deduction No Deduction
	One spouse covered – for covered spouse	$64,999 or less $65,000 – $74,999 $75,000 or more	$69,999 or less $70,000 – $79,999 $80,000 or more	Full Deduction Partial Deduction No Deduction
	One spouse covered – for non-covered spouse	$149,999 or less $150,000 – $159,999 $160,000 or more	$149,999 or less $150,000 – $159,999 $160,000 or more	Full Deduction Partial Deduction No Deduction

Uniform Life Table

For Calculating Required Minimum Distributions from Qualified Plans and Traditional IRAs

Current Age	Distrib. Period	Current Age	Distrib. Period
70	27.4	93	9.6
71	26.5	94	9.1
72	25.6	95	8.6
73	24.7	96	8.1
74	23.8	97	7.6
75	22.9	98	7.1
76	22.0	99	6.7
77	21.2	100	6.3
78	20.3	101	5.9
79	19.5	102	5.5
80	18.7	103	5.2
81	17.9	104	4.9
82	17.1	105	4.5
83	16.3	106	4.2
84	15.5	107	3.9
85	14.8	108	3.7
86	14.1	109	3.4
87	13.4	110	3.1
88	12.7	111	2.9
89	12.0	112	2.6
90	11.4	113	2.4
91	10.8	114	2.1
92	10.2	115 and older	1.9

Education Incentives

Coverdell Education Savings Accounts (Education IRAs): Contribution Limit $2,000

AGI Phaseout Range for Contributions to Coverdell Education Savings Accounts:
Married Filing Jointly: $190,000 – $220,000 **Single:** $95,000 – $110,000

Qualified Tuition Programs – Section 529 Plans
Distributions after 12/31/01 used for qualified higher education expenses are income tax free

Hope and Lifetime Learning Credits

Hope Credit – Up to $1,500 per student, for first 2 years of higher education tuition paid
Lifetime Learning Credit – Up to 20% of tuition paid; $2,000 max

AGI Phaseouts:	2004	2005
Married Filing Jointly	$85,000 – $105,000	unavailable from IRS
Others	$42,000 – $52,000	

Exclusion of U.S. Savings Bond Income

AGI Phaseouts:	2004	2005
Married Filing Jointly	$89,750 – $119,750	unavailable from IRS
Others	$59,850 – $74,850	

Student Loan Interest Deduction – Maximum Deduction: $2,500

AGI Phaseouts:	2004	2005
Married Filing Jointly	$100,000 – $130,000	unavailable from IRS
Single	$50,000 – $65,000	
Deductibility Period	No time Limit	

Deduction for Higher Education Expenses
Maximum Deduction (above the line) for 2002 – 2003 is $3,000; for 2004 – 2005 is $4,000

Taxpayers with AGI below the following amounts are eligible:
Married Filing Jointly: $130,000 Single: $65,000 All others: $0

Long-term Care Insurance

Max. Qualified LTC Premiums Eligible for Itemized Medical Deduction:

age	40 or less	41 – 50	51 – 60	61 – 70	Over 70
2004	$260	$490	$980	$2,600	$3,250
2005	$270	$510	$1,020	$2,720	$3,400

Qual. LTC contract per diem limit ($230 in 2004) ($240 in 2005)

APPENDIX 4

Income Taxes

2004: If Taxable Income Is: Over	But not more than	The Tax Is	Of the Amount Over	2005: If Taxable Income Is: Over	But not more than	The Tax Is	Of the Amount Over
Married Filing Jointly:							
$0	$14,300	$0 + 10%	$0	$0	$14,600	$0 + 10%	$0
14,300	58,100	1,430 + 15%	14,300	14,600	59,400	1,460 + 15%	14,600
58,100	117,250	8,000 + 25%	58,100	59,400	119,950	8,180 + 25%	59,400
117,250	178,650	22,787.50 + 28%	117,250	119,950	182,800	23,317.50 + 28%	119,960
178,650	319,100	39,979.50 + 33%	178,650	182,800	326,450	40,915.50 + 33%	192,800
319,100		86,328 + 35%	319,100	326,450		88,320 + 35%	326,450
Single:							
$0	$7,150	$0 + 10%	$0	$0	$7,300	$0 + 10%	$0
7,150	29,050	715 + 15%	7,150	7,300	29,700	730 + 15%	7,300
29,050	70,350	4,000 + 25%	29,050	28,700	71,950	4,090 + 25%	29,700
70,350	146,750	14,325 + 28%	70,350	71,950	150,150	14,652.50 + 28%	71,950
146,750	319,100	35,717 + 33%	146,750	150,150	326,450	36,548.50 + 33%	150,150
319,100		92,592.50 + 35%	319,100	326,450		94,727.50 + 35%	326,450
Estates & Trusts:							
$0	$1,950	$0 + 15%	$0	$0	$2,000	$0 + 15%	$0
1,950	4,600	292.50 + 25%	1,950	2,000	4,700	300 + 25%	2,000
4,600	7,000	985 + 28%	4,600	4,700	7,150	975 + 28%	4,700
7,000	9,550	1,627 + 33%	7,000	7,150	9,750	1,661 + 33%	7,150
9,550		2,468.50 + 35%	9,550	9,750		2,519 + 35%	9,750

Corporations: (2004)

Over	But not more than	The Tax Is	Of the Amount Over
$0	$50,000	$0 + 15%	$0
50,000	75,000	7,500 + 25%	50,000
75,000	100,000	13,750 + 34%	75,000
100,000	335,000	22,250 + 39%	100,000
335,000	10,000,000	113,900 + 34%	335,000
10,000,000	15,000,000	3,400,000 + 35%	10,000,000
15,000,000	18,333,333	5,150,000 + 38%	15,000,000
18,333,333		+ 35%	

Capital Gains Tax:	Short-Term	Long-Term
Taxpayer in:	<12 months	>12 months
10, 15% Bracket	ordinary rate	5%
Other Brackets	ordinary rate	15%

Kiddie Tax: (Under age 14 with unearned income)

	2004	2005	
First	$800	$800	No Tax
Next	800	800	10% Tax
Amounts Over	1,600	1,600	Parents' Rate

Standard Deductions

		Annual	Add'l Age 65 or Older or Blind
Married Filing Jointly	2004	$9,700	$950
	2005	$10,000	$1,050
Single	2004	$4,850	$1,200
	2005	$5,000	$1,250

Personal Exemptions[1]

		Exemption	AGI Threshold / Upper Limit
Married Filing Jointly	2004	$3,100	$214,050 / $336,550
	2005	$3,200	$218,950 / $341,450
Single	2004	$3,100	$142,025 / $265,200
	2005	$3,200	$145,950 / $268,450

[1] Personal exemptions are phased out by 2% for each $2,500 by which AGI exceeds threshold

Phaseout of Itemized Deductions

- Reduced by 3% of taxpayer's AGI in Excess of $142,700 in 2004 (145,950 in 2005)
- Reduction limited to 80%; does not affect investment interest, medical, or casualty losses

Child Tax Credit: 2004 – 2010
$1,000 per child; phases out $50 for each $1,000 of AGI over $110,000 (married filing joint), or $75,000 (single)

Estate & Gift Taxes

For Deaths/Gifts Occurring in 2004

If Taxable Estate Is: Over	But Not Greater Than	The Tax Is:	Of The Amount Over:
$0	$10,000	$0 + 18%	
10,000	20,000	1,800 + 20%	$10,000
20,000	40,000	3,800 + 22%	20,000
40,000	60,000	8,200 + 24%	40,000
60,000	80,000	13,000 + 26%	60,000
80,000	100,000	18,200 + 28%	80,000
100,000	150,000	23,800 + 30%	100,000
150,000	250,000	38,800 + 32%	150,000
250,000	500,000	70,800 + 34%	250,000
500,000	750,000	155,800 + 37%	500,000
750,000	1,000,000	248,300 + 39%	750,000
1,000,000	1,250,000	345,800 + 41%	1,000,000
1,250,000	1,500,000	448,300 + 43%	1,250,000
1,500,000	2,000,000	555,800 + 45%	1,500,000
2,000,000		780,800 + 48%	2,000,000

Subtract applicable credit below from calculated tax:

Estate	Exclusion Amount	Applicable Credit
2004 – 2005	1,500,000	555,800
2006 – 2008	2,000,000	780,800
2009	3,500,000	1,455,800
2010	Estate tax repealed; gift tax remains	
2011	1,000,000	345,800

Annual Gift Tax Exclusion: $11,000
Gift Tax Exclusion: $1,000,000
GST Tax Exemption: $1,500,000 (2004 and 2005)

Social Security

Base Amount Of Modified Adjusted Gross Income Causing Social Security Benefits to be Taxable:

	50% Taxable	85% Taxable
Married Filing Jointly	$32,000	$44,000
Single	$25,000	$34,000

Max. Earnings Before Soc. Sec. Benefits are Reduced:
Assumes full retirement age is 65

	2004	2005
Under age 65 *(lose $1 for every $2)*	$11,640	$12,000
Age 65 and over	No Limit	No Limit

Maximum Compensation Subject to FICA Taxes:

	2004	2005
OASDI (Soc. Sec. 6.2%) Maximum	$87,900	$90,000
HI (Medicare 1.45%) Maximum	No Limit	No Limit

* *OASDI tax rate: 12.4% self-employed, 6.2% employees*
* *HI tax rate: 2.9% self-employed, 1.45% employees*

Qualified Plans

	2004	2005
Maximum elective deferral to retirement plans, e.g., 401(k), 403(b)	$13,000	$14,000
Maximum elective deferral to SIMPLE IRA plans	$9,000	$10,000
Maximum elective deferral to 457 plans or tax-exempt employers	$13,000	$14,000
Limit on annual additions to SEP plans	$41,000	$42,000
Limit on annual additions to defined contribution plans	$41,000	$42,000
Maximum annual compensation taken into account for contributions	$205,000	$210,000
Annual benefit limit under defined benefit plans	$165,000	$170,000
Threshold amount for definition of highly compensated employees	$90,000	$95,000
Threshold amount for definition of key employee in top-heavy plans	$130,000	$135,000

Catch-Up Contribution Limits for Other Qualified Plan Types

	2004	2005	2006
401(k), 403(b), SAR-SEP and 457 Plans	$3,000	$4,000	$5,000
SIMPLE Plans	$1,500	$2,000	[illegible]

Saver's Tax Credit

Contributions to Employer Plans and IRAs
Maximum Credit $2,000; for 2002 and after; AGI limits below

Married Filing Jointly	Single	Credit
$0 – $30,000	$0 – $15,000	50% of contribution
$30,001 – $32,500	$15,001 – $16,250	20% of contribution
$32,501 – $50,000	$16,251 – $25,000	10% of contribution
Over $50,000	Over $25,000	Not Available

APPENDIX 5

TAXABLE EQUIVALENT YIELD TABLES
Taxable Equivalent Yields

2004 Tax Year
Federal and State Tax-Exempt Yields and
Equivalent Taxable Yields

Federal Tax Bracket	15%	25%	28%	33%	35%
Taxable Income Single Return ($)	7,151- 29,050	29,051- 70,350	70,351- 146,750	146,751- 319,100	319,101+
Taxable Income Joint Return ($)	14,301- 58,100	58,101- 117,250	117,251- 178,650	178,651- 319,100	319,101+
Federal & State Combined Tax Bracket	19.89%	29.31%	32.14%	36.85%	38.74%
Effective State Tax Bracket	4.89%	4.31%	4.14%	3.85%	3.74%
Tax-Exempt Yields (%)	Equivalent Taxable Yields (%)				
1.00	1.25	1.41	1.47	1.58	1.63
1.50	1.87	2.12	2.24	2.38	2.45
2.00	2.50	2.83	2.95	3.17	3.26
2.25	2.81	3.18	3.32	3.56	3.67
2.50	3.12	3.54	3.68	3.96	4.08
2.75	3.43	3.89	4.05	4.35	4.49
3.00	3.74	4.24	4.42	4.75	4.90
3.25	4.06	4.60	4.79	5.15	5.31
3.50	4.37	4.95	5.16	5.54	5.71
3.75	4.68	5.31	5.53	5.94	6.12
4.00	4.99	5.66	5.89	6.33	6.53
4.25	5.31	6.01	6.26	6.73	6.94
4.50	5.62	6.37	6.63	7.13	7.35
4.75	5.93	6.72	7.00	7.52	7.75
5.00	6.24	7.07	7.37	7.92	8.16
5.25	6.55	7.43	7.74	8.31	8.57
5.50	6.87	7.78	8.10	8.71	8.98
5.75	7.18	8.13	8.47	9.11	9.39
6.00	7.49	8.49	8.84	9.50	9.79

Information presented in this chart is not guaranteed but is believed to be correct based upon federal and state income tax rates effective 12/30/03. The effective state tax is based on the top state rate. No local income taxes are taken into consideration.

COMPLIANCE DEPARTMENT JM PRINCIPAL.
This information is approved for use with the public.
It is intended for informational purposes only. It is believed
to be reliable, but its accuracy and completeness are not guaranteed.

APPENDIX 6

TAXABLE EQUIVALENT YIELD TABLES
Taxable Equivalent Yields

2004 Tax Year
Tax-free Yields and
Equivalent Out-of-State Tax-Free Yields

Federal Tax Bracket	15%	25%	28%	33%	35%
Taxable Income Single Return ($)	7,151-29,050	29,051-70,350	70,351-146,750	146,751-319,100	310,101+
Taxable Income Joint Return ($)	14,301-58,100	58,101-117,250	117,251-178,650	178,651-319,100	319,101+
State Tax Bracket	5.75%	5.75%	5.75%	5.75%	5.75%
Effective State Tax Bracket	4.89%	4.31%	4.14%	3.85%	3.74%
Tax-Exempt Yields (%)	Equivalent Out-of-state Tax-free Yields (%)				
1.00	1.05	1.05	1.04	1.04	1.04
1.50	1.58	1.27	1.56	1.56	1.56
2.00	2.10	2.09	2.09	2.08	2.08
2.25	2.37	2.35	2.35	2.34	2.34
2.50	2.63	2.61	2.61	2.60	2.60
2.75	2.89	2.87	2.87	2.86	2386
3.00	3.15	3.14	3.13	3.12	3.12
3.25	3.42	3.40	3.39	3.38	3.38
3.50	3.68	3.66	3.65	3.64	3.64
3.75	3.94	3.92	3.91	3.90	3.90
4.00	4.21	4.18	4.17	4.16	4.16
4.25	4.47	4.44	4.43	4.42	4.42
4.50	4.73	4.70	4.69	4.68	4.67
4.75	4.99	4.96	4.96	4.94	4.93
5.00	5.26	5.23	5.22	5.20	5.19
5.25	5.52	5.49	5.48	5.46	5.45
5.50	5.78	5.75	5.74	5.72	5.71
5.75	6.01	6.01	6.00	5.98	5.97
6.00	6.27	6.27	6.26	6.24	6.23

The above illustrates the yield necessary on an out-of-state tax-free bond to have the same spendable income as a yield on an in-state tax-free bond. The effective state tax is based on the top state rate reduced for the effect of the federal deductibility of state income taxes paid and, in some cases, the cross deductibility of both federal and state taxes paid. The above table does not take into account any intangible tax, if applicable.

COMPLIANCE DEPARTMENT JM PRINCIPAL.
This information is approved for use with the public.
It is intended for informational purposes only. It is believed
to be reliable, but its accuracy and completeness are not guaranteed.

CHAPTER XII

THE GOOD LIFE

"The Best is Yet to Come"

"Youth is a silly vapid state:
Old Age with fears and ills is rife.
The simple boon I beg of fate-
A thousand years of middle life."-

—Carolyn Wells

This expresses what some people know about middle age. The word "middle age" may have bad connotations—fatigue, discontent and boredom. But as Harvey Allen in "Anthony Adverse" says, "Grow up as soon as you can." It pays. The only time you really live is from 30 to 60. The young are slaves of drams; the old, servants of regrets, only the middle-aged have all their five senses in the keeping of their wits. This is a distortion of the other ages in life but it bespeaks a fundamental truth. The middlescent is not troubled by the impetuosity of youth, which pulls it madly into life-traps; they are stronger than the old and wiser than the young. The middlescent usually has enough perspective to keep from being led astray by the shallow and glamorous and to search for the true and most valuable. He or she has time to assess his errors of the past, to adjust his sights and to fulfill the opportunities, which lie ahead.

There is a special synthesis in the middlescent found nowhere else in the stages of man's life. This period is one of maturity—neither green nor overripe. Here the experiences of life are welded together in sensible understandable patterns, from which meaning is drawn from life. In the earlier part of adult life, the preoccupation with immediate pleasure and demands has been tempered and the middlescent evaluates life in terms of what is worthy rather than what is worth. If middle age were reckless as the twenties or early thirties, we would change panaceas for solving social and economic ills so frequently we would bring chaos to our lives. On the other hand, if the middlescent years were caught in the framework of regression to memory like many of our old, society wouldn't move at all. Aside from these broad platitudes, what constitutes the "good life"? There are some assumptions that this is based upon, what are they? They are, that one possess reasonably good health, both physical and mental, have enough financial resources to sustain one's life with a modicum of adequacy. Without these, the freedom to be one's self and to be creative is clearly limited. Without money enough to survive and/or to be physically ill, a person may have a positive outlook, but still it would be stretching the definition of "good life" to say they were the same.

To talk about the "Good Life" may seem imposterous in the nations life today. The possibility of tranquility and normality that allows people to go about their lives as usual at the present time and the near future is gone. The terrorists attacks have changed our ways of living by disrupting transportation, our work lives, our mental health as we develop paranoid postures, ever watchful for impending doom and cues that puts fear that some plague is upon us or is impending like Damocles Sword hanging tentatively above our heads. On the other hand in a way greater than ever before the freedom we have, the open horizon for growth and opportunity to make our place in our land is now more precious, less taken for granted and it gives us courage to overcome whatever circumstances we find ourselves confronted, be it disease, sacrifice of luxury, greatly reduced standards of living and disruption of our society. Increasingly the aspects of the good life that I speak of will be more important than ever—the common enemy will make us feel closer to our neighbors and each others, force us to recognize the importance of work, to burgeon out all we can make of ourselves the commitment to a cause far beyond the mundane world that is our usually purview and the need love plays in our lives. Love which expressed itself from our earlier national days—first for freedom, then equality, then to provide for the poor, the halt and the blind—allowing the kind of environment that guarantees in our great country the right to express love as individuals and as a group to defy the enemies of our motherland.

We shall win the war with the terrorists because we are determined, pledged to give what is necessary to go on to victory. In the lives of the Islamic, Jewish or Christians who give allegiance to Christ we are united and can steadfastly echo from our hearts the well-known refrain:

In the beauty of the lilies Christ was born across the seas,
With the glory in his bosom that transforms you and me,
As he died to make men holy let us die to make men free,
His truth is marching on—Glory, glory hallelujah his truth is marching on!—

Over a hundred years ago the English clergyman, Charles Mildmay wrote, "Every duty brings its peculiar delight, every denial its appropriate compensation, every thought its recompense, every cross its crown; pay goes with performance as effect with cause." We plant our vineyards in the springtime of life and harvest in the summer and early fall. In the middlescent years our earlier sins bring remorse; still there is time to undo most of this and more important the good we've done, the credits we have amassed pay off in a fine harvest.

Sure there are problems in the in-between years—the "change of life," but many have denied the myths surrounding it by projecting increased confidence in their sexuality and maintaining their appearance, in looking their best and at the same time being mature. Increasingly the middlescent looks after his body, keeping trim, exercising, proscribing the overindulgence in smoking, drinking and use of drugs, all of this denial helps to give a vitality to enjoy life. It is true that many middle-aged persons are afflicted with some chronic health problem, but they have found a way to stabilize it. The problem of diabetes or a heart problem can be a blessing in disguise in that one is saved from the brink and having done this can reconstruct their lives in more healthy productive ways. Having been able to manage one's life and have good health means that the anxieties, depressions and emotional upsets of the middle years will finally be rewarded with tranquility and equanimity. The notion that we are failures with our partners, our children and careers takes on new perspectives when having muddled through we arrive at a maturity level we thought impossible. Though we are divorced, our children have left the nest or are getting ready to leave and we are shakingly beginning a new career and/or marriage; we are hopeful and not without resources. Father Time does not have us in a bind, for now we are free from the "nattering nabobs of negatism"—that there is no time. At 35, 45, even 55, we can do something worthwhile in our lives—plan an adequate retirement, remarry, have a new career and change our life styles. The frantic drive for success no longer plagues us; we know we have time to do our own thing! And though we mourn the loss of our past selves—as the best looking woman in the room, the club Tennis Champion, when we were slim and trim and had fewer aches and pains we understand the illusion of our childhood, the destructive form of our urgency (Id.). We are at peace now more than ever. The good life beckons. Duke University Longitudinal Studies shown life satisfaction to be the best in middle age peaking at 55. Though it drops from then until 65 it rises for then into the seventies.

There are those like F. Scott Fitzgerald who declared: "There are no second acts in American lives." Maybe he was right, in a sense that we can't recreate our lives—be young again, have energy to spare, look like we did twenty years ago and attract men or women physically like we did at an earlier time. If we have been sensationally successful like Fitzgerald was following the publication of the novel, Tender Is the Night, perhaps we have no second act. But he was wrong too, in a sense, for millions of Americans or Europeans are beginning second acts in the middlescent years with verve and purpose. The good life begins and finds its basis in the first act and what happens in the second act depends on the first. The same with the third act. Dr. Taylor Morgan in his book of yesteryear, Welcome to the Middle Years, suggests that those who have had good first acts in their lives can expect to have some special gifts which come by being favored by the gods in their middle years. These are the things we get as payoff for our past investments in giving effort and by persevering. Morgan lists:

1. Seasoned maturity—it comes from having succeeded in one's job, you've gained an expertise on the job so now you can enjoy it.
2. Personal Respect—this goes hand in hand with maturity; you are recognized for knowing your field, or it is said of her, "she's tops in her field," others seek your counsel.
3. Tranquility at Home—all our wives' bad habits have been corrected along with ours; we have learned to live together. The period of adjustment is over, we can relax and be at peace with our spouses and others.
4. Financial Security—the saving and hard work we've done begins to pay off. The fruit of our labor bears a good harvest. We can burn the mortgage at some time during this period and have additional money to invest for retirement or to spend on ourselves.
5. Creature Comforts—with children gone and home ownership finalized an additional room—club or den—can be added; we can take a trip—California, Hawaii or Europe, or add some luxury item you want.
6. Personal Freedom—as middlescents we are no longer troubled with feverish search for a career as the young adult is; in many cases our

time is our own as we can adjust it to suit our needs. We have time to follow what beckons in new horizons.

You say this is not hardly the expectation of the younger middlescent? True and is more likely to be reserved to those in their late forties and fifties, which is precisely those Morgan, is writing about. But they do apply, even to the person in their late thirties. The thing that is important here is that it is possible to construct a better life and to have the "good life" even before all the ultimate rewards are obtained like those from earlier investments and when the children are grown up allowing for more time and less responsibility.

The "good life" has many definitions or synonyms, depending upon whom you ask about it. For many one word—money or leisure or fame, health, love, power or sex—characterizes the "good life." The "good life" is much broader than those isolated aspects of life and it is greater in its impact than a single-handed one could ever be. Adults in our time are driven to be "self actualized"—that is, to reach their ultimate potential. They seek kinetic happiness constantly agitating for change to achieve it. Increasingly, men and women are recognizing that adult life is not a stagnation or a plodding passage across an endless plateau but a matter of negotiation with ourselves, with our families, our work, spouses and friends. We also know that life consists of many ups and downs and the changing of direction. In most cases there is a consensus that adult development embraces, in the young adult period, the getting of a job and marrying. About thirty, for men, maybe earlier for women, a period of discontent and self-analysis begins which sometimes heralds divorce or a first time marriage and change of careers. Following this comes a period of "settling down." This phase usually ends by the time one is forty (man) or earlier for women with a stage in which they become one's "own man." During the forties and fifties changes occur which lead to greater fulfillment in the lives of many; for some, women for instance, will enter the labor market for the first time, divorce and find new men. Many men will marry for the second time and some will begin a new work life. Both men and women will usually enter after 65, into a period of transition—the young-old 65 75 (Bernice Neugarten's category) and later adulthood after 75. If you look at a number of people in the middlescent years, you will find a variety of differences. They are different in looks and health, the state of their mind, the family life, their work life and expectantly their views about life, certainly of what is "good" and important in life. So you undoubtedly find different emphasis on what constitutes the "good life."

The Good Life

I believe the "good life" consists of an amalgam of work, play, love, and a cause (worship). although adults with varying backgrounds will give these different weights, for it seems obvious that our value systems were built from those of our parents and though they are modified still remain much the same and reflect their views. That the "good life" consists of a balance between work, play, love and a cause seems deceptively simple. They do not of themselves bring happiness. I think happiness is a by-product of leading effective and ordered lives that are infused with the liking for work—the need to do it; to enjoy play—to be creative in it; to love—someone and others as much as we love ourselves; and to dedicate ourselves to a cause—commitment to something higher and beyond ourselves. You do not aim directly at being happy for it grows out of a number of things but not the satisfaction of something specific such as money. You think that will solve all your problems. Errant nonsense, it might well be the beginning of them! On the other hand, even the presence of work, play, love and a cause cannot insure we will reach the Elysian Field where the sirens will provide a soothing of our problems and a fulfillment of all our wishes. There is a structure upon which this mix is based. This, we should note, resolves upon our parents—their (our) value systems, life styles and commitment to work, play, love and a cause, all of which have to some degree internalized from them. All of our prospects for the "good life" come from them initially.

WORK

In the case of work, which is the first necessary ingredient of the good life, there are two aspects: (1) the method in which we handle our obligations (work) to family and children, and (2) the attention and effectiveness we give to our jobs, our professions and occupations. On the first point, you may object to my calling family obligation work (it may not be for many men and some women) but it is not just a matter of love, or loving to do it—keeping house, washing clothes, disciplining, waiting and worrying—it's routine and sheer hard, sacrificing work and devotion to duty.

As parents the important responsibility most of us will ever undertake is the raring of our children. Fathers and mothers have to be dedicated to the task of homemakers. A successful home is the early schooling for love. Children need to be loved from infancy through their growing years, for how else can they learn to love others and become happy adults. But love is not enough, for children need discipline if they are to develop as competent adults. Discipline is love in action! Those parents who do not persevere in rearing their children are leaving them free to develop on their own, letting other children and youth shape their views and habits or the media, principally television and the movies, do the job of rearing your children.

Requirements of a work or chore routine for children is appropriate in teaching that value is that which is worth saving for, working for, sacrificing for. It brings enjoyment in exactly the terms of energy expended. Even the development of security depends in children on guidelines laid down by parents—that limits are set on their activities in which they receive commendation and out of which they receive censure.

The work involved in family obligation is not simply dealing with the routine responsibilities of children and housework but dealing with the principals of the home—mother and father. In this one doesn't have to be routine, for that smacks of work in the most derogatory way, but consistent attention should be given to the other, in recognition of special events, their particular needs, and their valuableness. A pleasurable kind of work, enjoyed but constant and effective. The same sort of thing should be given to our larger families and kin, for they too are a part of our lives usually in increasing proportions. Maintaining good relations with our friends and neighbors is also of great importance. When we work at this task at the lowest level, we will find we touch everything higher up in our regard.

The jobs we hold and the service we give through them are of signal importance because they serve our economic needs in purchasing the necessities of life. Beyond this, the satisfactory work life is the hub virtually of our entire lives. The most successful people obviously are busy people, the most happy appear to be busy people—in short people who are busy, work and usually they work very hard. John Gardner says the best kept secret in America today is that people would rather work hard for something they believe in than enjoy a pampered idleness. Other satisfactions relate to and certainly the good life hinges upon the work life! For without the work world, there could be no effective play. Play is the offset from the routine, it gives relief from the tiring physical exertion and debilitating mental strain which often accompanies our work, it also allows us to unwind, it reduces the ennui that has set in and prepares us to enjoy recreation and leisure. This may be worked at as much as our occupations and professions, but it renews the spirits, settles the nerves and gives us strength to continue our work. Our work when it is done well has predictable fall-out allowing a plus to living and improving our lives contravening the old cliche "when poverty comes in the door love flies out the window." It provides the feeling of security, relaxation and worthiness through giving a plus to 'just getting by.'

According to William Shannon writing in *New York Times* magazine, "Work in the best sense is an expression of a person's intellectual powers, artistic sensibility or physical strength or personality. If one's work does not provide any kind of distinctive outlet, though Voltaire said it saves us from three great evils: boredom, vice and need, it may still provide the psychic rewards of being a member of a group with its own elan and cohesiveness." Those organizations that implement these outlets and rewards like family, schools, communities, recreation programs and churches are allies in building the "good life" for the future.

PLAY

In the chapter on "Leisure and Recreation," I devoted a section on how to get started with play. It sounds foolish to suggest that adults do not know how to play. But one should not confuse "playing around," "doing nothing," "goofing off," as play. It can be play without organizing it but it can be organized requiring as much energy as work, and as demanding in skill. Whatever the nature of play, as middlescents we should have it and enjoy the kind we have. A number of activities are categorized under play—travel, social life, entertainment, hobbies, and sports. Play in the sense of activity which is contrived on the spur of the moment is also valuable. All serve to be refreshing. Recreation refers to any activity that is both creative and re-creative, giving emotional satisfaction to the person involved. Of the categories of play listed above, travel is one of the most desired by the middlescent. Many have never been able to play or travel as they wished because of the obligations of the work and home life, which interfered. Now since our children are older we have this opportunity. We can arrange more time for vacation, therefore travel. We know also that the slower you travel the more you can see. Travel represents a field of civilized human activity in which maturity has real and tangible advantages over youth. It provides a sense of leisure that comes with maturity, leisure to travel slowly and to savor the mood, the flavor, and the atmosphere of the places you visit as you go.

Social life is another promising aspect of play. For many, this is the only outlet which allows persons to relax, to let off steam and enjoy other people. Most middlescent people would rather socialize than nearly anything else. The number of clubs, ladies aid societies, social organizations attest to this. The only drawback here is the fact that we often under exercise and overeat on these occasions. Nothing, in fact, is better than eating and drinking when we are in our middle years—we have learned to like many things, varieties we could not stomach in our earlier years—now we have this spice of life, we become gourmets. Card games for some, dancing for others, cocktail parties, camping and traveling together or just visiting friends or relatives satisfies others. Social life can be arranged with little effort and hardly any cost. For many of you who have never had a party at your home or apartment, you ought to try it. It will cost something, to be sure, but it's worth it. You can do it as a single or a married person, with little or no formality—it's a gesture of generosity and reveals you a person of sociability.

Entertainment for leisure and enjoyment is frequently invigorating—the theater, the movie, television, athletic events, concerts, art exhibits can all be great. I have found that a steady diet of television viewing gets stale in a hurry, even though I watch often while I read, sports, news, movies, special events, etc. I like a variety of programs found on the Public Broadcasting Television Stations—commentaries, debates, concerts, educational and travel presentations. The television programs provide considerable entertainment and relaxation; it even has some other attributes—my daughter, when she was very young, a few years ago told me the television was a comforter. For many it serves as complete relaxation—sleep—as the controlled noise is like rain on a tin roof. We should offset viewing the television with in person attendance at concerts, football and basketball games, and the festivals our towns and cities organized around themes—October Fest, Harbor Fests, Smoky Mountain Blue Grass Sing, Gasparilla Week, Mardi Gras, Centennials, etc. Some of them leave you gagging perhaps, but we should support them and argue for their improvement. Participation is the thing, not just passive listening or viewing. Increasingly we have paid entertainment and this provides us opportunity many times to be titillated when otherwise we could not be. We should not, however, depend upon this entirely forgetting what we can do to enliven our lives and others with our own locally arranged fun.

Hobbies can be the most fun and joy many people can have. It can be exclusively ours beyond public inspection. True it takes us from people, but for those who work constantly with people, this provides a good counteracting activity. It tends to slow the stimuli we constantly receive and allows a slower ingestion of it. Hobbies range from sewing, modeling, to reading. Hobbies can be an excellent avocation—many begun for fun become the fun way to make a living. More importantly hobbies provide a release of emotion from in us, they allow the aesthetic to be explored and experienced. Age is no drawback for those interested in painting, music, stamp collecting, embroidery, craft work and the like. A hobby is something we can become engrossed in, allowing us to shut out the mundane things giving us something to look forward to hope and delight, whether it's gardening or fixing old furniture or toys. If you don't have a hobby, you need one!

Athletic and sports activity is a marvelous source of play for many. I like it—that is, swimming, tennis (played since 8 years of age), running, pick-up games, formerly touch football and softball. You don't have to be twenty years old to enjoy and play these games. What I like about sports and exercising games is that the benefit is great for keeping your weight down, the sugar and cholesterol in check, and there are social accruals also. The body's muscle tone is much better when exercise is regular, allowing greater enjoyment for anything else you wish to do. The chance to work off tensions, reconstruct your feeling by reducing the charge up animus of the viscera, and finally to have a comfortable relaxed tingling sensation after you have exercised. Hopefully we can make our exercise play and fun. I try this but don't always succeed for some days I can't swim, play tennis or dance, so I have to jog—it's tough on hard earth and impossible on the street for it jolts my legs and joints after a couple of sessions. Nevertheless I get with it—it's better than stationary running or floor exercises, for me anyway. It's work, sometimes, and not play like at the beach for when you run there you can enjoy the scenery! Find some exercise that is fun—bicycle rides, take walks, hikes, but don't overlook the possibility of play even here.

LOVE

The songster said, "love makes the world go round." This is inexorably true! It gives meaning to our work, it enables play to be enjoyable, it ennobles our compassion for others and humane causes. Love is something we learn beginning in childhood; we are loved and in turn we love others besides mother and father, our first teacher, perhaps our first playmate. We come to understand that occasionally we lose people we love—through moving, through death and just because it can't always be permanent. The fact is when we get to be adults we sometimes wonder about whether there is any permanence or not. That we need to love and be loved we usually do not doubt. The truth is that no two people reach adulthood with the same capacity to give and receive love. If we have been loved in our early years, we usually feel secure with giving love to others. Our success in love, marriage, parenthood and to an extent in our work, our job or professional, depend on understanding these kinds of variations between people. Freud suggested that our earlier loves influence the way we love presently. The boy who suffers an unrequited love affair will bring to the next love a certain distrust or caution. The child who is the product of a family where all their affectional energy is utilized to sooth bruised egos may have upon reaching adulthood have little love to give or demands too much for himself. The quality of early love—enjoyed or suffered—affects later love. Allan Fromme says we usually think of love as attachment to someone. Broadening this definition we suggest that love is any kind of attachment to a person, an idea, a place, an object, activity or even to oneself. This provides a more profitable way, I believe, of looking at love. It suggests that the way we relate ourselves each day to people, places and events is an integral part of our life. Our capacity to love is gauged and is affected by our relationships, not alone by the romantic one we set apart as sufficient to call love. Love is a concept that applies to many things, friendship, patriotism, kinship, romance, brotherhood, parental and aesthetic appreciation. Many experts say that love is the main characteristic of normalcy and health—most agree that the ability to love is intimately tied to maturity. The "good life" requires maturity. Abraham Maslow, Psychiatrist, suggests maturity means the following:

1. Comfortable relations with the reality.
2. Acceptance of self, others, nature and spontaneity.
3. Problem centering—detachment, has need for privacy, friendship and attachments to family which are not of the possessive variety.
4. Independence of culture and environment—continued freshness of appreciation and limitless horizons.
5. Social feeling—deep by selective social relationships; democratic character structure (respect for humans as humans), ethical certainty, unhostile sense of humor and creativeness.

This is a large order, I'm afraid. There are not too many of us who fulfill all the requirements for being mature. Certainly the "good life" requires that we measure up or approach this ideal. Hugh Downs, a television personality, in addressing the "Congress on the Quality of Life" a few years back said that "if we look closely at the characteristics of maturity (as in the above list), they fit into two broad categories: work and love."

What he is saying is that our work should not be thought of as drudgery, that we should find pleasure in it, be committed to it. Work is fundamental and doing nothing but lying under the breadfruit tree absorbing nourishment from what drops into your mouth is not happiness. Maybe Mr. Downs has had the kind of stimulation, adulation and constant ego stroking which allows work to be play that we love and to which we are committed. Sometimes the last thing I need is to have an appointment with one more student about a thesis (the culminating aspect of their degree work). Their egos are intimately tied to completing their research, their goal and development. My work in suggesting, correcting, guiding, encouraging is frequently fraught with difficulty and sensitivity, it is accompanied with energy debilitation and ennui. This has to be balanced by recreation and leisure. Rituals are also important.

The ritual nature of play, religion or work enables most of us to function regularly and gives a feeling of being a part of the wider world. Our aspirations are listed in the solemn routine of church going, alms giving and confession of sins. The routine, the ritual makes us feel comfortable and safe, it relieves anxiety. I believe that ritual in the psychological sense is fundamental to living securely and well. The ritual has its place for it reduces fear, desensitized our irritabilities through habituation and serves to organize a pattern to our lives. The ritual of reflection, our fantasies and daydreams release tensions unrealizable in motor activity and life's events; it also conjures up the good from the past through memories and prospect for the future through our imagination. In worship the bowed head, the prayer book, the communion cup, the litany, all serve to impart a stimulus for the promise of a better and good life.

Love is respect not just consideration for others but for ourselves, it is not self-denial per se. In a little volume I discovered several years ago—"How to Be Your Own Best Friend" by two psychoanalysts, Newman and Berkowitz, the authors contend that adults are an admixture of the child and the mature person. Some selfishness remains with us, and within limits should, for as the authors of the above they suggest to me, doing what makes you feel good yourself is the opposite of self-indulgence. The Bible says, "Love they neighbor as thyself," not better than thyself! Self-denial in and of itself is not love; it may be duty or habit, but not love. Self-denial is one of the worst kinds of self-indulgence. It is the feeding of the part of you that feels worthless. This doesn't mean you can't decide to give up things or sacrifice for children or others, but that is a choice you make—it is done out of self-regard not self-hatred. It is existential. Charity begins at home, as Polonius suggested in Hamlet, a line quoted before but which I think indicates the sort of balance that is needed, when he said to his son, "to thine own self be true, and it must follow as the night the day, thou canst not then be false to any man." Self-love and egocentricity are not the same things nor are they mutually exclusive. Learning to savor your own success is important.

A Cause-A Commitment

We can have causes or be committed to something or someone, but it may be mostly self-love—we support someone, some charity, some church, some organization, some foundation for it is tied closely to our egos or allows us to shine in some reflected glory. These are not causes but ego trips. A worthy cause is one where we are required to give of ourselves through sacrifice, through direct energy application, the commitment of time and reflection to a project. I know that much good comes from the guilt with which we find ourselves strapped. Perhaps Freud was right when he suggested that progress in civilization and humanism (founding of hospitals, orphanages, etc.) came from the sickening feeling of sin brought about by religion. Religion which sensitizes our conscience. We need not make light of the matter that is sin, however way it produces good. But we must recognize that the "good life" comes from sorting out our motives; what we join as a cause should take us out of ourselves. Institutionalized giving and busy work should take us a step beyond the superficial do-gooding—"it makes us feel good if I've given my fair share." We should have a cause, which we want to have for ourselves depending upon a mature choice and our existential concern.

Causes grow out of our recognition of need—to be involved in helping others—of course to help ourselves. A good cause is one that demands our best—our best intelligence, our best ethics and our best ability in making a contribution. This is not unlike our jobs and work life, which should be characterized by the same devotion. Certainly our contribution can be quiet and unassuming. In fact I am struck by the numbers of persons working very hard for charities, etc., yet not wishing or allowing any publicity. It is not all due to fear of discovery and attempts to forego multiple requests for help for many of these have little money. We are essentially only what we give—our time, resources, our ideas, and hopes. Charity is a good, mature defense mechanism used by some, you do not need a million to be a volunteer, a contributor, a giver at least only time and energy. The anxiety ridden middlescent striving but never making it to a part of success often finds charity as an antidote and humor as a companion when surveying the valuable in their life.

Causes (what is worth most?) should involve us in the reflection of our life—"the unexamined life is not worth living." In the in-between years we have matured enough, seen enough of life—experienced its tragedies and the thrill of victory—to seek that part of us that connects us with the greater universe of purpose and peace. Many find their ultimate feeling of purpose to be rooted in the religious and the organized church. They worship paying tribute to the immutable, acknowledging man's and God's place in the scheme of things. Through faith they bind themselves to the cause of God or its idea—give to educational institutions, missionary work, homes for children and the elderly. As a consequence, communities, large and small, are better places to live because of them. Worship relates to wonderment, not of people but ideas about eternity and the essential nature of life. For most of us who "live lives of quiet desperation" as Thoreau wrote, the reverie, the philosophical is a boon! It is the renewal of curiosity seen in the children who ask "What makes it go?" It is a revival of that lost art, curiosity which makes us ask, what makes it go? Meditation helps bring order to our frantic lives.

Causes are not just religious or for charitable purposes. Causes also relate to organizations seeking to insure better life for others. The drive to create new parks and to protect lands is a worthy cause, to get passage of legislative programs, increased consideration for the elderly is another, as is also the caring for kin who are incapacitated—crippled, have chronic and/or terminal illness. These causes can be short termed so we may be involved in many such as these. We all need to be committed to something bigger than ourselves.

The final cause that we all must concern ourselves with is morality, mainly our own. Whether this is related to the morality of the church or to some other code of ethics, morality serves as the cement of our lives. We are counterfeit if we are not honest—it's hard to be for we have so many roles to play and masters to serve. A self-analysis sorting out the truth of our lives and the nature of ourselves is in order. The man who owes no allegiance to anyone or thing or has no faith or hope for improvement has forfeited the prospect of the good life—he has nothing left for which to live.

In our day of moral relativism, I suppose we would change the fact of right and wrong if we could. We certainly seem to act on this premise. For we know all too well that right and wrong varies in different cultures and times, situational ethics provides a rationalization, but nothing has validated the slow-learned wisdom that mankind has accumulated from ancient times. To kill, to steal, to lie, or to covet another person's possessions still leads to varying degrees of misery. As we must learn to eat the right things to sustain our physical health, we must learn to do the right thing to sustain moral health for in the Twenty-First Century we have found no way to repeal the Ten Commandments. Materialism has affected our civilization's ability to enjoy life. A material object which should be cherished at age 16 because it has been earned by odd jobs on Saturdays is nowadays a broken castoff when a child is half that age.

The "good life" of the mature years comes from arriving there with a healthy body (or with limited disabilities) respect for others, recognition that work is good, making leisure time and play desirable, and that the love that binds comes from commitment to some cause and to others. The "good life" for the in-between years is a compound of work, play, love and worship. Simple, cornball, illusory you say, certainly for Americans who regard frustration as ranking higher than cholera on the scale of human afflictions! There is more to life than work you say! You should work to live and not live to work. The Western World is racked by the insatiable demand for less work, more pay. Work is seen as something that wears you down, that produces stress, and stress is known to take a heavy toll. Dr. Hans Selye, expert on stress, says "it is true that biologic stress is involved in many common diseases such as ulcers, high blood pressure, etc. But does this mean that we should avoid stress whenever possible?" Certainly not. Stress is the spice of life!! It is associated with all types of activity and we could avoid it by never doing anything. No one would enjoy a life of "no runs, no hits, no errors"! To function normally, man needs work as he needs air, food, sleep, social contacts and sex. Our aim should be not to avoid work but to find the kind that suits us best. Work wears you out mainly through the frustration of failure. Each period of stress, especially if it results from unsuccessful struggles leaves scars. Now we have trials and tribulations, which forbid the knowledge of the future uncertainty plagues the future but the essentials, are work, play, love and wonderment. As Americans we need to pull together and support each other and create a bond of united effort against those seeking to do us harm. Successful activity, no matter how intense, leaves virtually no scars. Instead, it provides you with the exhilarating feeling of youthful strength, even at very advanced age. Short hours are a boon only for those underprivileged who are not good at anything, have no particular taste for anything, and no hunger for achievement. These are the true paupers of mankind! George Bernard Shaw suggested that the great elixir of life is to be thoroughly worn out before being discarded—"a force of nature, instead of a feverish, selfish, clod of ailments and grievances."

As important as work is, play—leisure and avocational pursuits are equally crucial to enjoyment in life. It is the antidote for emotional and routine aspects of life. Americans feel guilty about having nothing to do, so those who can just "do nothing" should develop a hobby, learn new sports or games. Nothing renews life as well as just good play. The need to slow down and change the rhythm of life is a constant one. With work and play there must be love and commitment to a cause. It suffuses all of life, for without love, life is hollow. We must give and receive it. When we come to our middlescent years with health and strong values, then work, play and love can make the good life. Eric Fromme proclaimed that "happiness is proof of partial or total success in the art of living." With some luck and careful planning, you can enjoy the good life!

978-0-595-36864-8
0-595-36864-6

Printed in the United States
38269LVS00003B/4-30